Clinical Laboratory Science
The Basics

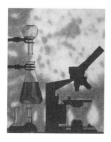

Clinical
Laboratory Science
THE BASICS

Jean Jorgenson Linné, B.S., M.T.(A.S.C.P.)

Assistant Professor,
Department of Laboratory Medicine and Pathology,
University of Minnesota Medical School,
Minneapolis, Minnesota

Karen Munson Ringsrud, B.S., M.T.(A.S.C.P.)

Assistant Professor,
Department of Laboratory Medicine and Pathology,
University of Minnesota Medical School,
Minneapolis, Minnesota

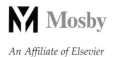 Mosby

An Affiliate of Elsevier

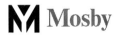
Mosby

An Affiliate of Elsevier

Editor: Janet Russell
Developmental Editor: Sarahlynn Lester
Project Managers: Mark Spann, Patricia Tannian
Production Editor: Steve Hetager
Book Design Manager: Judi Lang
Interior Designer: Jeanne Wolfgeher
Cover Designer: Jeanne Wolfgeher

Printed in the United States of America.

Composition by Top Graphics
Printing/binding by Maple-Vail Book Mfg. Group

Mosby, Inc.
11830 Westline Industrial Drive
St. Louis, Missouri 64146

ISBN 0-323-00759-7

05 06 07 08 / 9 8 7 6 5

Reviewers

Mary Breci-Swendrzynski, M.A., B.S.M.T.
Program Director,
Medical Laboratory Technology,
Midlands Technical College,
Columbia, South Carolina

Margaret L. Charette, M.Ed.,
M.T.(A.S.C.P.)S.C.
Program Director, MLT-AD,
MaineGeneral Medical Center,
Augusta, Maine

Judith A. Cowan, B.S., R.N, C.M.A.
Medical Assisting Program,
Kirkwood Community College,
Cedar Rapids, Iowa

Patrick Debold
Concord Career Colleges,
Kansas City, Missouri

Patricia Etnyre-Zacher, Ed.D.,
C.L.S.(N.C.A.), M.T.(A.S.C.P.)
Associate Professor,
Program in Clinical Laboratory Sciences,
School of Allied Health Professions,
Northern Illinois University,
Dekalb, Illinois

Jeanne M. Isabel, M.S.Ed., C.L.Sp.H.,
M.T.(A.S.C.P)
Assistant Professor,
Program in Clinical Laboratory Sciences,
School of Allied Health Professions,
Northern Illinois University,
Dekalb, Illinois

Beverly J. Philpott, B.Sc., C.M.A.
Assistant Professor,
Medical Assisting Program,
Kirkwood Community College,
Cedar Rapids, Iowa

George D. Smith, M.T.(A.S.C.P.)
Consultant,
Anderson Continuing Education,
Sacramento, California

To David, David, and Jonathan
Peter and Erik

Preface

Close to thirty years have passed since the publication of the first edition of our textbook *Clinical Laboratory Science: The Basics and Routine Techniques*. In these years, much has changed in the practice of clinical laboratory science. It is interesting to note, however, that although technology has produced drastic changes in how clinical laboratory tests are done, many of the techniques and procedures used today continue to be based on theory and practice that have been in place for many years. The clinical laboratory will continue in this evolution, with procedures changing for carrying out the tests, while the fundamentals are left intact. Because introductory information is necessary for anyone engaged in performing laboratory tests, a thorough understanding of basic concepts and general background material continues to be an essential first step in the practice of clinical laboratory science, regardless of the technology or specific procedural steps required in a given laboratory setting.

The third edition of our textbook, which was titled *Basic Techniques in Clinical Laboratory Science,* was divided into two parts, "Fundamentals of the Clinical Laboratory" and "Divisions of the Clinical Laboratory." Because there was a demand for a book containing only the material in Part I, this book, *Clinical Laboratory Science: The Basics,* has been published. A new fourth edition of the entire textbook (Parts I and II) is also available and is now entitled *Clinical Laboratory Science: The Basics and Routine Techniques.*

This abbreviated version, *Clinical Laboratory Science: The Basics,* includes general background material on regulation of clinical laboratories and professional issues, safety in the laboratory, collection and processing of laboratory specimens, systems of measurement and general laboratory equipment, use of the microscope, photometry, laboratory mathematics, quality assurance, automation in the clinical laboratory, and laboratory computers. All of this fundamental information is needed for performing laboratory procedures in each of the many divisions of the clinical laboratory. We have tried to retain from our earlier books the writing style, organization, and level of presentation so that the material can be used by students and laboratorians of many levels.

The expanded version of this book, *Clinical Laboratory Science: The Basics and Routine Techniques,* fourth edition, includes "Fundamentals of the Clinical Laboratory" as Part I and "Divisions of the Clinical Laboratory" as Part II. Routine laboratory assays are included in Part II for the areas of chemistry, hematology, coagulation and hemostasis, urinalysis, microbiology, immunology and serology, immunohematology, and, in a new chapter, examination of extravascular fluids and miscellaneous specimens. New pedagogy, including learning objectives, review questions (and answers), and, where applicable, case studies, has been added to both books.

We would like to thank our colleagues and friends at the University of Minnesota who have given us both technical and moral support in this endeavor. We appreciate the support of the Department of Laboratory Medicine and Pathology at the University of Minnesota, Leo T. Furcht, M.D., Professor and Head.

We once again acknowledge the unconditional support of our families during the process of completing these textbook revisions—no project of this magnitude can be undertaken without this support. We are thankful to our husbands, David Linné and Peter Ringsrud, and to our children, who have, in these almost thirty years, gone from infants to adults.

Jean Jorgenson Linné

Karen Munson Ringsrud

Brief Contents

Detailed Contents

Clinical Laboratory Science
The Basics

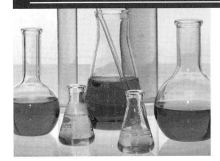

Introduction to Clinical Laboratory Science

Learning Objectives

From study of this chapter, the reader will be able to:

➤ Understand the organization of a clinical laboratory and its various parts, purposes, and personnel.

➤ Compare and contrast the uses of various sites for laboratory testing—central laboratory, point of care, physician office laboratory, reference laboratory.

➤ Appreciate the importance of federal, state, and institutional regulations concerning the quality and reliability of work being done—become familiar with the terms OSHA, CLIA '88, HCFA, JCAHO, NCCLS, and CAP.

➤ Understand the CLIA '88 regulations in particular and the concept of classification of laboratory testing by complexity of the test—waived, moderately complex, highly complex, and provider-performed microscopy.

➤ Understand the purpose of participation in CLIA '88–mandated proficiency testing programs and how they relate to quality assurance.

INTRODUCTION TO THE CLINICAL LABORATORY

The goal of medical practice is to resolve the problems presented to the physician by the patient. This includes establishing or ruling out a diagnosis, deciding on a management plan for the particular diagnosis and patient, giving the patient the prognosis for the presenting problem, and monitoring any follow-up therapy needed. Included in the process a physician uses is an interview with the patient and an organized analysis of the patient's presenting problem. This process includes the taking of a complete history, a physical examination, and the ordering of appropriate laboratory or other diagnostic tests. The findings are sorted and expanded where necessary, to make a diagnosis, formulate a prognosis, and decide on a course of management. Abnormal laboratory findings constitute only one aspect of the patient's problems, and any action taken because of these findings should be predicated on how this action will affect the patient as a whole. The ultimate goals of medical practice should be relief of patient suffering and prolonging the general well-being of the patient.

Laboratory Medicine or Clinical Pathology

Laboratory medicine or **clinical pathology** is the medical discipline by which clinical laboratory science and technology are applied to the care of patients. Several different disciplines make up this practice—chemistry, hematology, microbiology, urinalysis, immunology, and blood banking, to name the more traditional ones. Many changes are taking place in the clinical laboratory, and these are already affecting the types of tests being offered. A possible system for the organization of a clinical laboratory is seen in Fig. 1-1. In addition to the traditional areas already mentioned, the disciplines of cytogenetics, toxicology (often a part of the chemistry laboratory), and other specialized divisions are present in the larger laboratories. Molecular pathology diagnostics and the use of polymerase chain reaction (PCR), DNA probes, and other genetic testing are evident in many laboratories.

Another change is to move from tests being done in a centralized laboratory setting to point-of-care testing (POCT). Alternative testing sites, such as at the bedside of the patient, in the operating rooms or recovery areas, or even in the home of the patient, should be a part of any discussion of the clinical laboratory and its organization. Automation has already changed the way in which testing is done, and more changes are likely to come. The diversity available in the clinical laboratory is necessary to provide the clinicians seeing patients with the best, most appropriate information for the total care of their patients.

Utilization of the Clinical Laboratory

The appropriate utilization of the clinical laboratory is of the utmost importance in the practice of laboratory medicine. It is important that the laboratory serve to educate the physician and other health care providers so that the information available through the results reported for the various tests ordered can be utilized in an appropriate manner. When tests are being ordered, the clinical laboratory should assume a role of leadership and education in assisting the physician to understand the most useful pattern of ordering, for example, to serve the best interest of the patient, the clinical decision-making process for the physician, and the costs involved. Continuing education is always a part of any laboratory's program for ensuring high-quality service as well as for maintaining the morale of the laboratory staff.

Hundreds of different laboratory tests are readily available in the larger laboratories, but it is often the case that only a percentage of these tests are routinely ordered. Only 50 to 60 tests of the hundreds available account for 70% of the results generated by a modern hospital clinical laboratory.[5] The implication of these data is that common diseases are investigated by using common laboratory tests. When the results of these common tests are utilized appropriately in the

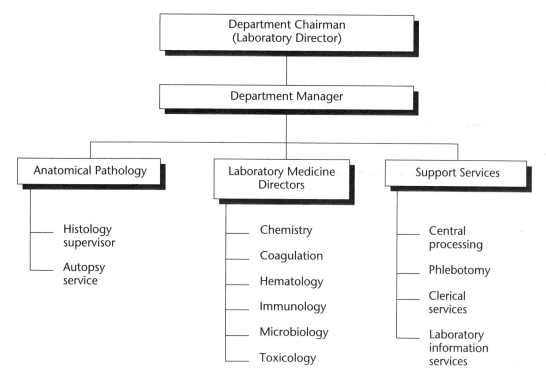

FIG 1-1. Organization of a clinical laboratory. (From Kaplan LA, Pesce A: *Clinical Chemistry: Theory, Analysis, and Correlation,* ed 3. St Louis, Mosby, 1996, p 49.)

context of the patient's clinical case, physical examination findings, and the medical history, clinical decision making will be improved. It is unusual that the results from a single laboratory assay will make a diagnosis. Certain additional laboratory tests may be needed to take decision making to the next step. Generally a small number of appropriately chosen laboratory tests may be sufficient to confirm, or rule out, one or more of the possibilities in a differential diagnosis.

Future Directions for Laboratory Medicine

Biotechnology is a fast-growing discipline of the diagnostic laboratory. Molecular biology or the discipline of **molecular diagnostics** utilizes this technology. Molecular pathology applies the principles of basic molecular biology to the study of human diseases. New approaches to human disease assessment are being developed by clinical laboratories because of the new information about the molecular basis of disease processes in general. The use of traditional laboratory analyses gives results based on a description of events currently going on in the patient—blood cell counts, infectious processes, blood glucose concentration. Molecular biology introduces a predictive component: findings from these tests can be used to anticipate events that may occur in the future, when patients may be at risk for a particular disease or condition. This predictive component reinforces, more than ever, the importance of how laboratory test results are utilized and emphasizes ethical considerations and the need for use of genetic counseling. Genetic counseling has gained an important status in the utilization of the laboratory results obtained from molecular biologic tests. Nucleic acids form the chemical basis for transmission of genetic information, and genetic information is sustained as sequences of nucleic acids. Chromosomes contain DNA as a primary component, and genetic traits can be transmitted through DNA.

Patient Specimens

Clinical laboratorians work with many types of specimens. Blood and urine specimens are probably the ones most often tested, but tests are also ordered on body tissues and other body fluids, such as synovial, cerebrospinal, peritoneal, and pericardial fluids. Since the purpose of the clinical laboratory is to provide information regarding the assay results for the specimens analyzed, it is most important that the specimens be properly collected in the first place. In the testing process, analytes or constituents are measured by using only very small amounts of the specimens collected, but in interpreting the results, it is assumed that the results obtained do represent what the actual concentrations of the analytes are in the patient. It is only by use of the various quality assurance systems discussed later in this book that the reliability of results can be ensured. No matter how carefully a laboratory assay has been carried out, valid laboratory results can be reported only when preanalytical quality control has also been ascertained. Special patient preparation considerations for some specimen collections, along with proper transportation to and handling in the laboratory prior to the actual analytical assay, are very important. Appropriate **quality assurance programs** must be in place in the laboratory to make certain that each patient specimen is given the very best analysis possible and that the results reported will benefit the patient in the best possible way.

REGULATION OF THE CLINICAL LABORATORY

In current laboratory settings, many governmental regulations, along with regulations and recommendations from professional, state, and federal accreditation agencies and commissions of various types, govern the activities of the laboratory, all of which must be explicitly understood and followed. Many of these groups are working toward similar goals, two primary ones being (1) ensuring that the quality of work being done in the laboratory is such that reliable results are reported to the physician who is treating the patient and (2) assuring the laboratory workers that the workplace provided to them is safe and healthful. Adhering to the regulatory mandates must constantly be balanced with also making certain that the testing of specimens and the results reporting are being done in a cost-effective manner. The regulations and standards are designed specifically to protect the people working in the laboratory, other health care personnel, the patients being treated in the health care facility, and society as a whole. **Federal regulations** exist to meet these objectives. Certain regulatory mandates have been issued externally, such as the **Clinical Laboratory Improvement Amendments of 1988 (CLIA '88)**, others are internal, and some are combinations of both.[2 4] Many of the factors governing the standards and their resulting regulations are associated with laboratory-acquired infections or accidents involving hazards in the workplace. These are discussed in Chapter 2.

A laboratory that wishes to receive payment for its services from Medicare or Medicaid must be licensed under the **Public Health Service Act**. To be licensed, the laboratory must meet the conditions for participation in those programs. The **Health Care Financing Administration (HCFA)** has the administrative responsibility for both the Medicare and CLIA '88 programs. Facilities accredited by approved private accreditation agencies, such as the College of American Pathologists, must also follow the regulations for licensure under CLIA '88. States with equivalent CLIA '88 regulations are reviewed individually as to possible waiver for CLIA '88 licensure.

The Health Care Financing Administration, under the U.S. **Department of Health and Human Services (HHS),** has also established regulations to implement CLIA '88. Any facility performing quantitative, qualitative, or screening test procedures or examinations on materials derived from the human body is regulated by CLIA '88. This includes hospital laboratories of all sizes; physician office laboratories; nursing home facilities; clinics; industrial laboratories; city, state, and county laboratories; pharmacies, fitness centers, health fairs; and independent laboratories.

The leaders and managers of the clinical laboratory must be certain that all legal operating regulations have been met and that all persons working in the laboratory setting are fully aware of the importance of compliance with these regulations. Those in leadership positions in a clinical laboratory must be well grounded in their expertise in medical, scientific, and technical areas in addition to fully understanding the regulatory matters. All laboratory personnel must be aware of these regulatory considerations, but it is up to the management to make certain that this information is communicated to everyone who needs to know.

Quality Assurance Requirements

Quality assurance programs are now also a requirement in the federal government's implementation of CLIA '88. The standards mandated are for all laboratories, with the intent that the medical community's ability to provide good-quality patient care will be greatly enhanced. Included in the CLIA '88 provisions are requirements for quality control and quality assurance, for the use of proficiency testing, and for certain levels of personnel to perform and supervise the work in the laboratory (see also Chapter 8).

External Regulations

Much of how the work of the clinical laboratory is carried out is delineated by federal regulations or other external regulations. The Clinical Laboratory Improvement Amendments of 1988 govern most of the activities of a particular laboratory.[2] The goals of these amendments are to ensure that the laboratory results reported are of high quality regardless of where the testing is done—small laboratory, physician's office, large reference laboratory, or something in between.

CLIA '88 regulations include aspects of proficiency testing programs, management of patient testing, quality assurance programs, the use of quality control systems, personnel requirements, inspections and site visits, and consultations. Several federal agencies govern practices in the clinical laboratory. These regulatory agencies or organizations are primarily concerned with setting standards, conducting inspections, and imposing sanctions, when necessary. External standards have been set to ensure that all laboratories provide the best, most reliable information to the physician and the patient. It was to this end, primarily, that CLIA '88 was enacted.

In addition to the CLIA '88 regulations, other state and federal regulations are in place to regulate chemical waste disposal, use of hazardous chemicals, and issues of laboratory safety for the personnel working there; safety issues include the handling of biohazardous materials and the application of standard precautions (see Chapter 2).

Based on the complexity of tests performed by a laboratory, a tiered grouping has been devised, with varying degrees of regulation for each level. The law contains a provision to exempt certain laboratories from standards for personnel and from quality control programs, proficiency testing, or quality assurance programs. These laboratories are defined as those that perform only simple, routine tests, which, as determined by HHS, have an insignificant risk of an erroneous result. These laboratories receive a "certificate of waiver." Another category based on complexity of testing is provider-performed microscopies (PPM); generally it is the physician himself or herself who is performing the testing in the office setting. The PPM category is also exempt from some of the CLIA requirements. The moderate-complexity and high-complexity levels are more regulated, with some minimal personnel standards required, as well as proficiency testing and quality assurance programs. The level to which the laboratory is assigned depends on the complexity of the tests performed. The criteria for classification include risk of harm to the patient, likelihood of erroneous results, type of testing method used, degree of independent judgment and interpretation needed, and availability of the particular test in question for home use. A panel of experts will periodically review the test complexity criteria for the categories and make suggestions for any changes needed.

External standards have been set to ensure quality of results reported—quality assurance, as imposed by CLIA '88 and administered by the Health Care Financing Administration. A clinical laboratory must be certified by HCFA, by a private certifying agency, or by a state regulatory agency that has been given approval by HCFA. Once certified, the laboratory is scheduled for regular inspections to determine that there has been compliance with the federal regulations, including CLIA '88. Two certifying agencies, the **College of American Pathologists (CAP)** and the **Joint Commission on Accreditation of Healthcare Organizations (JCAHO)**, have been given *deemed status* to act on the federal government's behalf. From an external source, guidelines and standards have also been set to govern safe work practices in the clinical laboratory (see also Chapter 2). Through labor laws and environmental regulations, assurance has been given to laboratory workers that they are in a safe atmosphere and that every precaution has been taken to maintain that safe atmosphere. The **Occupational Safety and Health Administration (OSHA)** has been involved in setting these practices into motion, and it is through OSHA that the mandates have come to be a part of the daily life of the laboratory workplace. Other external controls include standards mandated by public health laws and reporting requirements via the **Centers for Disease Control and Prevention (CDC)** and via certification and licensure requirements issued by the **Food and Drug Administration (FDA)**. State regulations are imposed by Medicaid agencies, state environmental laws, and state public health laws and licensure laws. Local regulations include those determined by building codes and fire prevention codes.

Independent agencies also have influence over practices in the clinical laboratory through accreditation policies or other responsibilities. These include groups such as the College of American Pathologists, the Joint Commission on Accreditation of Healthcare Organizations, and other specific proficiency-testing programs.

Internal Regulations

Local, internal programs must be in place to carry out the external mandates. Internal regulation also comes from the need to ensure quality performance and reporting of results for the many laboratory tests being done—a process of quality assurance. It is the responsibility of the clinical laboratory, to both patient and physician, to ensure that the results reported from that laboratory are reliable and also to provide the physician with an estimate of what constitutes the reference range or "normal" for an analyte being measured. Internal monitoring programs are concerned with **total quality management (TQM), quality assurance (QA),** or **continuous quality improvement (CQI),** each of which is designed to monitor and improve the quality of services provided by the laboratory.

CLIA '88: Federal Regulation of the Clinical Laboratory

Regulation of clinical laboratories in general began at about the same time as the Medicare law in 1965. Since then, the federal government has been moving closer to regulation of all types of clinical laboratories, beginning with larger hospital and reference laboratories engaging in interstate commerce, and including physician office laboratories (POLs) with the implementation of CLIA '88. Until 1988, regulation applied only to hospitals and independent laboratories under the Clinical Laboratory Improvement Act of 1967 (CLIA '67). This act provided for licensing of laboratories that accepted specimens for testing from across state lines (interstate commerce). In addition, Medicare law provided for inspection and accreditation of laboratories (hospital and independent) that performed tests on and were billed for reimbursement of Medicare patients. These two laws generally did not apply to smaller laboratories such as physician office laboratories.

On October 31, 1988, Congress passed the Clinical Laboratory Improvement Amendments of 1988 in response to a series of newspaper articles about poor Pap smear testing in the Washington, D.C., area. According to federal law, under CLIA '88, a laboratory is now defined as " . . . a facility for the biological, microbiological, serological, chemical, immunohematological, hematological, biophysical, cytological, pathological, or other examination of materials derived from the human body for the purpose of providing information for the diagnosis, prevention, or treatment of any disease or impairment of, or the assessment of the health of human beings."[2] As a result of CLIA '88, any facility that performs testing on material derived from humans for the purpose of diagnosis, assessment, or treatment is subject to federal regulation. Proposed regulations implementing CLIA '88 were published on May 21, 1990. These were met with more than 60,000 comments and protests. On February 28, 1992, the Secretary of Health and Human Services published the final rules implementing CLIA '88.[2] These regulations replaced the Medicare, Medicaid, and CLIA '67 standards and apply to almost all laboratory testing of human specimens. The regulations set standards for laboratory personnel, quality assurance and quality control, and proficiency testing, which are based on test complexity and risk factors. In addition, the regulations establish application procedures and fees for CLIA certification, plus enforcement procedures and sanctions if laboratories fail to meet standards. The regulations were generally effective (implemented) on September 1, 1992, although some parts of the regulations were effective at a later date and modifications are ongoing.[3,4]

CLIA Categories Based on Complexity of the Tests Done by the Laboratory

CLIA regulations divide laboratories into groups based on the "complexity" of the tests being per-

formed: **waived, moderately complex,** and **highly complex test** categories. Included in the moderately complex category are two subcategories: (1) **provider-performed microscopies (PPM),** specific microscopies (wet mounts) usually performed by a physician or provider for his or her own patients, and (2) **accurate and precise technology (APT),** or "easy," automated quantitative tests or easy qualitative tests such as agglutination patterns or color change end points. Most laboratory tests are classified as moderately complex. Tests are categorized by the federal government on the basis of the analyte tested and the method or instrumentation used to perform the test. For example, reagent strip or tablet urine tests are categorized as waived tests when results are read visually, but as moderately complex when results are read by instrumentation. The microscopic analysis of the urine sediment is categorized as a moderately complex test, unless performed by a physician or provider, in which case it falls under the PPM category.

Waived Tests. As currently defined, waived laboratory tests or procedures are those cleared by the Food and Drug Administration (FDA) for home use, which employ methodologies that are so simple that the likelihood of erroneous results is negligible and which pose no reasonable risk of harm to the patient if a test is performed incorrectly.

Procedures in the Waived Test Category. Waived tests listed in the April 1995 Federal Register regulations (with revisions in February 1996) are: dipstick or tablet reagent urinalysis (nonautomated) for bilirubin, glucose, hemoglobin, ketone, leukocytes, nitrite, pH, protein, specific gravity, and urobilinogen; fecal occult blood; ovulation tests—visual color comparison tests for human luteinizing hormone; urine pregnancy tests—visual color comparison tests; erythrocyte sedimentation rate—nonautomated; hemoglobin—copper sulfate, nonautomated (an extremely outdated testing methodology); blood glucose by glucose monitoring devices cleared by the FDA specifically for use at home; spun microhematocrit; hemoglobin by single analyte instruments with self-contained or component features to perform specimen-reagent interaction, providing direct measurement and readout; blood cholesterol test by cholesterol monitoring device approved by the FDA for use at home; and Cholestech L*D*X System for total cholesterol, HDL cholesterol, triglycerides, and glucose.[3] As technology changes, this list may be expanded.

Provider-Performed Microscopy. To meet the criteria for being in this category, procedures must follow these specifications: the examination must be personally performed by the practitioner (defined as a physician, a midlevel practitioner under the supervision of a physician, or a dentist), the procedure must be categorized as moderately complex, the primary instrument for performing the test is the microscope (limited to brightfield or phase-contrast microscopy), the specimen is labile, control materials are not available, and there is limited specimen handling.

Procedures in the PPM Category. As currently defined, all direct wet mount preparations for the presence or absence of bacteria, fungi, parasites, and human cellular elements in vaginal, cervical, or skin preparations, all potassium hydroxide (KOH) preparations, pinworm examinations, fern tests, postcoital direct, qualitative examinations of vaginal or cervical mucus, urine sediment examinations, nasal smears for granulocytes (eosinophils), fecal leukocyte examinations, and qualitative semen analysis (limited to the presence or absence of sperm and detection of motility) are included in the PPM category.

Other Regulatory or Accreditation Agencies and Organizations

In addition to CLIA '88 regulations, other agencies and private organizations that regulate or provide accreditation to clinical laboratories include the following:

Occupational Safety and Health Administration (OSHA)

Environmental Protection Agency (EPA)

Food and Drug Administration (FDA)

State agencies (such as state departments of health)

College of American Pathologists (CAP)

Commission on Office Laboratory Accreditation (COLA)

Joint Commission on Accreditation of Healthcare Organizations (JCAHO)

National Committee for Clinical Laboratory Standards (NCCLS)

Americans with Disabilities Act (ADA)

Commission on Office Laboratory Accreditation

As of December 29, 1993, the HCFA approved the accreditation program developed by the **Commission on Office Laboratory Accreditation (COLA)** for the physician office laboratory. This means that COLA accreditation requirements are recognized by HCFA as being equivalent to those established by CLIA. The COLA accreditation established a peer-review option in place of the CLIA regulatory requirements. COLA-accredited laboratories are surveyed every two years to see that they meet requirements developed by their peers in family practice, internal medicine, or pathology.

National Committee for Clinical Laboratory Standards

The **National Committee for Clinical Laboratory Standards (NCCLS)** is a nonprofit, educational organization created for the development, promotion, and use of national and international laboratory standards. It was founded in 1968 and accredited by the American National Standards Institute. It employs voluntary consensus standards that are intended to maintain the performance of the clinical laboratory at the high level necessary for quality patient care. Participants include individual laboratories, laboratory professional associations, industries, and agencies of the federal and state governments. NCCLS guidelines and standards are cited throughout this text when applicable. NCCLS recommendations, guidelines, and standards follow the CLIA '88 mandates and therefore serve to inform and assist the laboratory in following the federal regulations.

Americans with Disabilities Act

The **Americans with Disabilities Act (ADA)** of 1990 (signed into law in 1992) prohibits employment discrimination against qualified persons who have disabilities, in both the public and the private sectors. Under this Act, specific plans must be developed for any known disabled person working in the laboratory to make certain that he or she is working in a safe atmosphere.

QUALITY ASSURANCE UNDER CLIA REGULATIONS

According to CLIA '88 regulations, quality assurance (QA) activities in the laboratory must be documented and be an active part of the ongoing organization of the laboratory. It is essential that all persons working in the clinical laboratory be totally committed to the concepts of the quality assurance process as it is defined by their institution. The dedication of sufficient planning time to the topic of quality assurance and the implementation of the program in the total laboratory operation are critical. All persons working in the clinical laboratory must be willing to work together to make the quality of service to the patient their top priority. It is not a system meant to penalize the laboratory staff but a means of giving self-confidence to the persons performing tests. Because the total laboratory staff must be involved in carrying out any quality assurance process, it is important to develop a comprehensive program to include all levels of laboratorians. See also Chapter 8.

Continuous Quality Improvement

The ongoing process of making certain that the correct laboratory result is reported for the right patient in a timely manner and cost is known as Continuous Quality Improvement, or CQI. This is a process of assuring the clinician ordering a test that the testing process has been done in the best possible way to provide the most useful information in diagnosing or managing the particular patient in question.

Proficiency Testing

According to CLIA '88, a laboratory must establish and follow written quality control procedures for monitoring and evaluating the quality of the analytical testing process of each method, to ensure the accuracy and reliability of patient test results and reports. **Proficiency testing (PT)** is a means by which quality control between laboratories is maintained. Provisions of CLIA '88 require enrollment in an external proficiency testing program for laboratories performing moderately complex or highly complex tests. Only the waived tests under CLIA '88 are exempt from proficiency testing regulations. The PT program being used must be approved by CLIA. Proficiency testing programs are available through the CAP, the Centers for Disease Control and Prevention, and the health departments in some states.

Laboratories enrolled in a particular PT program test samples for specific analytes and send the results to be tabulated by the program managers. Results of the assays are graded for each participating laboratory according to designated evaluation limits, and the results are compared with those of other laboratories participating in the same PT program.

If a laboratory performs only waived tests, it is not required to participate in a proficiency testing program. However, it must apply for and be given a certificate of waiver from the United States Department of Health and Human Services. If a laboratory performs moderate- or high-complexity tests for which no proficiency testing is available, it must have a system for verifying the accuracy and reliability of its test results at least twice a year.

LABORATORY DEPARTMENTS OR DIVISIONS

The organization of a particular clinical laboratory will depend on factors of size, numbers of tests done, and the facilities available. Larger laboratories tend to be departmentalized; there is a separate area designated for each of the various divisions. There is a trend currently to have a more open design, in which personnel can work in any of several areas or divisions. Aspects of cross-training are important considerations in the open model. There is more chance for cooperation and interfacing when the open model is used. As consultation and cooperation are encouraged in health care in general, this trend would appear to be supported by use of the open model for the clinical laboratory. With either the more traditional divisions by separate areas or the open model, there are still several distinct departments or divisions to the organization of the clinical laboratory. Some of these are hematology, coagulation, urinalysis, blood bank (immunohematology), chemistry, immunology/serology, and microbiology.

Hematology

Hematology is the study of blood. The formed elements of the blood, or blood cells, include erythrocytes (red blood cells, RBC), leukocytes (white blood cells, WBC), and thrombocytes (platelets). The routine hematology screening test for abnormalities in the blood is the complete blood count, or CBC. This test includes several parts; the following are included in most CBCs: RBC count, WBC count, platelet count, hemoglobin concentration, hematocrit, and a percentage differential of the white blood cells present. The results of the CBC are useful in diagnosing anemias, in which there are too few red blood cells or too little hemoglobin, in leukemias, in which there are too many white blood cells, and in infectious processes of several etiologies, in which changes in white cells are noted. These tests are done in most hematology laboratories by use of an automated instrument. Many of these automated cell counters also provide automated white cell differential analyses, separating the types of white cells present by size, maturity, and nuclear and cytoplasmic characteristics. Cell counts for other body fluids, such as cerebrospinal fluid or synovial fluid, are also performed in some hematology laboratories. There is also a microscopy

component to work done in the hematology laboratory, as microscopic assessment of a stained blood film is done as part of some CBCs, especially when automated instrumentation is not readily available or when a more complete morphologic examination is necessary.

Other tests done in hematology laboratories are reticulocyte counts and erythrocyte sedimentation rate measurements. Examination of bone marrow is done in special hematology divisions where trained hematopathologists and technologists are present to examine the slides. The process of obtaining the bone marrow from the patient is done by a trained physician.

Coagulation

Work done in the coagulation laboratory assesses bleeding and clotting problems. In some laboratories, hematology and coagulation tests are part of the same laboratory department. The two most commonly performed tests in the coagulation laboratory are prothrombin time (PT) and activated partial thromboplastin time (aPTT). These tests can be used to identify potential bleeding disorders and to monitor anticoagulant therapy. Patients who have had a heart attack or stroke, both due to formation of blood clots, are given medications that anticoagulate their blood or slow the clotting process and must be monitored because too large a dose of these drugs can lead to bleeding problems.

Urinalysis

In this laboratory division, the routine urine screening tests are done. The routine urinalysis was one of the earliest laboratory tests performed, historically, and it still serves to give valuable information regarding the detection of disease related to the kidney and urinary tract. By evaluating the results of the three component parts of the urinalysis—observation of the physical characteristics of the urine specimen itself, such as color, clarity, and specific gravity; screening for chemical constituents such as pH, glucose, ketone bodies, protein, blood, bilirubin, urobilinogen, nitrites, and leukocyte esterase; and microscopic examination of the urinary sediment—metabolic diseases such as diabetes mellitus, kidney diseases, or infectious diseases of the urinary bladder or kidney can be diagnosed and monitored.

Clinical Chemistry

The clinical chemistry laboratory performs quantitative analytic procedures on a variety of body fluids, but primarily on serum or plasma that has been processed from whole blood collected from the patient. Tests are also done on urine or, less frequently, on body fluids such as cerebrospinal fluid. Several hundred analytes can be tested in the chemistry laboratory, but a few tests are used much more often in the aid of diagnosis of disease. Probably the most common chemistry tests done are for blood glucose, cholesterol, electrolytes, and serum proteins. Blood glucose tests are used to diagnose and monitor diabetes mellitus. Cholesterol is a test that is part of a battery of tests to monitor the lipid status of the patient. Electrolytes affect many of the metabolic processes in the body; among these processes are maintenance of osmotic pressure and water distribution in various body compartments, maintenance of pH, regulation of the functioning of heart and other muscles, and oxidation-reduction processes. Elevated protein levels can indicate disease states of several types. Serum enzyme tests are done to identify damage to or disease of specific organs, such as heart muscle damage or liver cell damage. Tests to monitor drug therapy and drug levels, toxicology, are also performed in chemistry laboratories. Most routine chemistry testing is done by automated methods, using computerized instruments that are very sophisticated and fast and that provide reliable results. Persons working in chemistry laboratories will be using automated analytic equipment, and having a good working knowledge of the various types of methodologies and instrumentation used is essential.

Blood Bank (Immunohematology)

When blood is donated for transfusion purposes, it must undergo a rigorous protocol of testing to make certain that it is safe for transfusion. Proper sample identification is particularly crucial in blood banking procedures, as a mislabeled specimen could result in a severe transfusion reaction or even death for the recipient. Most of the testing done in the blood bank laboratory is based on antigen-antibody reactions. In the specific tests performed in the blood bank laboratory, the antigens are specific proteins that are attached to the red and white blood cells. The nature of these antigens determines the blood group assigned, whether it is group A, B, O, or AB: group A red cells have antigen A, group B have antigen B, group AB have both antigens A and B, and group O have neither antigen A nor antigen B. Rh typing is also done, with blood being classified as Rh positive or Rh negative. Donated blood is also screened for any unusual antibodies present and for the presence of infectious antibodies such as hepatitis virus or human immunodeficiency virus. The donor blood must be matched to that of the prospective recipient to ensure that the recipient will not suffer any ill effects from the transfusion as a result of incompatible antibodies. When a blood transfusion is ordered, it is extremely important that only properly matched blood is transfused.

Blood banks are also engaged in the practice of transfusion medicine using components of blood or blood products. A patient does not usually need the whole unit of blood, only a particular part of it, such as the red blood cells, platelets, or specific clotting factors. By use of blood component therapy, one unit of donated blood can help several different patients who have different needs. The blood bank laboratorian will separate the donated unit into its components and store them for transfusion at a later time.

Immunology/Serology

The normal immune system functions to protect the body from foreign microorganisms that may invade it. When foreign material—that is, something that the body does not already have as part of itself—enters the body, the immune system works to eliminate the foreign material. This foreign material can be bacteria, viruses, fungi, or parasites, for example. The body's defensive action is carried out by its white blood cells—lymphocytes, monocytes, and other cells—by which the invading organism is eliminated or controlled. As in the blood bank laboratory, many of the immunology/serology laboratory's procedures are based on antigen-antibody reactions. When foreign material (antigen) is introduced into the body, the body reacts by means of its immune system to make antibodies to the foreign antigen. The antibodies formed can be measured in the laboratory.

In the evaluation of certain infectious diseases, the detection of antibodies in the serum of the patient is an important step in making and confirming a diagnosis and in the management of the illness. The use of serologic testing is based on the rise and fall of specific antibody titers in response to the disease process. In many instances serologic testing is done retrospectively, as the disease must progress to a certain point before the antibody titers will rise—often it takes several days or weeks for the antibody titer to rise after the first symptoms appear. In general, serologic testing is most useful for infectious organisms that are difficult to culture, cause chronic conditions, or have prolonged incubation periods.

In addition to its use in the diagnosis of infectious disease, the immunology laboratory can identify normal and abnormal levels of immune cells and serum components. Immune cellular function can also be determined.

Microbiology

In the microbiology laboratory, microorganisms that cause disease are identified; these are known as pathogens. Generally, the common bacteria, viruses, fungi, and parasites are identified in a typical clinical laboratory. Specimens sent to the microbiology laboratory for culture include swabs from the throat or wounds, sputum, vaginal excretions, urine, and blood. It is important that the microbiology laboratorian be able to differentiate the normal flora—those organisms which are part of the normal constituents of the host—from the pathogenic flora. Various differential testing is done, from the inoculation and incubation of the classic culture plate to observe an organism's growth characteristics, to the use of Gram staining techniques to separate gram-positive from gram-negative organisms. Once a pathogen is suspected, more testing is done to confirm its identity. Rapid testing methods have been developed to identify routine pathogens. For example, immunologic tests have been devised using monoclonal antibodies to identify the streptococcal organism causing pharyngitis or "strep" throat.

Another task for the microbiology laboratory is to identify the appropriate antibiotic to use for treatment of the offending pathogen. The pathogen is tested by using a panel of antibiotics of various types and dosages to determine the susceptibility of the organism to the various antibiotics. By doing this, the most effective antibiotic along with its correct dosage can be used to treat the specific patient's pathogenic organism in the most cost-effective and beneficial way.

PERSONNEL IN THE CLINICAL LABORATORY

Physicians generally do not perform the needed laboratory tests themselves but rely on trained laboratory personnel to do this for them. Clinical laboratorians, persons working in clinical laboratories, are an important component of the medical team. This clinical laboratory team generally is made up of the medical director, or pathologist, medical technologists/clinical laboratory scientists, laboratory assistants, phlebotomists, and specialists in the various laboratory disciplines, such as chemists, microbiologists, and hematologists. The categories of laboratory personnel and their titles vary from facility to facility. Generally the more highly trained persons will do the more complex work and administrative tasks, leaving the routine work to others. Many clinical laboratories are highly automated, and the job duties will reflect this. In some laboratories personnel are cross-trained to work in all disciplines; in others there may be specialists in certain areas such as clinical chemistry or microbiology. The size and work load of the laboratory may determine the organization of the work load for the personnel.

CLIA Requirements for Personnel

The personnel section of the CLIA regulations defines the responsibilities of persons working in each of the testing sites where tests of moderate or high complexity are done, along with the educational requirements and training and experience needed. Minimum education and experience needed by testing personnel to perform the specific laboratory tests on human specimens are also regulated by CLIA '88. These job requirements are listed in the CLIA '88 final regulations, along with their amendments published from 1992 to 1995.[2-4] There are no CLIA regulations for testing personnel who work at sites performing only the waived tests or the PPMs. For laboratories where only tests of moderate complexity are performed, the minimum requirement for testing personnel is a high school diploma or equivalent, as long as there is documented evidence of an amount of training sufficient to ensure that the laboratorian has the skills necessary to collect, identify, and process the specimen, and to perform the laboratory analysis itself. For tests of the highly complex category, the personnel requirements are more stringent. Anyone who is eligible to perform highly complex tests can also perform moderate-complexity testing. The Occupational Safety and Health Administration requires that training in handling chemical hazards, as well as training in handling infectious materials (standard precautions), be included for all new testing personnel. The laboratory director is ultimately responsible for all personnel working in the laboratory.

Pathologist

Most clinical laboratories are operated under the direction of a **pathologist**. The clinical laboratory can be divided into two main sections: clinical pathology and anatomic pathology. Many pathologists have training in both anatomic and clinical pathology. The anatomic pathologist is a licensed physician trained, usually for an additional four to five years after graduating from medical school, to examine (grossly and microscopically) all of the surgically removed specimens from patients, which include frozen sections, tissue samples, and autopsy specimens. Examination of Pap smears and other cytologic and histologic examinations are also generally done by an anatomic pathologist.

A clinical pathologist is also a licensed physician, with additional training in clinical pathology or laboratory medicine. As described earlier, laboratory medicine is the medical discipline by which clinical laboratory science and technology are applied to the care of the patient. Under the direction of the clinical pathologist, many common laboratory tests are performed on blood and urine, including assays such as blood cell counts and white cell differentials, urinalysis, common chemistry tests for blood sugar and cholesterol, microbiologic cultures of throat swabs and urine, coagulation studies such as prothrombin time tests, and immunoassays of various types. With training and advanced education in the use of various laboratory assays of the patient's blood, urine, tissue, or other body fluids or excretions, and with the effective utilization of these findings to present an informative result report to the patient's attending clinician, the clinical pathologist fulfills his or her role in the practice of laboratory medicine. The interpretation of laboratory findings in a timely and useable fashion is very important. Consultation with clinicians along the course of this process is also important; any and all information gained concerning the patient's case is actually the result of collaborative activity between the laboratory and the attending physician.

The pathologist will perform only certain of the services, such as examination of the surgical specimens, which is done primarily by the anatomic pathologist. Other work, such as the routine tests for blood cell counts and urinalysis, will be performed by trained laboratory personnel with various levels of education and experience, under the pathologist's responsibility and supervision.

Other Laboratory Personnel

Depending on the size of the laboratory and the numbers and kinds of laboratory tests performed, various levels of trained personnel are needed. CLIA '88 regulations set the standards for personnel, including their levels of education and training. Generally, the level of training or education of the laboratorian will be taken into consideration in the roles assigned in the laboratory and the kinds of laboratory analyses performed. In addition to the categories described below, various specialist categories are available to laboratorians; specific extra training and education will earn certification in areas such as blood banking or chemistry, for example. Other specialized training includes that for cytotechnologists, histotechnologists, and phlebotomists.

Laboratory Supervisor/Manager/Chief Technologist

Typically, a laboratory has a supervisor or manager who is responsible for the technical aspects of management of the laboratory. This person is most often a clinical laboratory scientist (also known as a medical technologist) with additional experience and skills in administration. In very large laboratories, a chief technologist may be in place to supervise the technical aspects of the facility (matters dealing with assay of analytes), including quality control programs and maintenance of the laboratory instruments. In addition, a business manager may be hired specifically to handle administrative details. The supervisor or administrative manager may also be the chief technologist in the case of smaller laboratories. Section-supervising technologists are in place as needed, depending on the size and work load of the laboratory. A major concern of administrative technologists, no matter what the job titles are called, is making certain that all federal, state, and local regulatory mandates are being followed by the laboratory. Persons in

leadership and management positions in the clinical laboratory must be certain that all legal operating conditions have been met and that they are balanced with the performance of work in a cost-effective manner.

It is important that the people serving in a supervisory position be able to communicate in a clear, concise manner, both to the persons working in their laboratory settings and to the physicians and other health care workers who utilize the services of the laboratory.

Clinical Laboratory Scientist

Medical technologists (MT), now also known as **clinical laboratory scientists (CLS)**, usually have earned a bachelor of science degree in medical technology or clinical laboratory science. Responsibilities vary; among other things, they may perform laboratory assays, supervise other laboratorians, or teach. Some are engaged in research. An important aspect of the training for a clinical laboratory scientist is to understand the science behind the tests being performed so that problems can be recognized when they occur and solutions undertaken. Troubleshooting is a constant consideration in the clinical laboratory. Because of his or her in-depth knowledge of technical aspects, principles of methodology, and instrumentation used for the various laboratory assays being done, the clinical laboratory scientist is able to correlate and interpret the data. Once educational requirements have been met at an accredited institution, certification for this level of laboratorian is offered through examination by the **Board of Registry of the American Society of Clinical Pathologists (ASCP)** and the **National Certification Agency for Medical Laboratory Personnel (NCA)**, an independent nonprofit certification agency.

Medical Laboratory Technician, Clinical Laboratory Technician, Clinical Laboratory Assistant

These laboratorians generally have some limitations in what work they can do in the laboratory and have different titles according to where they trained and in which health care facility they are employed—**medical laboratory technician (MLT), clinical laboratory assistant (CLA), clinical laboratory technician (CLT)**. These titles (and possibly others) indicate laboratorians with similarities. These laboratory personnel generally have a lesser amount of formal education or training than the clinical laboratory scientist. They usually possess some formal training; some have completed associate degrees, while others have a certificate of completion from a technical school or other vocational program. Much of the general, routine laboratory testing is done by these persons. Their work is usually done under the supervision of a clinical laboratory scientist or a pathologist. The CLT, MLT, or CLA collects, processes, and tests specimens (mostly blood and urine specimens) for the many routine, high-volume, repetitive tests done in a clinical laboratory. He or she is trained to seek help when a problem arises. Certification for CLT or MLT is offered through examination by ASCP and NCA.

SITES OF TESTING

Central Laboratory Testing vs. Point-of-Care Testing (Decentralization of Laboratory Testing)

The traditional setting for performance of diagnostic laboratory testing has been a centralized location in a health care facility (hospital) where specimens from patients are sent to be tested. The **centralized laboratory** setting remains in many institutions, but the advent of near-testing, bedside testing, or **point-of-care testing (POCT)** has changed the organization of many laboratories. In the POCT concept of testing, the laboratory testing actually comes to the bedside of the patient. Any changes to implement the use of POCT should show a significant improvement in outcome for the patient and should also show a total financial benefit to the patient and the institution and not just a reduction in the costs of equipment and supplies.

Point-of-Care Testing

Decentralization of testing away from the traditional laboratory setting can greatly increase the interaction of laboratory personnel with patients and with other members of the health care team. POCT is an example of an interdisciplinary activity that crosses many boundaries in the health care facility. POCT is not always performed by laboratorians, however. Other health care personnel, such as nurses, respiratory therapists, anesthesiologists, operating room technologists, and physician assistants, often are the ones doing the testing. However, the CLIA '88 regulations associated with clinical laboratory testing must also be followed for POCT, even if nonlaboratorians are actually performing the tests. These CLIA regulations are considered "site neutral," meaning that all laboratory testing must meet the same standards for quality of work done, personnel, proficiency testing, quality control, and so on, regardless of where the tests are performed—in a central laboratory or at the bedside of the patient. Test complexity is also considered for POCT, and the categories described earlier in this chapter, under Regulation of the Clinical Laboratory (waived tests, tests of moderate complexity, tests of high complexity, and provider-performed microscopies) also apply in regulations for POCT. If these tests are performed in a facility that is JCAHO or CAP accredited, they are regulated in essentially the same way as tests done in a centralized laboratory.

Qualifications for POCT personnel are also set by federal, state, and local regulations.[1,2] The level of training varies with the analytical system being employed and with the background of the individual involved—this can range from a requirement for a high school diploma with no experience to a bachelor of science degree with two years of experience. The director of the laboratory is responsible for setting additional requirements, as long as the federal CLIA '88 regulations are also being followed.

With the immediate reporting of results being available and with the patient's case management depending on the result, it is essential that POCT devices have built-in quality control and quality assurance systems to prevent erroneous data from being reported to the physician. POCT has been found to provide cost-effective improvement of medical care. In a hospital setting, POCT provides immediate assessment and management of the critically ill patient—this is its most significant use for this setting. Tests commonly included in POCT are ones based on criteria of immediate medical need; these include blood gases, electrolytes (Na^+, K^+, Ca^{++}), prothrombin time (PT), partial thromboplastin time (PTT) or activated clotting time (ACT), hematocrit or hemoglobin, and glucose. POCT attempts to meet the demands of intensive care units, operating rooms, and emergency departments for the faster reporting of test results. Other possible benefits of POCT are improved therapeutic turnaround times, less trauma and more convenience for the patient (when blood is collected and analyzed at the bedside), decreased preanalytical errors (errors formerly due to specimen collection, transportation, and handling by the laboratory), decreased manpower (the use of cross-training, whereby nurses can perform the laboratory analysis, eliminating a laboratorian for this step), more collaboration of clinicians with the laboratory, and shorter intensive care unit stays. Certain tests, such as the fecal screen for blood and the routine chemical screening of urine by reagent strips, can often be done more easily on the nursing unit, as long as the tests are properly performed and controlled using quality assurance protocol.

POCT in outpatient settings provides the ability to obtain test results during the patient's visit to the clinic or the physician's office, enabling diagnosis and subsequent case management in a more timely manner.

When central laboratory testing is compared with POCT, consideration must be given to which site of testing will provide the most appropriate testing mechanism. Centralized laboratories can provide "stat" testing capabilities, which can report results in a very timely manner. Sometimes laboratories will develop a laboratory satellite that is set up to function at the point of need—a laboratory located near or in the operating room, for example, or a laboratory that is portable and can be transported on a cart to the point of need.

Reference Laboratories

When a laboratory performs only routine tests, specimens for the more complex tests ordered by the physician must be sent to a **reference laboratory** for analysis. It is often more cost-effective for a laboratory to actually perform only certain common, repetitive tests and to send out the others for another laboratory to perform. These reference laboratories can then perform the more complex tests for many customers, giving good turnaround times—this is their service to their customers. It is important to select a reference laboratory where the mechanisms for specimen transport and results reporting are managed well. The turnaround time is important, and it often is a function of how well the specimens are handled by the reference laboratory. There must be a good means of communication between the reference laboratory and its customers. The reference laboratory should be managed by professionals who recognize the importance of providing quality results, and information about the utilization of the results when needed, to the patient's clinician. Messengers or couriers are engaged to transport or drive specimens within a fixed, reasonable geographic area. The various commercial delivery systems are used for transport out of the area.

Physician Office Laboratories

A **physician office laboratory (POL)** is a laboratory where the tests performed are limited to those done for the physician's own patients coming to the practice, group, or clinic. Because of the concern that some of these laboratories were lacking in quality of work done, the CLIA '88 regulations included POLs also. Prior to CLIA '88, the POLs were largely unregulated. Most POLs perform only the waived tests or provider-performed microscopy, as set by the CLIA. For a description of the tests included in the waived test category and for those in the PPM category, see CLIA Categories Based on Complexity of the

Tests Done by the Laboratory, earlier in this chapter. Tests most commonly performed in POLs are reagent strip urinalysis, blood glucose, occult fecal blood, rapid strep A in throats, hemoglobin, urine pregnancy, cholesterol, and hematocrit.

The convenience to the patient of having laboratory testing done in the physician's office is a driving force for a physician to include a laboratory in his or her office or clinic. Manufacturers of laboratory instruments have accommodated the clinic or office setting with a modern generation of instruments that require less technical skill on the part of the person using them. The improved turnaround times for test results and patient convenience must be balanced, however, with cost-effectiveness and the potential for the physician to be exposed to problems that may be outside the realm of his or her expertise or training. Laboratorians, including pathologists, must be available to act as consultants when the need arises.

A physician office laboratory must submit an application to the Department of Health and Human Services or its designee. On this application form, details about the number of tests done, the methodologies used for each measurement, and the qualifications of each of the testing personnel employed to perform the tests are included. Certificates are issued for up to two years, and any changes in tests done or methodologies used, personnel hired, and so forth, must be submitted to HHS within 30 days of the change. This application may also be made through an accreditation agency whose requirements are deemed by HHS to be equal to or more stringent than the HHS requirements. Accreditation requirements from the Commission on Office Laboratory Accreditation have been recognized by the HCFA as being equivalent to the CLIA requirements. See Regulation of the Clinical Laboratory, earlier in this chapter.

When a POL performs only waived tests or PPM tests, there are no CLIA personnel requirements. The physician is responsible for the work done in the POL. When moderately or highly complex testing is done in a POL, the more stringent CLIA personnel requirements must be followed for the testing personnel; these POLs must also adhere to a program of quality assurance, including programs of proficiency testing.

MEDICAL-LEGAL ISSUES

Informed Consent

For laboratories, an important responsibility is that of obtaining informed consent from the patient. **Informed consent** means that the patient is aware of, understands, and agrees to the nature of the testing to be done and what will be done with the results reported. Generally, when a patient enters a hospital, there is an implied consent to the many routine procedures that will be performed while he or she is there. Venipuncture is one of the routine tests that carries this implied consent. The patient must sign specific consent forms for more complex procedures, such as bone marrow aspiration, lumbar puncture for collection of cerebrospinal fluid, or fine-needle biopsies, and for nonurgent transfusion of blood or its components. The patient should be given sufficient information about the reasons why the informed consent is needed and must be given the opportunity to ask questions. In the event the patient is incapable of signing the consent form, a guardian should be obtained—for example, when the patient is a minor, legally not competent, physically unable to write, or hearing impaired, or does not speak English. Health care institutions have policies in place for handling these situations.

Confidentiality

Any results obtained for specimens from patients must be kept strictly confidential. Any information about the patient, including the types of measurements being done, must also be kept in confidence. Only authorized persons should have access to the information about a patient, and any release of this information to non–health care persons, such as insurance personnel, lawyers, or friends of the patient, can be done only when authorized by the patient. It is important to speak about a particular patient's situation only in the confines of the laboratory setting and not in any public place, such as elevators or hospital coffee shops.

Chain of Custody

Laboratory test results that could potentially be used in a court of law—at a trial or judicial hearing—must be handled in a specific manner. For evidence to be admissible, each step of the analysis, beginning with the moment the specimen is collected and transported to the laboratory, to the analysis itself and the reporting of the results, must be documented—a process known as maintaining the **chain of custody.** The links between specimen collection and presentation in court must establish certainty that the material or specimen tested had not been altered in any way that would change its usefulness as admissible evidence. Any specimen that has potential evidentiary value should be labeled, sealed, and placed in a locked refrigerator or other suitable secure storage area. Specimens that provide alcohol levels, specimens collected from rape victims, specimens for paternity testing, and specimens submitted from the medical examiner's cases are the usual types requiring the "chain of custody" documentation. See also Chapter 3.

REFERENCES

1. Ancillary (Bedside) Testing in Acute and Chronic Care Facilities, Approved Guideline. Villanova, Pa, National Committee for Clinical Laboratory Standards, 1994, NCCLS Document C30-A.
2. Department of Health and Human Services, Health Care Financing Administration: Clinical Laboratory Improvement Amendments of 1988. *Federal Register*, February 28, 1992. CLIA '88; Final Rule. 42 CFR. Subpart K, 493.1201.
3. Department of Health and Human Services, Health Care Financing Administration: Clinical Laboratory Improvement Amendments of 1988. *Federal Register*, April 24, 1995, vol 60, no 78. Final rules with comment period.
4. Department of Health and Human Services, Health Care Financing Administration: Clinical Laboratory Improvement Amendments of 1988. *Federal Register,* September 15, 1995, vol 60, no 179. Proposed rules.
5. Tietz NW (ed): *Applied Laboratory Medicine.* Philadelphia, W.B. Saunders Co., 1992, p 1.

BIBLIOGRAPHY

Clerc JM.: *An Introduction to Clinical Laboratory Science.* St Louis, Mosby, 1992.

Henry JB (ed.): *Clinical Diagnosis and Management by Laboratory Methods*, ed 19. Philadelphia, WB Saunders Co., 1996.

Kaplan LA, Pesce AJ: *Clinical Chemistry: Theory, Analysis, and Correlation*, ed 3. St Louis, Mosby, 1996.

Laboratory Design, Proposed Guideline. Villanova, Pa, National Committee for Clinical Laboratory Standards, 1994, NCCLS Document GP18-P.

NCCLS: *Clinical Laboratory Technical Procedure Manuals: Approved Guideline,* ed 3. Villanova, Pa, 1996, National Committee for Clinical Laboratory Standards, NCCLS Document GP2-A3.

NCCLS: *CLIA-NCCLS Index (A Collection of Documents).* Villanova, Pa, National Committee for Clinical Laboratory Standards, NCCLS Document X2-R.

NCCLS: *CLIA Specialty Collection (A Collection of Documents).* Villanova, Pa, National Committee for Clinical Laboratory Standards, NCCLS Document SC11.

NCCLS: *Continuous Quality Improvement: Essential Management Approaches and their Use in Proficiency Testing: Proposed Guideline.* Villanova, Pa, 1997, National Committee for Clinical Laboratory Standards, NCCLS Document GP22-P.

NCCLS: *Point-of-Care Testing (A Collection of Guidelines).* Villanova, Pa, National Committee for Clinical Laboratory Standards, NCCLS Document SC17-L.

NCCLS: *Training Verification for Laboratory Personnel: Approved Guideline.* Villanova, Pa, 1995, National Committee for Clinical Laboratory Standards, NCCLS Document GP21-A.

Physician Office Laboratory Policy and Procedure Manual. Northfield, Ill, College of American Pathologists, 1993.

Physician Office Laboratory Series. Commonwealth of Pennsylvania, Department of Health, Bureau of Laboratories, 1988.

STUDY QUESTIONS

1. Which of the following acts, agencies, or organizations was created to make certain that the quality of work done in the laboratory is reliable?

   A. Healthcare Finance Administration (HCFA)
   B. Occupational Safety and Health Administration (OSHA)
   C. Clinical Laboratory Improvement Amendments of 1988 (CLIA '88)
   D. Centers for Disease Control and Prevention (CDC)

2. Match each of the following agencies or organizations (1 to 5) with the best description of its purpose pertaining to the clinical laboratory (A to E):

   1. Healthcare Financing Administration (HCFA)
   2. Joint Commission on Accreditation of Healthcare Organizations (JCAHO)
   3. College of American Pathologists (CAP)
   4. Commission on Office Laboratory Accreditation (COLA)
   5. National Committee for Clinical Laboratory Standards (NCCLS)

   __4__ A. Sets accreditation requirements for physician office laboratories (POLs).
   __1__ B. Administers both the CLIA '88 and Medicare programs.
   __2__ C. HCFA has given it *deemed status* to act on the government's behalf to certify clinical laboratories.
   __5__ D. A nonprofit, educational group that establishes consensus standards for maintaining a high-quality laboratory organization.
   __3__ E. Accredits health care facilities and sets standards for quality assurance programs in those facilities.

mod complex, waived

3. Name the categories of laboratory tests based on the complexity of the test performed, as established by CLIA '88.

4. Laboratories performing which of the following types of tests must be enrolled in a CLIA-approved Proficiency Testing Program? (More than one of the answers may be correct.)

   A. Waived
   B. Moderately complex
   C. Highly complex
   D. Provider-performed microscopies

5. Match the following terms (1 to 4) with the descriptive statements (A to D) that follow:

   1. Proficiency testing (PT)
   2. Quality assurance (QA)
   3. Provider-performed microscopies (PPM)
   4. Point-of-care testing (POCT)

   _____ A. A continuing process of evaluating and monitoring all aspects of the laboratory to ensure accuracy of test results.
   _____ B. Specific microscopies (wet mounts) performed by a physician for his or her own patients.
   _____ C. A means by which quality control between laboratories is maintained.
   _____ D. A process of performing the laboratory testing at the bedside of the patient; a means of decentralizing some of the laboratory testing.

CHAPTER 2

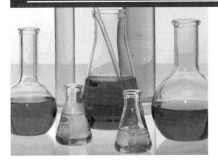

Safety in the Clinical Laboratory

Learning Objectives

From study of this chapter, the reader will be able to:

➤ Know the general safety regulations governing the clinical laboratory, including components of the OSHA-mandated plans for chemical hygiene and for occupational exposure to blood-borne pathogens, the importance of the safety manual, and generic emergency procedures.

➤ Know the basic aspects of infection control policies, including how and when to use personal protective equipment or devices (gowns, gloves, goggles), and the reasons for using standard precautions.

➤ Know the importance of a safety program in the laboratory.

➤ Know how to take the necessary precautions to avoid exposure to the many potentially hazardous situations in the clinical laboratory, including biohazards and chemical, fire, and electrical hazards, along with dangers in using certain supplies and equipment (broken glassware, for example)—the successful implementation of the "right to know" rule.

➤ Know the pre-exposure and post-exposure prophylactic measures for handling potential occupational transmission of certain pathogens, namely hepatitis B and human immunodefiency viruses (HBV and HIV).

➤ Know how to properly decontaminate a work area when a hazardous spill has occurred and, in general, how to keep the workplace clean.

➤ Know how to properly segregate and dispose of the various types of waste products generated in the clinical laboratory, including the use of sharps containers for needles and lancets.

➤ Know the basic steps of first aid.

IMPORTANCE OF LABORATORY SAFETY

The importance of safety and correct first-aid procedures cannot be overemphasized to anyone working in the clinical laboratory. Students as well as laboratory personnel should be constantly reminded of safety precautions. Many accidents do not just happen—they are caused by carelessness or lack of proper communication. For this reason, the practice of safety should be uppermost in the mind of anyone working in a clinical laboratory.

Most laboratory accidents are preventable by the exercise of good technique and by the use of common sense. There are many potential hazards in the laboratory, but most can be controlled by taking simple precautions. In every medical institution, the administration supplies the laboratory with safety devices for equipment and personal use, but it is up to the individual to make use of them. Safety is personal, and its practice must be a matter of individual desire and commitment. Real appreciation for safety requires a built-in concern for the other person, for an unsafe act may harm the bystander without harming the person who performs the act.

SAFETY MANUAL

Each laboratory should have a **safety manual** readily available that covers all safety practices and precautions. The safety manual should be updated frequently with additional or new information as it becomes available and should also include regulations covering the proper use of laboratory equipment and the handling of all hazardous or infectious materials. Anything that poses a potential safety hazard for persons in the laboratory should be described in the safety manual. All persons in the laboratory setting should be familiar with the location and the contents of this manual.

EMERGENCY PRECAUTIONS

A posted **plan for evacuation** of the laboratory in the event of an emergency must be readily available. Routes for exiting the room and the building must be made known to all persons working in that setting, as well as the locations of the various safety devices—fire extinguishers, emergency showers, eye washers, fire blankets, and other equipment such as respirators or goggles. Implementation of periodic unannounced safety drills may motivate the laboratory personnel to become familiar with current safety practices.

SAFETY STANDARDS AND GOVERNING AGENCIES

Safety standards for clinical laboratories are initiated, governed, and reviewed by several agencies or committees. These include the U.S. Department of Labor's **Occupational Safety and Health Administration (OSHA);** the **National Committee for Clinical Laboratory Standards (NCCLS),** a nonprofit educational organization providing a forum for development, promotion, and use of national and international standards; the Centers for Disease Control and Prevention (CDC), a part of the U.S. Department of Health and Human Services' Public Health Service; and the College of American Pathologists (CAP).[5,6,9,12]

To ensure that workers have safe and healthful working conditions, the United States government created a system of safeguards and regulations under the **Occupational Safety and Health Act of 1970.**[7] This system touches almost every person working in the United states today. It is especially relevant to discuss the meaning of the act in terms of safety in the clinical laboratory, where there are special problems with respect to potential safety hazards. Diseases or accidents associated with preventable causes cannot be tolerated.

The Occupational Safety and Health Act regulations apply to all businesses with one or more employees and are administered by the U.S. Department of Labor through OSHA. The programs deal with many aspects of safety and health protection, including compliance arrangements, inspection procedures, penalties for noncompliance, complaint procedures, duties and responsibilities for administration and operation of the system, and how the many standards are set. Responsibility for compliance is placed on both the administration of the institution and the employee.

The **OSHA standards**, where appropriate, include provisions for warning labels or other appropriate forms of warning to alert all workers to potential hazards, suitable protective equipment, exposure control procedures, and implementation of training and education programs—all for the primary purpose of ensuring safe and healthful working conditions for every American worker.

A person who understands the potential hazards in a clinical laboratory and knows the basic safety precautions can prevent accidents. The Occupational Safety and Health Act requires a **safety program** in every clinical laboratory. Identification of potential hazards is an important part of any such program. Although many hazards are commonly found throughout the clinical laboratory, the specific type of hazard may be slightly different in the various departments. Two programs have been mandated by OSHA to ensure the safety of persons working in a clinical laboratory. One covers occupational exposure to chemical hazards; the other covers occupational exposure to blood-borne pathogens.[5,6] Both of these programs will be discussed in subsequent sections of this chapter.

LABORATORY HAZARDS

Biological Hazards and Infection Control

Because many hazards of the clinical laboratory are unique, a special term, **biohazard**, was devised. This word is posted throughout the laboratory to denote infectious materials or agents that present a risk or even a potential risk to the health of humans or animals in the laboratory. The potential risk can be either through direct infection or through the environment. Infection can occur during the process of specimen collection, or from handling, transporting, or testing the specimen. Biological infections are frequently caused by accidental aspiration of infectious material, accidental inoculation with contaminated needles or syringes, animal bites, sprays from syringes, aerosols from the uncapping of specimen tubes, or centrifuge accidents. Some other sources of laboratory infections are cuts or scratches from contaminated glassware, cuts from instruments used during animal surgery or autopsy, and spilling or spattering of pathogenic samples on the work desks or floors. Persons working in laboratories on animal research or other research involving biologically hazardous materials are also susceptible to the problems of biohazards. The symbol shown in Figure 2-1 is used to denote the presence of biohazards.

One precaution that can be taken is to see that all containers are properly labeled. Labeling may be the simplest and the single important step in

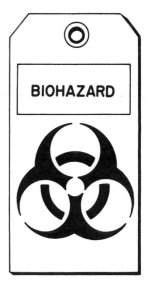

FIG 2-1. Biohazard symbol.

the proper handling of any hazardous substance. A label for a container should include a date and the contents of the container. When the contents of one container are transferred to another container, this information should also be transferred to the new container.

Laboratories must make every effort to implement a **program for infection control**. This can start with prevention of contamination when specimens are collected and when they are delivered to the laboratory. A large percentage of the specimens sent to a laboratory contain blood, and their safe collection and transportation must take top priority in any discussion of safety in the laboratory (see also Chapter 3).

Infection Control Programs

Since the clinical laboratory performs assays on various biological specimens from patients, one of the most important OSHA regulations covers exposure to biological hazards. Protection from **blood-borne pathogens** is of major importance. The OSHA-mandated program, Occupational Exposure to Bloodborne Pathogens, must be in place, and has been a law since March 1992.[5] Clinical specimens received from patients pose a potential hazard to laboratory personnel because of infectious agents they may contain. In addition, the CDC recommends safety precautions concerning the handling of all patient specimens. These are known as standard precautions (or universal blood and body fluid precautions), formally known as universal precautions; they are published by the Centers for Disease Control and Prevention as a guideline for hospital infection control practices and also published in *Morbidity and Mortality Weekly Report* (MMWR) which is a series of recommendations from the CDC to protect health care workers and others from infection by blood-borne pathogens.[2,10]

Recommendations from OSHA include an infection control plan, engineering and work practice controls, personal protective clothing and equipment, sufficient education and training, signs and labels, provision of hepatitis B virus (HBV) vaccination, and medical follow-up

after exposure incidents. The CDC provides recommendations for chemoprophylaxis after occupational exposure to HIV.[1] The NCCLS has also issued guidelines for the laboratory worker in regard to protection from blood-borne diseases spread via contact with patient specimens.[9]

Together, these agencies are working to lessen the risk of exposure of health care workers to blood-borne pathogens. An infectious disease program must be in place in any health care facility to ensure the safety of the people working there. The U.S. Department of Labor (under OSHA) has developed standards of practice for health care institutions. The CDC has issued guidelines for implementation of these standards. The College of American Pathologists offers a voluntary accreditation program for clinical laboratories. The requirements include safe work practices, which, in turn, include biosafety measures.

Standard Precautions

The term **standard precautions** refers to a system of infectious disease controls that assumes that every direct contact with body fluids is infectious. These controls include personal protective devices, good work practices, and the proper implementation of engineering controls. They require that every employee who has direct contact with patients and with their body fluids be protected as though such body fluids contained an infectious pathogen such as **hepatitis B virus (HBV)** or **human immunodeficiency virus (HIV)**. Since not all patients carrying blood-borne pathogens are identified prior to the handling of their specimens, all persons who handle patient specimens or who come in contact with patients in a health care setting should exercise certain consistent precautions on a routine basis. These standard precautions recognize the infectious potential of any patient specimen. The CDC recommendations also recognize that although all patients are potentially infectious, not all types of specimens pose the same degree of risk for health care personnel.

Blood and certain body fluids pose the greatest risk for those persons whose activities involve contact with them. Body fluids included in this classification are semen and vaginal secretions, tissues, cerebrospinal fluid, synovial fluid, peritoneal fluid, and amniotic fluid. For the purposes of prudent laboratory practice, however, adherence to standard precautions for the handling of all biological patient specimens is recommended. Through the use of these precautions, both the prevention of cross-transmission of infectious disease to patients and the protection of laboratory personnel from infected patients will be addressed. In most health care institutions, all patient specimens and body substances encountered during patient care are regarded as infectious and are handled by using the standard precautions policy.

The essence of any standard precautions policy is the avoidance of direct contact with patient specimens in general. When contact with any patient specimen is anticipated, health care workers should use the appropriate barrier precautions to prevent cross-transmission and exposure of their own skin and mucous membranes.

Protection from Specimen-Borne Pathogens

Precautions against exposure to possible specimen-borne infection focus mainly on HBV, HIV, and human T cell lymphotropic viruses (HTLV). Focus on HBV and HIV transmission is emphasized, owing to the severity of illnesses due to hepatitis B and acquired immunodeficiency syndrome (AIDS)—risks to health care workers that have grave consequences.[12] There are other viruses of concern to laboratory workers; **hepatitis C virus (HCV)**, formerly known as hepatitis non-A non-B virus, is one example. It is believed, however, that the standard precautions recommended for HBV and HIV are sufficient for most pathogens in general.

Virus Transmission. The major infectious pathogens, HBV and HIV, may be transmitted in the laboratory directly by three main routes:

1. Percutaneous: parenteral inoculation of blood, plasma, serum, or body fluids, which can occur by accidental needle sticks, scalpel cuts, and so forth, and by transfusion of infected blood or blood products

2. Nonintact skin: transfer of infected blood, plasma, serum, or body fluids in the absence of overt punctures of the skin, through the contamination of preexisting minute cuts, scratches, abrasions, burns, weeping or exudative skin lesions, and so forth

3. Mucous membranes: contamination of mucosal surfaces with infected blood, plasma, serum, or body fluids, as may occur with mouth pipetting, splashes, spattering, or other means of oral or nasal mucosal or conjunctival contact

HBV and HIV can be transmitted indirectly from such common inanimate surfaces as telephones, test tubes, laboratory instruments, and work surfaces that have been contaminated with infected blood or certain body fluids to areas of broken skin or mucous membranes by hand contact. HIV has been isolated from blood, semen, vaginal secretions, saliva, tears, breast milk, cerebrospinal fluid, amniotic fluid, and urine. However, only blood, semen, vaginal secretions, and breast milk have been implicated in the transmission of HIV. Hepatitis B is of special concern in laboratories of hospitals where organ transplants are done, where large volumes of blood and blood products are used. Personnel most heavily exposed to these large amounts of blood, such as blood from renal transplant patients—for example, through accidental inoculation, ingestion of blood, or inhalation of blood aerosols during laboratory work on these samples—are at the greatest risk of infection.

Hepatitis B and C viruses cause the most frequent laboratory-associated infections. As a precautionary measure against potential exposure to HBV, a licensed inactivated vaccine (HB) is recommended. The CDC's Advisory Committee on Immunization Practices (ACIP) recommends the use of this vaccine as a precautionary step for persons who are at a substantially greater risk for HBV infection—clinical laboratorians, phlebotomists, and pathologists.[8]

Hepatitis B Virus Exposure. After skin or mucosal exposure to blood that is known to contain or might contain hepatitis B antigen, the ACIP recommends **immunoprophylaxis**, depending on several factors. If the worker has not been vaccinated against HBV, a single dose of hepatitis B immune globulin should be given as soon as possible, within 24 hours if practical, along with doses of HB vaccine at a later date. The specific protocol for these measures will rest with the institution's infection control division. Post-vaccination testing for the development of antibody to surface HB antigen (anti-HBsAg) for persons at occupational risk who may have had needle-stick exposures necessitating post-exposure prophylaxis should be done to ensure that the vaccination has been successful.

Hepatitis C Virus Exposure. After exposure to blood of a patient infected or suspected of being infected with HCV, immune globulin should be given as soon as possible. No vaccine is currently available.

Human Immunodeficiency Virus Exposure. Transmission of HIV is believed to result from intimate contact with blood and body fluids from an infected person. Casual contact with infected persons has not been documented as a mode of transmission. If there has been occupational exposure to a potentially HIV-infected specimen or patient, the antibody status of the patient or specimen source should be determined, if it is not already known. If the source is a patient, voluntary consent should be obtained, if possible, for testing for HIV antibodies as soon as possible. High-risk exposure prophylaxis includes the use of a combination of antiretroviral agents to prevent seroconversion. **Post-exposure prophylaxis (PEP)** guidelines from the CDC are based on the determined risks of transmission (stratified as highest, increased, and no risk). Highest

risk has been determined to exist when there has been occupational exposure both to a large volume of blood (as with a deep percutaneous injury or cut with a large-diameter hollow needle previously used in the source patient's vein or artery) and to blood containing a high titer of HIV (known as a high viral load), to fluids containing visible blood, or to specific other potentially infectious fluids or tissue, including semen, vaginal secretions, and cerebrospinal, peritoneal, pleural, pericardial, and amniotic fluids.[10]

An enzyme immunoassay (EIA) screening test is used to detect antibodies to HIV. Before any HIV result is considered positive, the result is confirmed by Western blot (WB) analysis. A negative antibody test for HIV does not confirm the absence of virus. There is a window period after infection with HIV during which detectable antibody is not present. In these cases, detection of antigen is important; a polymerase chain reaction (PCR) assay for HIV DNA can be used for this purpose, and a p24 antigen test is used for screening blood donors for HIV antigen.

If the source patient is seronegative, the exposed worker should be screened for antibody again at 3 and 6 months. If the source patient is at high risk for HIV infection, more extensive follow-up of both the worker and the source patient may be needed.

If the source patient or specimen is HIV positive (HIV antibodies, Western blot, HIV antigen, or HIV DNA by PCR), the blood of the exposed worker should be tested for HIV antibodies within 48 hours, if possible. Exposed workers who are initially seronegative for the HIV antibody should be tested again 6 weeks after exposure. If this test is negative, the worker should be tested again at 12 weeks and 6 months after exposure. Most reported seroconversions have occurred between 6 and 12 weeks after exposure. Post-exposure prophylaxis should be started immediately and according to policies set by the institution's infection control program. A policy of "hit hard, hit early" should generally be in place.

During the early follow-up period after exposure (especially the first 6 to 12 weeks), the worker should follow the recommendations of the CDC regarding the transmission of AIDS, including:[1]

1. Refrain from donating blood or plasma.
2. Inform potential sex partners of the exposure.
3. Avoid pregnancy.
4. Inform health care providers of their potential exposure, so that necessary precautions can be taken by them.
5. Do not share razors, toothbrushes, or other items that could become contaminated with blood.
6. Clean and disinfect surfaces on which blood or body fluids have spilled.

The exposed worker should be advised of and alerted to the risks of infection and evaluated medically for any history, signs, or symptoms consistent with HIV infection. Serologic testing for HIV antibodies should be made available to all health care workers who are concerned that they may have been infected with HIV.

Tuberculosis Control. For **tuberculosis control**, OSHA also now requires the use of certain types of masks and respirators for persons occupationally exposed to patients with suspected or confirmed cases of pulmonary tuberculosis.

Safe Work Practices

To eliminate the risk of transmitting infectious pathogens, those working with blood specimens in the laboratory must take several precautions. Washing the hands frequently is one of the most important ways of preventing contamination. At least one sink in the laboratory should be equipped with a foot pedal for operating the faucets, and it should also have a foot pedal dispenser with a detergent solution for the hands.

Hand Washing. **Hand washing** is the most important means of interrupting transmission of infectious pathogens. Immediately after any accidental skin contact with blood, body fluids, or tissues, hands or other skin areas must be thoroughly washed. If the contact occurs through breaks in gloves, the gloves must be removed immediately and the hands thoroughly washed according to established procedure for the laboratory. It is also good practice to wash the hands any time there is visible contamination with blood or any body fluid, after completion of laboratory work and before leaving the laboratory, after removing gloves, and before any activities that involve contact with mucous membranes, eyes, or breaks in the skin.

Hand Washing Procedure (Procedure 2-1). Washing with soap and water is recommended, although any standard detergent product acceptable to the personnel may be used. Except in a unique situation, the use of hand towelettes and cleansing foams is not recommended, because they do not provide the necessary dilution and detergent action with the proper rinsing action to follow. No additional benefit has been established for washing with antiseptic soaps or solutions. Any product that disrupts the integrity of the skin should be avoided. Moisturizing hand creams or lotions may reduce skin irritation caused by the frequent hand washing that is so necessary.

Food and Drink Restrictions. Since the safety of the laboratory personnel is the reason for such scrutiny in the handling of specimens and other items, previously discussed, it is only prudent that there be no eating, drinking, smoking, or application of cosmetics in the laboratory. Hands may be contaminated with infectious organisms, which can easily be spread to the mouth during the above-mentioned activities.

Personal Protective Equipment

Personal protective equipment, including that for eyes, face, head, and extremities, protective clothing, respiratory devices, and protective shields and barriers, are to be provided to laboratory personnel whenever necessary by reason of the potential hazards of processes or environment. This equipment not only should be pro-

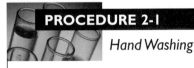

PROCEDURE 2-1

Hand Washing

1. Wet both hands and wrists with warm water only; do not use very hot or very cold water.

2. Apply soap from a dispenser to the palms first (about one teaspoonful).

3. Lather well and wash hands and wrists, fingernails, and between the fingers. Do this for a minimum of 10 seconds.

4. Rinse well with warm water and dry completely.

5. If the sink being used is not equipped with foot- or knee-operated controls, turn off the hand faucets with a paper towel to avoid recontamination of clean hands.

---

vided but also should be maintained in a sanitary and reliable condition. OSHA requires that institutions provide their personnel with personal protective equipment.[5]

Barrier Precautions

As discussed previously, precautions for exposure to possible specimen-borne infection focus mainly on HBV and HIV. With the emergence of multidrug-resistant strains of the bacteria causing pulmonary tuberculosis, OSHA now also requires the use of special types of masks or respirators when there will be exposure to patients with known or suspected pulmonary tuberculosis. **Protective devices** and **barrier precautions** will prevent transmission of most infectious disease if compliance is strictly maintained.

In the laboratory, the skin (especially when scratches, abrasions, dermatitis conditions, or lesions are present) and the mucous membranes of the eye, mouth, nose, and possibly the respiratory tract can be considered potential pathways for entry of infectious pathogens. Puncture with needles, sharp instruments, broken glass, or other sharp objects must be avoided. The handling and discarding of these objects must be done carefully and in a consistent manner. Constant vigilance and care must be exercised in the handling of infected cell-culture liquid or other virus-containing materials. Barrier precau-

tions are implemented to prevent exposure to infectious pathogens.

Gloves. Protective gloves must be worn by all persons who engage in procedures that involve direct contact of skin with biological specimens. The implementation of standard precautionary practices is recommended for handling clinical specimens, body fluids, and tissues from humans or from infected or inoculated laboratory animals.

Gloves must be manufactured from the appropriate material, usually intact latex, of the appropriate quality for the procedures required, and of the appropriate size for each health care worker. Gloves should be thrown away and not washed and used again. Since barrier protection is the ultimate goal, gloves must be discarded if they are peeling, cracking, or discolored (indications of deterioration), or if they have tears or punctures. Proper discarding of used gloves is necessary.

Gloves are worn during phlebotomies and during the processing of body fluid and blood specimens in the laboratory. After the gloves are removed and discarded, the hands must be washed immediately.

Gowns. All laboratory workers should wear a long-sleeved laboratory coat or gown with a closed front. Gowns and coats worn in the laboratory should be removed when the worker leaves. If personnel desire to wear a laboratory coat out of the laboratory, it is recommended that they have coats of different colors—one color to be worn in the laboratory (considered to be contaminated) and a different color to be worn outside the laboratory (considered to be noncontaminated).

When splashes to the skin or clothing are likely to occur, a special protective gown, apron, or laboratory coat must be worn. This protective clothing should be manufactured of fluid-proof or fluid-resistant material and should protect all areas of exposed skin.

Masks and Eye Protectors. When contamination of mucosal membranes (mouth, eyes, or nose) is likely to occur, the use of masks and protective eye wear or face shields is required. Such contamination can occur with body fluid splashes or aerosolization. Protective eye wear should be worn for transferring blood from a collection syringe into the specimen container, for example. Potential splashes can also occur when chemicals are being used. Certain laboratory reagents are known to be especially caustic to the mucosa. Broken glassware projectiles and vapors from some chemicals can also cause serious eye injuries. The eyes should always be protected with goggles when glassware is being cleaned with analytic cleaners and when laboratory reagents are being prepared from strong acids or bases or any other hazardous material.

Respirators or Masks for Tuberculosis Control. A person must be exposed to the tuberculosis bacterium to be infected. This occurs through close contact over a period of time, when contaminated droplet nuclei from an infected person's respiratory tract enter another person's respiratory tract. A commonsense way to control transmission of these contaminated droplets is to cover the mouth during coughing and to use tissues. In addition, certain specialized types of masks or respirators are now OSHA-mandated for use by persons who are occupationally exposed to patients with suspected

or confirmed cases of pulmonary tuberculosis. A "Special Respiratory Precautions" sign should identify rooms where there are patients fitting this criterion. Health care personnel caring for these patients must be fitted with and trained to use the proper respirator.

Protection From Aerosols

Biohazards are generally treated with great respect in the clinical laboratory. The adverse effects of pathogenic substances on the body are well documented. The presence of pathogenic organisms is not limited to the culture plates in the microbiology laboratory. Airborne infectious particles, or **aerosols**, can be found in all areas of the laboratory where human specimens are used.

Biosafety Cabinets. Biosafety cabinets are protective workplace devices used to control the presence of infectious agents in the air. Microbiology laboratories selectively utilize biological safety cabinets for performing procedures that generate infectious aerosols. Several common procedures in the processing of specimens for culture—grinding, mincing, vortexing, centrifuging, and preparation of direct smears—are known to produce aerosol droplets. Air containing the infectious agent is sterilized by heat or ultraviolet light or, most commonly, by passage through a high-efficiency particulate air (HEPA) filter. Biosafety cabinets not only remove air contaminants through a local exhaust system but provide an added measure of safety by confining the aerosol contaminant within an enclosed area, thereby isolating it from the worker.

Specimen Processing Protection. Specimens should be transported to the laboratory in plastic leak-proof bags. Protective gloves should always be worn for handling biological specimens of any kind.

Substances can become airborne when the stopper (cap) is popped off a blood-collecting container, a serum sample is poured from one tube to another, or a serum tube is centrifuged. When the cap is being removed from a specimen tube or a blood collection tube, the top should be covered with a disposable gauze pad or a special protective pad. Gauze pads with an impermeable plastic coating on one side can reduce contamination of gloves. The tube should be held away from the body and the cap gently twisted to remove it. Snapping off the cap or top can cause some of the contents to aerosolize. When not in place on the tube, the cap should still be kept in the gauze and not placed directly on the work surface or counter top.

Specially constructed plastic splash shields are used in many laboratories for the processing of blood specimens. The tube caps are removed behind or under the shield, which acts as a barrier between the person and the specimen tube. This is designed to prevent aerosols from entering the nose, eyes, or mouth. Laboratory safety boxes are commercially available and can be used for unstoppering tubes or doing other procedures that might cause spattering. Splash shields and safety boxes should be periodically decontaminated.

When specimens are being centrifuged, the tube caps should always be kept on the tubes. Centrifuge covers must be used and left on until the centrifuge stops. The centrifuge should be allowed to stop by itself and not be manually stopped by the worker.

Another step that should be taken to lessen the hazard from aerosols is to exercise caution in handling pipettes and other equipment used to transfer human specimens, especially pathogenic materials. These materials should be discarded properly and carefully.

Other Hazards

The fact that clinical laboratories present many potential hazards simply because of the nature of the work done there cannot be overemphasized. In addition to biological hazards, open flames, electrical equipment, glassware, chemicals of varying reactivity, flammable solvents, and toxic fumes are but a few of the other hazards present in the clinical laboratory.

BOX 2-1

Seven Rules for Biosafety in the Laboratory

1. Never mouth-pipette.
2. Treat infectious fluids carefully to avoid spills and to minimize aerosolization.
3. Restrict use of needles and syringes to procedures in which there is no alternative; use needles, lancets, and other "sharps" carefully to avoid self-inoculation; dispose of sharps in leak- and puncture-resistant containers.
4. Use protective laboratory coats and gloves.
5. Wash hands frequently: after all laboratory activities, after removing gloves, and immediately after contact with infectious materials.
6. Decontaminate work surfaces before and after use; wipe up any spills immediately.
7. Never eat, drink, store food, or smoke in the laboratory.

Flammable Substances

One serious hazard in laboratory work is the potential for fire and explosion when flammable solvents such as ether and acetone are used. These materials should always be stored in special safety containers in an appropriate storage cabinet. Even with proper storage of these materials, there is always some release of flammable vapors in a working laboratory. A good ventilation system for the room and vent sites for the storage area will help to eliminate some of the potential hazard. When flammable materials are being used, proper precautions must be taken; for instance, flammable liquids should be poured from one container to another slowly, they should never be used when there is an open flame in the room, and they should be kept in closed containers when they are not being used.

Chemical Hazards

Other sources of injury in the laboratory are poisonous, volatile, caustic, or corrosive reagents, such as strong acids or bases. Chemicals and reagents can present different types of hazards. Some are dangerous when inhaled (sulfuric acid), some are corrosive to the skin (phenol), some are caustic (acetic acid), some are volatile (many solvents), and some combine these hazards. Acids and bases should be stored separately in well-ventilated storage units. When not in use, all chemicals and reagents should be returned to their storage units. Bottles of particularly volatile substances should not be left open for extended periods.

OSHA is also involved in setting standards directed at minimizing occupational **exposures to hazardous chemicals** in laboratories. The OSHA hazard communication standard (the **employee "right-to-know" rule**) is designed to ensure that laboratory workers are fully aware of the hazards associated with chemicals in their workplaces.[6] This OSHA-mandated program became law in January 1991. The occupational exposure to chemical hazards law necessitates the development of comprehensive plans at each work site to implement safety measures throughout the laboratory insofar as the use of laboratory chemicals is concerned. A **chemical hygiene plan** for each laboratory must outline the specific work practices and procedures that are necessary to protect workers from any health hazards associated with hazardous chemicals. Information and training regarding hazardous chemicals must be provided to all workers in the laboratory setting. The individual states have also enacted "right-to-know" laws to ensure that available information is disseminated at the local level.

Information about signs and symptoms associated with exposure to hazardous chemicals used in the laboratory must be communicated to all. Reference materials for this information are included in the **material safety data sheets (MSDS)** provided by all chemical manufacturers and suppliers. This information concerns hazards, safe handling, storage, and disposal of hazardous chemicals used in the laboratory.

Material Safety Data Sheets. Information is provided by chemical manufacturers and suppliers about each chemical. This information is to accompany the shipment of all chemicals and should be available for anyone to review. Each laboratory must have on file all MSDSs for the hazardous chemicals used in that laboratory. Use of MSDSs is a common way that potential product hazard information is made available, and OSHA requires their provision by all chemical manufacturers. The health care facility, in turn, is required to provide this information to its workers in the laboratory.

Each MSDS contains basic information about the specific chemical or product. Trade name, chemical name and synonyms, chemical family, manufacturer's name and address, emergency telephone number for further information about the chemical, hazardous ingredients, physical data, fire and explosion data, and health hazard and protection information are included for each chemical.

Protection. When any potentially hazardous solution or chemical is being used, protective equipment for the eyes, face, head, and extremities, as well as protective clothing or barriers, should be used. Volatile or fuming solutions should be used under a fume hood. In case of accidental contact with a hazardous solution or a contaminated substance, quick action is essential. The laboratory should have a safety shower where quick, all-over decontamination can take place immediately. Another safety device that is essential in all laboratories is a face or eye washer that streams aerated water directly onto the face and eyes to prevent burns and loss of eyesight. Any action of this sort must be undertaken immediately, so these safety devices must be present in the laboratory area.

Measures to limit exposure to hazardous chemicals must be implemented. Appropriate work practices, emergency procedures, and personal protective equipment are to be employed by all. Many of the measures taken are also those needed for protection from biological hazards, as discussed previously (see under Personal Protective Equipment). These measures include the use of gloves, keeping the work area clean and uncluttered, the proper and complete labeling of all chemicals, and the use of proper eye protection, fume hood, respiratory equipment, and any other emergency or protective equipment as necessary.

Chemical waste must be deposited in appropriately labeled receptacles for eventual disposal.

Specific Hazardous Chemicals. Some specific chemicals that must be handled with care, and some potential hazards in their use, are as follows:

- *Sulfuric acid:* at a concentration above 65% may cause blindness; may produce burns on the skin; if taken orally may cause severe burns, depending on the concentration.
- *Nitric acid:* gives off yellow fumes that are extremely toxic and damaging to tissues; overexposure to vapor can cause death, loss of eyesight, extreme irritation, smarting, itching, and yellow discoloration of the skin; if taken orally can cause extreme burns, may perforate the stomach wall, or cause death.
- *Acetic acid:* severely caustic; continuous exposure to vapor can lead to chronic bronchitis.
- *Hydrochloric acid:* inhalation of vapors should be avoided; any acid on the skin should be washed away immediately to prevent a burn.
- *Sodium hydroxide:* extremely hazardous in contact with the skin, eyes, or mucous membranes (mouth), causing caustic burns; dangerous even at very low concentrations; any contact necessitates immediate care.
- *Phenol (a disinfectant):* can cause caustic burns or contact dermatitis even in dilute solutions; wash off skin with water or alcohol.

- *Carbon tetrachloride:* damaging to the liver even at an exposure level where there is no discernible odor.
- *Trichloroacetic acid:* very severely caustic; respiratory tract irritant.
- *Ethers:* cause depression of central nervous system.

Select Carcinogens. These are substances regulated by OSHA as carcinogens. **Carcinogens** are any substances that cause the development of cancerous growths in living tissue; they are considered hazardous to people working with them in laboratories. When possible, substances that are potentially carcinogenic have been replaced by ones that are less hazardous. If necessary, with the proper safeguards in place, potentially carcinogenic substances can be used in the laboratory. Lists of potential carcinogens used in a particular laboratory must be available to all who work there. These lists can be long.

Hazard Warning. A hazard identification system was developed by the National Fire Protection Association.[4] This system provides at a glance, in words, symbols, and pictures, information on the potential health, flammability, and chemical reactivity hazards of materials used in the laboratory. This information is provided on the labels of all containers of hazardous chemicals.

The hazard identification system consists of four small, diamond-shaped symbols grouped into a larger diamond shape (Fig. 2-2). The top diamond is red and indicates a flammability hazard. The diamond on the right is yellow and indicates a reactivity-stability hazard. These materials are capable of explosion or violent chemical reactions. The diamond on the left is blue and indicates a possible health hazard. The diamond on the bottom is white and provides special hazard information. It can provide information about radioactivity, special biohazards, and other dangerous elements. The system also indicates the severity of the hazard by using numerical designations from 4 to 0, with 4 being extremely hazardous and 0 being no hazard.

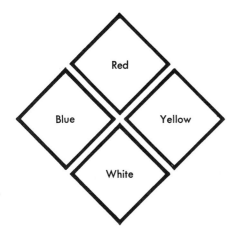

FIG 2-2. Identification system of the National Fire Protection Association. (From Kaplan LA, Pesce AJ: *Clinical Chemistry: Theory, Analysis, and Correlation,* ed 3. St Louis, Mosby, 1996.)

Electrical Hazards

Shocks from electrical apparatus in the clinical laboratory are a common source of injury if one is not aware of the potential hazard. This may be one of the most serious hazards in the laboratory. The important thing to understand with respect to danger to the human body is the effect of an electrical current. Current flows when there is a difference in potential between two points, and this knowledge is used in determining the approach to safety in the use of electrical equipment. Grounding of all electrical equipment is essential. If there is no path to ground, such a path might be established through the human in contact with the apparatus, resulting in serious injury. Attempts to repair or inspect a disabled electrical device should be left to someone who is trained to do this work.

Hazards With Glassware

The use of many kinds of glassware is basic to work in the clinical laboratory. Caution must be used to prevent unnecessary or accidental breakage. Some types of glassware can be repaired, but most glassware used today is discarded when it is broken. Any broken or cracked glass-

ware should be discarded in a special container for broken glass, and not thrown into the regular waste container. Common sense should be used in storing glassware, with heavy pieces being placed on the lower shelves and tall pieces being placed behind smaller pieces. Shelves should be placed at reasonable heights; glassware should not be stored out of reach. Broken or cracked glassware is the cause of many lacerations, and care should be taken to avoid this laboratory hazard.

Fire Hazards

Various types of fire-extinguishing agents must be available and their use must be understood. Fire in clothing should be smothered with a fire blanket or heavy toweling, or the flame should be beaten out; it should not be flooded with water. Everyone in the laboratory should know the correct use of the fire alarm and the procedure to follow in the event of a fire (see under Emergency Precautions).

Pipetting Safeguards: Automatic Pipetting Devices

It is a generally accepted rule that all pipetting must be done by mechanical means, either mechanical suction or aspirator bulbs. This procedure guards against burning the mouth with caustic reagents and against contamination by pathogenic organisms in samples. All specimens of human origin that are used in the laboratory (blood, urine, spinal fluid, stools, and so on) should be considered potentially infectious. To eliminate the use of aspirator bulbs and to provide increased pipetting accuracy, a form of automatic pipetting device is frequently used. Such devices offer fast, accurate ways of dispensing repetitive volumes. They can be set to deliver volumes in different ranges, depending on the device used. In general, a syringe reservoir is filled with the reagent to be measured, the volume to be delivered is determined by setting the dispenser dial, and the dispensing button is depressed to deliver the amount selected. The syringe mechanisms are usually autoclavable, and the pipette tips are disposable. Another device, a bottle top dispenser, can be used to deliver repetitive aliquots of reagents. Such a device is designed as a bottle-mounted system that can dispense repetitive selected volumes in an easy, precise manner. It is usually trouble free and requires a minimum of maintenance.

DECONTAMINATION

It is important to keep the laboratory workplace in a clean and sanitary condition. Cleaning and **decontamination** of the working surfaces after contact with blood or other potentially infectious materials are of prime importance. Most disinfectants are less active in the presence of high concentrations of protein. Because blood and other body fluids contain high concentrations of protein, these specimens, if spilled, should first be absorbed as completely as possible with disposable towels or gauze pads prior to disinfection. After absorption of the liquid, all contaminated materials (paper towels, etc.) should be discarded as **biohazard waste**. After absorption, the spill site should be cleaned with an aqueous detergent solution, and then disinfected with a high-level hospital **disinfectant** such as a dilution of **household bleach**.

Use of Bleach

Sodium hypochlorite, liquid household bleach, is often used as an intermediate-level disinfectant. Dilutions of bleach—a 0.5% solution made from a 5% solution (one part 5% sodium hypochlorite and nine parts water)—should be made up fresh weekly to prevent the loss of germicidal action during prolonged storage.

To clean up the laboratory work area, a strong bleach solution can be used for any spills of biological materials. Desk tops can be cleaned daily with a dilute solution of bleach. Any contaminated laboratory ware that must be reused cannot be cleaned with bleach, because it corrodes stainless steel containers and coagulates proteins. A strong detergent solution such as 3% phenolic

detergent can be used before autoclaving. Contaminated pipettes should be placed in long horizontal covered trays that are deep enough to minimize the chance of spilling when they are transported to the autoclave.

Autoclaves

Material that is to be autoclaved should be loosely packed so the steam can circulate freely around it. Autoclaving depends on humidity, temperature, and time. Under pressure, steam becomes hotter than boiling water and kills bacteria much more quickly. Autoclaves must be used with caution.

Autoclaves should be monitored regularly for their performance in adequately sterilizing the materials to be decontaminated. This monitoring procedure should be part of the ongoing quality assurance program for the laboratory.

LABORATORY WASTE DISPOSAL

OSHA standards provide for the implementation of a **waste disposal program**.[11] Receptacles used for the disposal of medical wastes should be manufactured from leak-proof materials and be maintained in a sanitary condition. The purpose of waste disposal control is to confine or isolate any possible hazardous material from all workers—laboratory personnel as well as custodial and housekeeping personnel. The NCCLS has also published guidelines on management of clinical laboratory waste.[3]

Infectious Waste

OSHA has defined **infectious waste** as blood and blood products, contaminated sharps, pathologic wastes, and microbiological wastes. Infectious waste is to be packaged for disposal in color-coded containers and should be labeled as such with the universal symbol for biohazards. Final disposal is by incineration or autoclaving.

Containers for Waste

Containers must be easily accessible to personnel needing them and must be located in the laboratory areas where they are commonly used. They should be constructed in such a manner that their contents will not be spilled if the container is tipped over accidentally.

Sharps Containers

After use, disposable syringes and needles, scalpel blades, and other sharp items should be placed in puncture-resistant **sharps containers** for disposal. The most widespread control measure required by OSHA and NCCLS is the use of puncture-resistant sharps containers.[5,9] The primary purpose of using these containers is to eliminate the need for anyone to transport needles and other sharps while looking for a place to discard them. Sharps containers are to be located in the patient areas as well as being conveniently placed in the laboratory. Use of the special sharps container permits quick disposal of a needle without recapping. This supports the recommendation against recapping, bending, breaking, or otherwise manipulating any sharp needle or lancet device by hand. Most needlestick accidents have occurred during recapping of a needle after a phlebotomy. If a needle must be recapped, it should be done in a one-handed fashion with one hand held behind the back. Injuries also can occur to housekeeping personnel when contaminated sharps are left on a bed, concealed in linen, or disposed of improperly in a waste receptacle. Most accidental disposal-related exposures can be eliminated by the use of sharps containers.

Biohazard Containers

Body fluid specimens, including blood, must be placed in well-constructed **biohazard containers** with secure lids to prevent leakage during transport and for future disposal. Contaminated specimens and other materials used in laboratory tests should be decontaminated before reprocessing for disposal or should be placed in special impervious bags for disposal in accordance with established waste removal policies. If outside contamination of the bag is likely, a second bag should be used.

Hazardous specimens and potentially hazardous substances should be tagged and identified as such. The tag should read "biohazard," or the biological hazard symbol should be used. All persons working in the laboratory area must be informed about the meaning of the tags and about what precautions should be taken for each.

Contaminated equipment must be placed in a designated area for storage, washing, decontamination, or disposal. With the increased use of disposable protective clothing, gloves, and so forth, the volume of waste for discard will be on the increase.

Biohazard Bags

Plastic bags are appropriate for disposal of most infectious waste materials, but rigid, impermeable containers should be used for disposal of sharps and broken glassware. Plastic bags with the biohazard symbols and lettering prominently visible can be used in secondary metal or plastic containers. These containers can be decontaminated or disposed of on a regular basis or immediately when visibly contaminated. These biohazard containers should be used for all blood, body fluids, tissues, and other disposable materials contaminated with infectious agents and should be handled with gloves.

Final Decontamination of Waste Materials

Final decontamination of materials in bags or containers is done by either incineration or autoclaving, either off or on site.

Disposal of medical waste should be done by licensed organizations that will ensure that no environmental contamination or anything aesthetically displeasing occurs. Congress has passed various acts and regulations regarding the proper handling of medical waste to assist the Environmental Protection Agency (EPA) to carry out this process in the most prudent fashion.

BOX 2-2

General Rules for Safety in the Clinical Laboratory

1. Know where the fire extinguishers are located, the different types for specific types of fires, and how to use them properly.

2. Pipette all solutions by using mechanical suction or an aspirator bulb. Never use mouth suction.

3. Handle all flammable solvents and fuming reagents under a fume hood. Store in a well-ventilated cabinet.

4. Use an explosion-proof refrigerator to store ether. Never use ether near an open flame. It is highly flammable.

5. Do not use any flammable substance near an open flame.

6. Wear gloves when handling infectious substances or toxic substances such as bromine or cyanide.

7. Mercury is poisonous. Contact supervisor; institution-specific protocol for cleanup of mercury is necessary.

8. If glass tubing is to be cut, hold the tubing with a towel to prevent cuts of the hands. This precaution also applies to putting a piece of glass tubing through a rubber stopper.

9. Use extreme caution when handling laboratory glassware. Broken glass is probably the greatest source of injury in the laboratory. Immediately discard cracked or broken glassware in a separate container, not with other waste.

10. If strong acids or bases are spilled, wipe them up immediately, using copious amounts of water and great care. Keep sodium bicarbonate on hand to assist in neutralizing acid spillage.

11. Plainly label all laboratory bottles, specimens, and other materials. When a reagent bottle is no longer being used, store it away in its proper place.

12. Put away safely or cover any equipment that is not being used.

13. Replace covers, tops, or corks on all reagent bottles as soon as they are no longer being used. Never use a reagent from a bottle that is not properly labeled.

14. If water is spilled on the floor, wipe it up immediately. Serious injuries can result from falls caused by slipping on a wet floor.

15. Never taste any chemical. Smell chemicals only when necessary and then only by fanning the vapor of the chemical toward the nose.

16. When handling blades or needles, use extreme caution to avoid cuts and infections. Dispose of all blades and needles in sharps containers.

17. Always pour acid into water for dilution. Never pour water into acid. Pour strong acids or bases slowly down the side of the receiving vessel to prevent splashing.

18. Use standard precautions when obtaining any specimen from a patient. Handle blood, serum, plasma, cerebrospinal fluid, urine, or any other patient specimen carefully, as if it were infectious. Severe infections and illnesses can result from handling specimens carelessly.

19. Wear gloves when handling any biological specimen.

20. Wash hands frequently while working in the laboratory, especially after handling patient specimens or reagents. Always wash hands before leaving the laboratory.

BOX 2-2

General Rules for Safety in the Clinical Laboratory—*cont'd*

21. Wear safety goggles when preparing reagents with strong chemicals. Some states (e.g., Minnesota) have enacted laws that require students, teachers, and visitors in educational institutions who are participating in or observing activities in eye-protection areas (areas where work is performed that is potentially hazardous to the eyes) to wear devices to protect their eyes.

22. In case of severe fire or burns, know where the safety shower is located and how to operate it.

23. Know the location of a fire blanket, which is used to smother flames in case of fire.

24. Most hospitals and teaching institutions have some type of warning signal and a procedure to follow in the event of a fire. This procedure should be understood thoroughly by anyone working in such an institution, whether as a student or as an employee. These institutions also have disaster plans, with which every worker must be thoroughly familiar.

25. When using burners and other heating devices, keep them far enough away from the working area that there is no possibility that anything will catch on fire.

26. Never lean over an open flame. Extinguish flames when not in use.

27. Learn the procedure used in the laboratory for discarding hazardous substances such as strong acids and bases.

28. Never pour volatile liquid or hazardous waste chemicals down a sink drain. Disposal of waste chemicals must be handled according to chemical hygiene protocol established by the facility.

29. To free a frozen glass stopper, run hot water over it, tap it lightly with a towel wrapped around it, or grasp it with a rubber glove or tourniquet.

30. Wear gloves when cleaning glassware, in case there is broken glass in the sink or soaking bucket.

31. Handle all hot objects with tongs, not hands. Extremely hot objects are to be handled with asbestos gloves.

32. If contaminated materials such as human specimens or bacterial agents are spilled on the work area, discard the contaminated material properly and wipe off the work area with bleach solution or other laboratory disinfectant.

33. Primary specimen (blood, primarily) collection tubes should be centrifuged with the caps left on them or by using sealed centrifuge cups for specimens without caps.

34. Cover all centrifuges to avoid flying broken glass and aerosols. Do not open centrifuges before they have stopped. Do not stop the centrifuge head by hand.

35. Be familiar with the OSHA rules and regulations, and be ready for an inspection by OSHA.

BASIC FIRST AID PROCEDURES

Since there are so many potential hazards in a clinical laboratory, it is easy to understand why a knowledge of **basic first aid** should be an integral part of any educational program in clinical laboratory medicine. The first emphasis should be on removal of the accident victim from further injury; the next involves definitive action or first aid to the victim. By definition, first aid is "the immediate care given to a person who has been injured or suddenly taken ill." Any person who attempts to perform first aid before professional treatment by a physician can be arranged should remember that such assistance is only a stop-

PROCEDURE 2-2

First Aid for Skin Puncture or Mucosal Contamination

1. For skin puncture or surface skin contamination, wash skin site with soap and water while encouraging bleeding. If appropriate, bandage the site. Report incident to supervisor.

2. For contaminated mucosal or conjunctival sites, wash with large amounts of water for an extended period of time. Report incident to supervisor.

gap—an emergency treatment to be followed until the physician arrives. Stop bleeding, prevent shock, and then treat the wound—in that order.

A rule to remember in dealing with emergencies in the laboratory is to keep calm. This is not always easy to do, but it is very important to the well-being of the victim. Keep crowds of people away, and give the victim plenty of fresh air. Because so many of the possible injuries are of an extreme nature and because in the event of such an injury immediate care is most critical, application of the proper first-aid procedures must be thoroughly understood by every person in the medical laboratory. A few of the more common emergencies and the appropriate first-aid procedures are listed below. These should be learned by every student or person working in the laboratory.

1. *Alkali or acid burns on the skin or in the mouth:* Rinse thoroughly with large amounts of running tap water. If the burns are serious, consult a physician.

2. *Alkali or acid burns in the eye:* Wash out thoroughly with running water for a minimum of 15 minutes. Help the victim by holding the eyelid open so that the water can make contact with the eye. An eye fountain is recommended for this purpose, but any running water will suffice. Use of an eyecup is discouraged. A physician should be notified immediately, while the eye is being washed.

3. *Heat burns:* Apply cold running water (or ice in water) to relieve the pain and to stop further tissue damage. Use a wet dressing of 2 tablespoons of sodium bicarbonate in 1 quart of warm water. Bandage securely but not tightly. In the case of a third-degree burn (the skin is burned off), do not use ointments or grease, and consult a physician immediately.

4. *Minor cuts:* Wash carefully and thoroughly with soap and water. Remove all foreign material, such as glass, that projects from the wound, but do not gouge for embedded material. Removal is best accomplished by careful washing. Apply a clean bandage if necessary (see Procedure 2-2).

5. *Serious cuts:* Direct pressure should be applied to the cut area to control the bleeding, using the hand over a clean compress covering the wound. Call for a physician immediately.

In cases of serious laboratory accidents, such as burns, medical assistance should be summoned while first aid is being administered. For general accidents, competent medical help should be sought as soon as possible after the first-aid treatment has been completed. In cases of chemical burns, especially when the eyes are involved, speed in treatment is most essential. Remember that first aid is useful not only in your working environment, but at home and in your community. It deserves your earnest attention and study.

REFERENCES

1. CDC update: provisional public health service recommendations for chemoprophylaxis after occupational exposure to HIV. *MMWR* 1996; 45:468-472.
2. Centers for Disease Control and Prevention (CDC): Hospital Infection Control Practices Advisory Committee (HICPAC), *Guidelines for Isolation Precautions in Hospitals,* 1996.
3. *Clinical Laboratory Waste Management: Approved Guideline.* Villanova, Pa, National Committee for Clinical Laboratory Standards, 1993, NCCLS document GP5-A.
4. National Fire Protection Association: *Hazardous Chemical Data.* Boston, National Fire Protection Association, 1975, no 49.
5. Occupational Safety and Health Administration (Department of Labor): Occupational exposure to bloodborne pathogens: final rule. *Federal Register* 29 CFR part 1910.1030(235), 64003-64182, Dec 6, 1991.
6. Occupational Safety and Health Administration (Department of Labor): Occupational exposure to hazardous chemicals in laboratories: final rule. *Federal Register* 29 CFR part 1910.1450, 55(21), 3327-3335, Jan 31, 1990.
7. Occupational safety and health standards. *Federal Register* 1978; 43(Oct 24, Nov 17).
8. Protection against viral hepatitis: recommendations of the Immunization Practices Advisory Committee. *MMWR* 1990; 39:1-23.
9. *Protection of Laboratory Workers from Infectious Disease Transmitted by Blood, Body Fluids, and Tissue: Tentative Guideline,* ed 2. Villanova, Pa, National Committee for Clinical Laboratory Standards, 1991, NCCLS document M29-T2.
10. Recommendations for prevention of HIV transmission in health-care setting. *MMWR* 1987; 36(suppl):3s.
11. Standards for the tracking and management of medical waste: interim final rule and request for comments. *Federal Register* 1989; 40(March 24): 12326.
12. Update: universal precautions for prevention of transmission of human immunodeficiency virus, hepatitis B virus, and other bloodborne pathogens in health-care settings. *MMWR* 1988; 37:377.

BIBLIOGRAPHY

Clinical Laboratory Safety: Approved Guideline. Villanova, Pa, National Committee for Clinical Laboratory Standards, 1996, GP17-A.

Henry JB (ed): *Clinical Diagnosis and Management by Laboratory Methods,* ed 19. Philadelphia, WB Saunders Co, 1996.

Kaplan LA, Pesce AJ: *Clinical Chemistry: Theory, Analysis, and Correlation,* ed. 3, St Louis, Mosby, 1996.

STUDY QUESTIONS

1. Which of the following acts, agencies, or organizations is primarily responsible for safeguards and regulations to ensure a safe and healthful workplace?

    A. Healthcare Finance Administration (HCFA)
    B. Occupational Safety and Health Administration (OSHA)
    C. Clinical Laboratory Improvement Act, 1988 (CLIA '88)
    D. Centers for Disease Control and Prevention (CDC)

2. The OSHA hazard communication standard, the "right to know rule," is designed for what purpose?

3. To comply with various federal safety regulations, each laboratory must have which of the following? (More than one of the answers may be correct.)

    A. A chemical hygiene plan
    B. A safety manual
    C. Biohazard labels in place
    D. An infection control plan

4. What is the essence of any standard precautions policy?

5. If it is likely that an employee has been exposed to blood or any other potentially HBV-infected material, to what preventive measure is the employee entitled free of charge?

6. What is the single most important procedure that can be performed to prevent the transmission of most infectious agents?

7. If a chemical spill occurs, what is one important source of information about the potential hazards resulting from exposure to that chemical? Explain how this source is used.

8. What is the main purpose of any waste disposal program in place in the laboratory?

CHAPTER 3

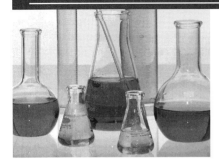

Collecting and Processing Laboratory Specimens

Learning Objectives

From study of this chapter, the reader will be able to:

➤ Appreciate the skills needed to interact with patients in the collection of specimens and the importance of the Patient's Bill of Rights.

➤ Understand the use of standard precautions and transmission-based precautions policies.

➤ Know the proper collection technique for venous blood.

➤ Know the proper collection technique for capillary or peripheral blood.

➤ Identify common anticoagulants and additives used to preserve blood specimens.

➤ Know the preferred urine specimen for a routine urinalysis, storage requirements for it, and the difference between the various types of urine collection—clean-catch, midstream, quantitative, and timed.

➤ Explain collection procedures for other body fluid specimens—cerebrospinal, pleural, synovial, and so forth.

➤ Collect a throat swab for culture.

➤ Collect feces for occult blood ("hidden" blood) tests and other tests.

➤ Know the importance of general specimen collection requirements prior to analysis—transport, processing, and storage.

GENERAL SPECIMEN REQUIREMENTS

The laboratory test can be no better than the specimen on which it is performed. If the specimen is improperly collected, not stored correctly, or mishandled in some way, the most quantitatively perfect determination is of no use because the results are invalid and cannot be used by the physician in diagnosis or treatment.

All samples sent to the laboratory must be processed according to certain established policies. Each division of the laboratory has unique requirements for specimens used in that division, but several general considerations apply to all specimens.

Quality Assurance Considerations

The term **quality assurance** is used to describe management of the treatment of the whole patient. As it applies to the clinical laboratory, quality assurance requires establishing policies that maintain and control, as much as possible, the many processes that involve the patient and any laboratory results for that patient. It includes properly preparing the patient for any specimens to be collected, collecting valid samples, correctly performing the laboratory analyses needed, validating the test results, correctly recording and reporting the test results, and getting those results into the patient's record. Another very important aspect of quality assurance is the policy regarding how records describing quality assurance practices and quality control measures used for laboratory analyses are documented, maintained, and made available, if needed, for review.

The purpose of a quality assurance policy is to make certain that over a long period of time, the laboratory provides reliable data that accurately reflect the status of the patient. Since physicians use laboratory test data to make diagnoses and to determine courses of therapy, it is essential that the results be reliable. As stated previously, the accuracy of a test result begins with the quality of the specimen received by the laboratory. The quality of a specimen depends on how it was collected, transported, and processed.

The person collecting any patient specimen has the responsibility of ensuring that the collection is done in the best manner possible. By following established policy and with training and experience, specimens can be collected that will yield valid results, thus ensuring high-quality patient care.

Patient Identification

Initial identification of the patient is extremely important. It is essential that a specimen from a particular patient be collected in the appropriate container and labeled for that patient. The patient's name, unique identification number and room number or clinic, and date and time of collection are commonly found on the label. All specimens sent to the laboratory must be properly labeled. For some tests, labels must include the time of collection of the specimen and the type of specimen. A properly completed request form should accompany all specimens sent to the laboratory.

Labels

Quality assurance policies are implemented in the clinical laboratory to protect the patient from any adverse consequences of errors resulting from an improperly handled specimen—beginning with the collection of that specimen. Laboratory quality assurance and accreditation require that specimens be properly labeled at the time of collection.

An unlabeled container or one labeled improperly should not be accepted by the laboratory. Specimens are considered improperly labeled when there is incomplete or no patient identification on the tube or container holding the specimen. Many specimen containers are transported in leak-proof plastic bags. It is not acceptable that only the plastic bags be labeled—the container actually holding the specimen must also be labeled. If the identification is illegible, the specimen is also unacceptable. In laboratories where computers are used, labels are computer generated, which assists in making certain that the proper identification information is included for each patient. Bar-coded labels facilitate this process. A specimen is unacceptable if the specimen container identification does not match exactly the identification on the request form for that specimen. Each laboratory has a specific protocol for the handling of mislabeled or "unacceptable" specimens.

All specimen containers must be labeled by the person doing the collection, to ensure that the specimen is actually collected from the patient whose identification is on the label.

USE OF STANDARD PRECAUTIONS AND TRANSMISSION-BASED PRECAUTIONS

With the use of **standard precautions** (formerly known as universal precautions), the need for the isolation category called "blood and body fluid isolation" (formerly referred to as "strict isolation") has been for the most part eliminated. The Centers for Disease Control and Prevention (CDC) recommends several disease-specific precautionary policies for patients known to be or suspected of being infected with certain pathogens.[6] With strict adherence to standard precautions, all sources of specimens (patients) are considered potentially pathogenic or infectious; that is, all specimens are treated in the same way. The use of proper personal protective equipment and barriers to prevent transmission of infectious agents is discussed in Chapter 2.

For known airborne pathogens (such as tuberculosis) or other highly communicable diseases that are spread by airborne or contact routes, specific additional **transmission-based precautions** should be taken for specimen collection. Respirators designed to control transmission of tuberculosis should be worn to enter the patient's room. CDC transmission-based precautions apply for patients (1) with known specific infection or suspected to be infected with specific microorganisms spread by air-borne, droplet, or contact routes of transmission and (2) during the incubation period of certain easily transmitted diseases. The individual health care

facility will initiate its specific precautions policies. Always follow the procedure of the hospital or patient care unit regarding transmission-based precautionary policies.

Contact precautions must be used for patients with volumes of drainage, skin infections, lice, scabies, cytomegalovirus infections, etc., when direct care is being given.

Protective Isolation

Protective isolation is used to protect the patient from infectious agents. For example, a burn patient is very susceptible to infection, so anyone entering the room of a burn patient must use protective isolation procedures. When specimens are collected from patients with leukemia or severe burns, or those who are immunosuppressed in preparation for receiving organ or bone marrow transplants, body radiation therapy, or plastic surgery, who must be protected from exposure to pathogens and other bacteria, a sterile gown, cap, gloves, and mask should be worn. Shoe coverings may also be required. With patients needing these extra measures, protective isolation techniques should be used for their sake, as well as the usual standard precautions being used for the sake of the health care worker.

TYPES OF SPECIMENS COLLECTED

Several different kinds of specimens are analyzed routinely in the clinical laboratory, but the specimen most often tested is blood. It is true that blood represents a large percentage of the specimens sent to the laboratory, but urine specimens are also sent in great numbers.

Many pathologic conditions may be associated with fluids that accumulate in the various cavities of the body. Laboratory examination of body cavity fluid may yield useful information regarding its formation and constituents. The physician can also be alerted to the type of disease process present by the information obtained from the laboratory analysis of a patient's various body cavity fluids—presence of infection, inflammation, tumor, etc. Some of the body cavity fluids examined in the laboratory are pleural, pericardial, peritoneal, synovial, amniotic, and cerebrospinal.

Fecal specimens and other miscellaneous specimens such as throat cultures and swabs from wound abscesses are also sent to the laboratory for analysis.

Blood: General Collection Information

Blood represents a large percentage of the specimens assayed in the clinical laboratory. Blood specimens are collected by several different types of health care personnel, depending on the facility. In some institutions, this work is done by the clinical laboratory scientists, medical technologists, or certified medical laboratory technicians. In other institutions, there are specially trained individuals who do the blood collecting. The person who practices this specialty is called a phlebotomist.

Circulation of Blood

Blood, although a liquid, can also be called a tissue. It circulates throughout the body, acting as a transportation system. As it circulates through the system of blood vessels (the vascular system), oxygen is transported from the lungs to the tissues of the body, products of digestion are absorbed in the intestine and carried to the various body tissues, and substances produced in various organs are transferred to other tissues for use. Cellular elements of the blood may also be transported to fight infection or aid in the coagulation of the blood. At the same time, waste products from the body tissues are picked up by the blood, and these end products of metabolism are then excreted through the skin, kidneys, and lungs.

The heart is the pump that forces the blood, under pressure, out through the arteries to all parts of the body. If an artery is cut, blood spurts out in small bursts each time the heart contracts. Near organs and muscles, the arteries branch out into smaller and smaller blood vessels called arterioles. Still smaller branches from the arterioles are called capillaries. In the tiny capillaries, the blood cells give up the oxygen they have been carrying and exchange it for the waste product from the body tissues, carbon dioxide. The capillary blood carrying carbon dioxide flows into larger vessels called venules, and then into still larger vessels called veins. The veins carry the blood back to the heart. As the blood flows through the capillaries, it gradually loses pressure. In the veins it has still less pressure. Therefore, if a vein is cut, the blood oozes out; it does not spurt out. After the veins have carried the blood back to the heart, the blood is pumped into the alveoli, or air sacs of the lung. In the alveoli the carbon dioxide is removed from the red blood cells, which take up oxygen in its place. The blood then returns to the heart to be pumped out to the body once again through the arteries. It is important to understand the basics of the blood circulation so that the proper sites for blood collection are used.

The chemical compound in the red blood cells that actually picks up the oxygen and exchanges it for carbon dioxide is hemoglobin. When hemoglobin is saturated with oxygen, it is bright red. When oxygen is replaced by carbon dioxide, the hemoglobin becomes darker red. When blood from an artery is compared with blood from a vein, the arterial blood is a visibly brighter red because of the nature of the hemoglobin compound.

The Phlebotomist

A professional **phlebotomist** has specific training in the technical skills of drawing blood. The phlebotomist is an important connection between the patient and the clinical laboratory. In addition to being skilled in obtaining blood by venipuncture, he or she is also trained to do capillary blood collections and perform special skin punctures, such as collecting specimens from infants in neonatal care units. Drawing specimens from indwelling lines is another collection specialty for those engaged in collecting blood.

Related areas of specimen transportation, handling, and processing must also be fully understood by the phlebotomist and by anyone who collects blood specimens. It is important therefore, to understand the proper means for collecting, preserving, and processing blood samples.

Approaching the Patient

Because it is relatively easy to obtain a blood sample, numerous studies are done on blood in diseased and normal states. Much valuable information is readily available at relatively low cost and with little discomfort to the patient. Certain routine blood studies are part of new hospital admissions. Many of these studies are carried out in the hematology and chemistry departments. Blood is also cultured in the microbiology department.

Anyone who plans to assume a duty or occupation in which contact with patients is required must consider several factors. These persons are providing a service to the patient. Adequate performance of this service involves not only technical knowledge but also sincere and concerned interest in people. This is a quality that, unfortunately, cannot be taught readily. It is a quality that a person must learn as a part of being engaged in a professional endeavor. Those in the medical laboratory field must be not only academically capable but also psychologically and socially responsible.

Patient's Bill of Rights. When blood specimens are collected, it is important that the rights of patients be kept in mind at all times. Being cognizant of these rights is consistent with good patient care. Phlebotomy involves direct patient contact, and it is essential that all people engaged in this aspect of laboratory work remember to serve the patient well.

Many hospitals have adopted a **patient's bill of rights** as declared by the Joint Commission on Accreditation of Healthcare Organizations (JCAHO). In some states, laws have been passed making patients' rights mandatory (California and Minnesota have these laws). Such a law could become the basis of litigation if a patient feels that his or her rights have been violated.

Box 3-1 is a summary of basic patient rights as endorsed by the JCAHO.

Patient Considerations. A patient in the hospital experiences several emotions, including anxiety and fear. The patient, separated from familiar surroundings, is also probably not feeling well, is concerned about his or her physical condition, and may be afraid of what is going to happen next. For these and other reasons, the patient's mental state is probably at its worst during hospitalization. It is extremely important that the patient be shown kindness and understanding. The collection of blood specimens is one area in which laboratory personnel have an opportunity to meet patients. It is essential, therefore, that those doing the blood collecting try to understand what the patient is feeling—to imagine what it would be like to be the patient—and act accordingly. Talking to the patient in a comfortable, friendly, pleasant, yet honest way is important.

When approaching a patient for the first time, there are certain procedures to remember. First, make certain that the patient on whom the test is being done is actually the right patient. Checking the identification number of the patient is essential. Check the wrist tag of the hospitalized patient to make certain that he or she is the right patient. For outpatients and for hospitalized patients, ask the patient's name—this is also a good way to start conversation. A mix-up in labeling tubes or drawing blood from the wrong patient can be disastrous. Always label the tubes of blood at the bedside of the patient or at the drawing site, as well as any slides, microcollection/capillary tubes, or other materials used for taking specimens. Proper and immediate labeling is essential.

Pediatric Patients. When working with a pediatric patient, one must first gain the patient's confidence. This may be the first time a child has had blood drawn. If this first experience is a bad one, it will be remembered and feared for years to come. It is therefore important to take some extra time to gain the child's confidence before

BOX 3-1

Patient's Bill of Rights

The patient has a right to:

1. Impartial access to treatment or accommodations that are available or medically indicated, regardless of race, creed, sex, national origin, or sources of payment for care.
2. Respectful, considerate care and treatment.
3. Confidentiality of all communications and other records and data which pertain to the care received by the patient.
4. Expect that any discussion or consultation involving the patient's case will be conducted discreetly and respectfully and that persons not directly involved in the case will not be present without the permission of the patient or guardian.
5. Expect reasonable personal safety in accord with the hospital practices and environment.
6. Know the identity and professional status of individuals providing service and to know which physician or other practitioner is primarily responsible for his or her care.
7. Obtain from the practitioner complete and current information about diagnosis, treatment, and any known prognosis, in terms which can reasonably be understood by the patient.
8. Reasonable and informed participation in decisions involving his or her health care. The patient shall be informed if the hospital proposes to engage in or perform human experimentation or other research or educational projects affecting his or her care or treatment. The patient has the right to refuse participation in such activity.
9. Consult a specialist at the patient's own request and expense.
10. Refuse treatment to the extent permitted by law.
11. Request and receive an itemized and detailed explanation of the total bill for services rendered in the hospital regardless of the source of payment.
12. Be informed of the hospital rules and regulations.

going ahead with the collection procedure. Get acquainted with the child by using a book or a toy, for example. Keep your equipment tray as inconspicuous as possible. Be frank with the child. Sometimes it may be possible to tell a story about what you are doing. It is important in working with pediatric patients to bolster their morale as much as possible. Ask for help in restraining a very small or uncooperative child.

Older children may be more responsive when permitted to "help," by holding the gauze, for example. Working with a child often involves working with the parents also. This is best accomplished by allowing the parents to know, by the professional attitude assumed, that the laboratorian or phlebotomist is kind but very defi-

nitely in charge of the situation. This attitude, which is so basic for laboratory personnel, can be developed only with practice.

In the nursery, each hospital will have its own rules, but a few general precautions apply. After working with an infant in a crib, the crib sides must be returned to the position in which they were found when the collection process was begun. If an infant is in an incubator, the portholes should be closed as much as possible. When oxygen is in use, do not forget to close the openings when the collection process is completed. Dispose of all waste materials properly.

Adult Patients. Adult patients must be told briefly what is expected of them and what the test involves. With adults as well as with children, complete honesty is important. It is unwise to say that a finger puncture will not hurt, when it really will. However, if possible, avoid dwelling on that aspect of the collection process.

The patient should be greeted in a friendly and tactful manner; without becoming overly familiar, a conversation can be started in a quiet, pleasant, and calm manner. The patient should be told about the purpose of the blood collection. Any personal information the patient relates is being told in confidence. Religious beliefs of the patient should be respected, laboratory reports kept confidential, and any personal information about the patient also kept in confidence. Information about other patients or physicians is always kept in confidence. If the same patient is seen frequently, it is possible to become familiar with his or her interests, hobbies, or family and to use these as topics of conversation. Many patients in the hospital are lonely and need a friend. Occasionally, especially with the extremely ill patient, he or she will not wish to talk at all; in this case, respect these wishes. It is important to be honest, but to attempt to boost the patient's morale as much as possible.

Even if the patient is disagreeable (and many are), the laboratorian should remain pleasant. A smile can often work miracles. It is important to be firm when the patient is unpleasant, to remain cheerful, and to express confidence in the work to be done. Young children who do not understand words seem pacified by the sound of a confident voice. Talking pleasantly to every patient is essential.

In a hospital setting, before leaving the patient's room, the area should be checked to see that everything is in place in the laboratory tray and that the room has been left as it was found. The tray holding the blood collection supplies and equipment should always be kept out of reach of the patient. This is especially important in working with children, but it applies to all patients.

Types of Collection Procedures

Any discussion concerning blood specimens must include collection procedures for blood—this applies to all areas of the clinical laboratory. There are two general sources of blood for clinical laboratory tests: peripheral, or capillary, blood and venous blood. The National Committee for Clinical Laboratory Standards (NCCLS) has set standards for the collection of both **capillary blood (skin puncture)** and **venous blood (venipuncture)**.[8,9] For small quantities of blood for some hematologic or microchemical determinations, capillary blood is suitable; it is obtained from the capillary bed by puncture of the skin (see Capillary or Peripheral Blood Collection by Skin Puncture, below). The tip of the finger is the site most commonly punctured. For larger quantities of blood, a puncture is made directly into a vein (phlebotomy), using a sterile syringe and needle collection system or evacuated tube and needle collection system (see Venous Blood Collection by Venipuncture, later in this chapter). A vein in the upper forearm (or antecubital fossa) area is most often chosen for venipuncture, as these veins are easily palpable and fairly well fixed.

Gloves. Before any contact with the patient is made, the phlebotomist must put on protective gloves to implement the necessary barrier protection required by the standard precautions policy.

Capillary or Peripheral Blood Collection by Skin Puncture

For the small quantities of blood required for most hematologic procedures and for microchemical techniques requiring serum or plasma, an adequate blood sample may be obtained from the capillary bed by puncture of the skin—a capillary puncture or skin puncture. The NCCLS has set standards for the collection of capillary blood by skin puncture.[8] (See Procedures 3-1 and 3-2.) From certain patients, such as babies, burned patients, very sick patients, or amputees, it may be

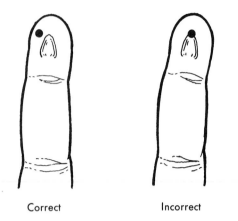

Correct   Incorrect

FIG 3-1.   Sites for finger puncture. (From Powers LW: *Diagnostic Hematology*. St Louis, Mosby, 1989, p 433.)

necessary or desirable to obtain only a very small amount of blood. This can be accomplished quite easily by means of capillary puncture. This blood is collected into suitable capillary tubes, pipettes, or microcontainers or used directly to prepare blood films.

Capillary blood is often used for point-of-care tests (POCT)—bedside testing for glucose using one of several available reading devices and the accompanying reagent strips being a common one. This same procedure is done at home by countless diabetics on their own blood to ascertain the level of blood glucose for maintenance of good glucose control.

In adults and older children, the tip of the finger is punctured (Fig. 3-1) (see Procedure 3-1). In infants, the plantar surface of the heel or the large toe is punctured (Fig. 3-2) (see also

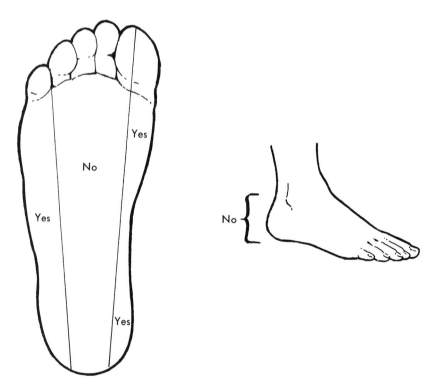

FIG 3-2.   Sites for heel puncture in infants. (From Powers LW: *Diagnostic Hematology*. St Louis, Mosby, 1989, p 435.)

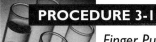

PROCEDURE 3-1

Finger Puncture

1. Assemble the necessary equipment: lancet device, alcohol pad, dry gauze, slides, and capillary tubes or other supplies necessary to receive the blood.

2. Be sure that the patient is seated comfortably.

3. Wash hands and put on gloves.

4. Choose an area for the puncture that is free from calluses, edema, or cyanosis. Warm the puncture site if it is cold by immersing it in warm water or by rubbing it.

5. Clean the skin of the puncture site on the third or fourth finger vigorously with a pad soaked in an alcohol solution. This will remove dirt and epithelial debris, increase the circulation, and leave the area relatively sterile. Allow the area to air-dry.

6. Grasp the finger firmly, and make a quick, firm puncture about 2 to 3 mm deep with a sterile disposable lancet or automated lancet device (see Fig. 3-4). This puncture should be made at right angles to the fingerprint striations on the patient's finger, midway between the edge and midpoint of the fingertip (see Fig. 3-1). The puncture should not be made too far down on the finger and should not be too close to the fingernail. A deep puncture hurts no more than a superficial one, and it gives a much more satisfactory flow of blood.

7. Discard the lancet in the sharps disposal container. Used lancets should never be left lying on the work area. They should be discarded immediately after use and should not be touched again.

8. Wipe away the first drop of blood, using a clean piece of dry gauze or tissue. This drop is contaminated with tissue fluid, which will interfere with some laboratory results. The succeeding drops are used for tests.

9. If a good puncture has been made, the blood will flow freely. If it does not, use gentle pressure to make the blood form a round drop. Excessive squeezing will cause dilution of the blood with tissue fluid.

10. Collect the specimens by holding a capillary tube to the blood drop or by touching the drop to a glass slide. Rapid collection is necessary to prevent coagulation, especially when several tests are to be done with blood from the same puncture site.

11. When the blood samples have been collected, have the patient hold a sterile, dry piece of gauze or cotton over the puncture site until the bleeding has stopped.

12. Remove gloves and wash hands.

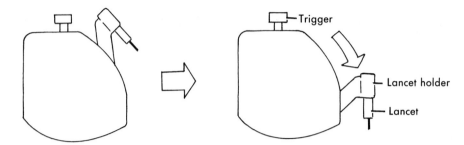

FIG 3-3. Automated lancet, spring-driven and trigger-activated (Autolet, Owen Mumford, Inc, Marietta, Ga.) (From Powers LW: *Diagnostic Hematology*. St Louis, Mosby, 1989, p 430.)

Procedure 3-2). In general, the ear lobe should be avoided for puncture because there is a slower flow of blood there and the concentrations of cells and hemoglobin will be greater. Blood obtained by skin puncture of these types is generally called capillary blood, but it is closer to arteriolar blood in its composition.

The results of tests from venous and capillary (fingertip) blood compare well if the capillary blood is free flowing. To ensure free flow of capillary blood, the finger must be warm.

Various types of disposable lancets or blades are used for skin puncture. Nondisposable lancets are not used, because of the risk of transmission of infectious pathogens. Lancets with safety gauges for depth of puncture are the best ones to use.

Precautions to Note When Obtaining Capillary Blood. If the patient's fingers are cold, slight rubbing may help to warm them. The finger or heel must not be squeezed excessively, because tissue fluid may dilute the blood sample or cause the blood to clot faster than it normally would. The first drop of blood is usually removed because it contains tissue fluid, alcohol, or perspiration, which will dilute the blood. Immediately after surgery, patients with low blood pressure and those in surgical shock may require more than one puncture. Only one sterile lancet is used at a time. The tip of the lancet should not touch anything until it punctures the skin of the patient. Contaminated lancets are discarded properly and new ones used. After the puncture is made, the

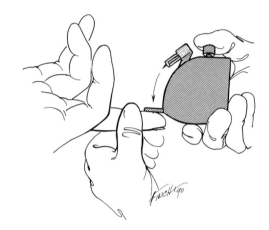

FIG 3-4. Finger puncture technique using automated lancet device (Autolet).

lancet is discarded immediately. Hand washing before and after each new patient is encountered, along with wearing gloves, is essential.

Skin Puncture Devices. A variety of automatic, **spring-activated skin puncturing devices** are commercially available. The NCCLS has set guidelines for skin puncture devices.[4] Clean, rapid incisions can be made of a consistent depth with the use of one of these devices. Devices such as the Autolet* have a lancet held in place by a cocking lever (Figs. 3-3 and 3-4). When released, the blade penetrates the skin to a depth of 2 to 3 mm, depending on the choice of platform used.

---

*Owen Mumford, Inc, Marietta, Ga.

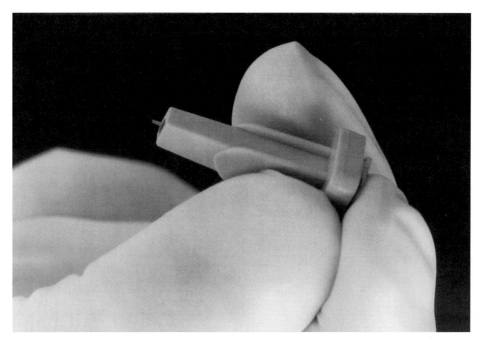

FIG 3-5. Microtainer Safety Flow Lancet. Courtesy Becton Dickinson & Co, Becton Dickinson VACUTAINER Systems, Franklin Lakes, NJ.)

The platform regulates the depth of the puncture. Disposable lancets/blades and platforms or guards are used with these devices. The device itself can be cleaned with a bleach or disinfectant solution. It is important that all used lancets and platforms be discarded in a container for sharps. Transmission of blood-borne infections must be prevented (see under Standard Precautions in Chapter 2).

Individual spring-activated lancet devices are also available, in which case the entire device is disposable. One such lancet system, the Microtainer Safety Flow Lancet,* is a sterile, self-contained spring-activated triggering device, containing a lancet housed in a protective plastic coating. These lancets are available in varying puncture depths (Fig. 3-5). To prevent accidental punctures once the device has been triggered, the lancet retracts into its protective covering once it has been used. Similar devices are available in a form used for neonatal heel punctures.

Procedure for Heel Puncture (Procedure 3-2). For infants under 3 months of age, the heel is the most commonly used site for obtaining a blood sample. Any wound-inflicting device can result in serious injury when excessive pressure and skin indentation accidentally allow the wound depth to reach the heel bone.

The foot must be held securely in place for the puncture (Fig. 3-6). The lateral or medial plantar surface of the foot should be used for the skin puncture (see Fig. 3-2). The site and depth of the puncture are of critical importance. The depth should not exceed 2.4 mm. The central portion and posterior curvature of the heel are not used, because the bone lies too close to the surface. Puncture of the heel bone (calcaneus) can result in osteochondritis or osteomyelitis. The NCCLS

---

*Becton Dickinson VACUTAINER Systems, Becton Dickinson & Co, Franklin Lakes, NJ.

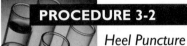

PROCEDURE 3-2

Heel Puncture

1. Wash hands and put on gloves.
2. Clean the puncture site with an alcohol sponge. Let it thoroughly dry.
3. Hold foot firmly to avoid sudden movement. Warm foot if needed.
4. Select lancet device with the appropriate depth for the size of the infant.
5. Perform the puncture on the most medial or most lateral portion of the plantar surface (see Figs. 3-2 and 3-5).
6. Puncture no deeper than 2.4 mm.
7. Do not perform punctures on the posterior curvature of the heel.
8. Do not puncture through previous sites, which may be infected.
9. Fill collection containers as needed.
10. When finished, elevate heel and place a piece of dry gauze on the puncture site. Keep pressure on the site until bleeding has stopped.
11. Discard used supplies in the appropriate waste containers. Notify nursing personnel that the procedure is complete.

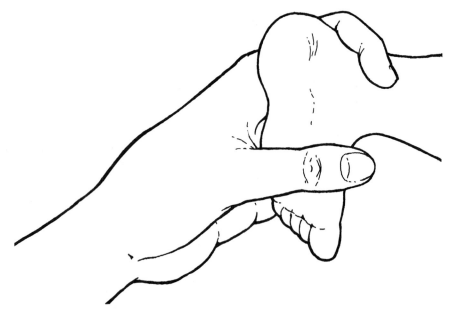

FIG 3-6. Holding an infant's heel for capillary puncture. (From Powers LW: *Diagnostic Hematology.* St Louis, Mosby, 1989, p 436.)

has established recommendations for heel punctures in neonates[8] (see Procedure 3-2).

A semiautomatic device for performing heel punctures, called tenderfoot,* makes an incision that is 1 mm deep and 2.5 mm wide, allowing free-flowing collection of up to 3 mL of blood (Fig. 3-7). A tenderfoot device with a depth of puncture specifically designed for premature infants is also available. The blade of the device automatically retracts following the skin incision, ensuring that neither the blood collector nor the infant is accidentally punctured. When compared with other puncturing devices, tenderfoot

---

*International Technidyne Corp, Edison, NJ.

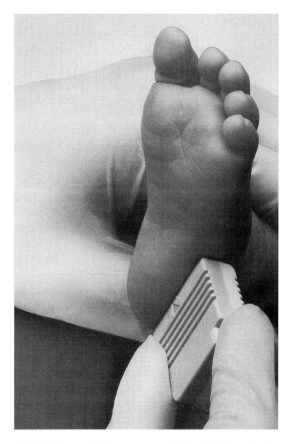

FIG 3-7. tenderfoot automated heel incision device for infant blood sampling. (Courtesy International Technidyne Corp, Edison, NJ.)

causes less hemolysis of the sample, requires fewer punctures to obtain the desired sample, and produces less physical trauma to the heel of the infant. It is a sterile, completely disposable device, reducing the possibility of introducing infection in the infant. The depth and width of the incision are controlled, thus eliminating the possibility of calcaneal puncture and osteomyelitis. The amount of sample collected and the free-flowing nature of the blood following the puncture make squeezing the foot unnecessary. The device reduces the number of heel punctures needed. The detailed procedure for using this device accompanies the product.

Blood Spot Collection for Neonatal Screening Programs. Most states have passed laws requiring that newborn infants be screened for certain diseases that can result in serious abnormalities, including mental retardation, if they are not diagnosed and treated early. These diseases include phenylketonuria (PKU), galactosemia, hypothyroidism, and hemoglobinopathies. The NCCLS has set standards for filter paper collection, or **blood spot collection**, of blood for these screening programs.[2] Blood should be collected 1 to 3 days after birth, before the infant is discharged from the hospital—at least 24 hours after birth and after ingestion of food for a valid PKU test. There is an increased chance of missing a positive test result when an infant is tested for PKU before 24 hours of age. When infants are discharged early, however, many physicians prefer to take a sample early rather than risk no sample at all.

In most **neonatal screening programs**, the specimen is collected onto filter paper and then sent to the approved testing laboratory for analysis. Special collection cards with a filter paper portion are supplied by the testing laboratory—these are kept in the hospital nursery or central laboratory. There is an information section on these cards, and all requested information must be provided—it is to be treated as any other request form. The filter paper section of the card contains circles designed to identify the portion of the paper onto which the specimen should be placed, where the filter paper will properly absorb the amount of blood necessary for the test.

Collection is usually done by heel puncture, following the accepted procedure for the institution. When a drop of blood is present, the circle on the filter paper is touched against the drop until the circle is completely filled. A large enough drop should be formed so that the process of filling the circle can be done in only one step. The filter paper is allowed to air dry and then is transported to the testing laboratory in a plastic transport bag or other acceptable container. The procedure established by the testing laboratory should be followed for the collection step.

Capillary Blood for Testing at the Bedside (Point-of-Care Testing). Capillary blood samples for glucose testing and for other assays are used frequently in many health care facilities for **bedside testing,** or **point-of-care testing (POCT).** Quantitative determinations for glucose are made available within 1 or 2 minutes, depending on the system employed. The NCCLS has set guidelines for these tests, as they are performed in acute care and long-term care facilities.[1] (POCT is also discussed in Chapter 1, under Sites of Testing.)

POCT for glucose is also performed at home by many outpatient diabetics, using their own blood and one of several glucose measuring devices. It is important for patients with diabetes, especially those with insulin-dependent diabetes mellitus, to monitor their own blood glucose levels several times a day and to be able to adjust their dosage of insulin accordingly to maintain good glucose control.

For the inpatient diabetes patient, POCT is also a valuable tool for management of the disease. The blood glucose level is often quite unstable in these patients, a situation that may necessitate frequent adjustments of insulin dosage. The POCT tests give results that are immediate, so dosages can be adjusted more quickly. Ordering and collecting venous blood speci-

mens for glucose tests done by a central laboratory with the necessary frequency and rapidity of reporting required are often impractical, thereby making the POCT tests much more useful. Good quality-control programs must be used to ascertain the reliability of the POCT results, however. Whole blood samples should be collected by puncture from the heel (for infants only), finger, or flushed heparinized line, using policies for standard precautions to protect against the transmission of blood-borne pathogens. Arterial or other venous blood should not be used, unless the directions from the manufacturer of the POCT device being used specify the appropriateness of these alternative blood specimens. The POCT instrument should be calibrated and the test performed according to the manufacturer's directions. Results should be recorded permanently in the patient's medical record in a manner that distinguishes between bedside test results and central laboratory test results.

It is critical to understand the limitations of each POCT detection system so that reliable results are obtained. The specific limitations described by each manufacturer must be considered. The use of a quality assurance program is mandatory to ensure reliable performance of these procedures. The use of POCT—bedside testing or self-testing for glucose—is intended for management of diabetes patients and not for initial diagnosis. It is not used to replace the standard laboratory tests for glucose, but only as a supplement.

Several commercial instruments are available, and with each product a meter provides quantitative determination of glucose present when used with a reagent strip that is designed to accompany the meter. A drop of capillary blood is touched to the reagent strip pad and, according to the specific procedure, read in the meter. The instrument provides an accurate and standardized reading when used according to the manufacturer's directions. The reagent strips must be handled with care and used within their proper shelf life. The strips are specific only for glucose.

The meters are packaged in convenient carrying cases and are small enough to be placed in a pocket or briefcase.

Capillary Blood for Slides. A finger or heel puncture is made and, after the first drop is wiped away, the glass slide is touched to the second drop formed. The slide is placed on a flat surface and a spreader slide used to prepare the smear. The slide is allowed to air dry, is properly labeled, and then is transported to the laboratory for examination.

Capillary Blood Specimen Containers. Once the skin has been punctured and the blood is flowing, the capillary sample can be collected into a variety of containers. For general purposes, glass tubes with or without heparin can be used and the blood allowed to flow into the tube by capillary action. For example, a heparinized capillary tube is used to collect blood for performing the microhematocrit test in the hematology laboratory.

Another capillary sampling device is called the Unopette* (Fig. 3-8). It consists of a disposable capillary pipette that measures a fixed volume and a reservoir of diluent appropriate to the test being performed. This pipette and diluent system can be used with either capillary or venous blood, and the general system has been adapted for several chemical and hematologic determinations.

Microcontainers are available to contain small volumes of blood. They consist of a small plastic tube with a blood drop collector as part of the lid (see Fig. 3-8). One such commercially available system is the Microtainer.* This allows the specimen to be collected by capillary action and results in a relatively large amount of specimen in a single container. When the collection is finished, the container can be properly capped and processed by centrifugation, if serum is to be obtained. These microcontainers are available with various additives, including serum separator gels.

---

*Becton, Dickinson & Co, Franklin Lakes, NJ.

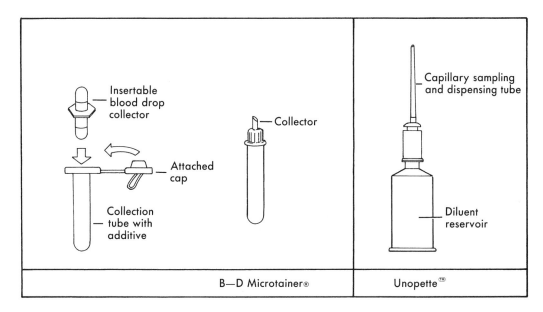

FIG 3-8. Types of microcontainer tubes and collecting devices. (From Powers LW: *Diagnostic Hematology.* St Louis, Mosby, 1989, p 431.)

Venous Blood Collection by Venipuncture

The veins that are generally used for venipuncture are those in the forearm, wrist, or ankle. The first choice for a venipuncture site is a vein in the forearm. Veins in this region are larger and fuller than those in the wrist, hand, or ankle. The wrist, hand, or ankle veins are used only if the forearm site is not available. Venipuncture must be performed with great care and technical skill. The NCCLS has set standards for the collection of venous blood.[9] The veins of the patient are the main source of blood for testing, and the entry point for medications, intravenous solutions, and blood transfusions. A patient has only a limited number of accessible veins, and it is important that everything possible be done to preserve their good condition and availability. Part of this responsibility lies with the person doing the blood drawing.

Blood may be obtained directly from a vein (phlebotomy) by using a sterile **syringe and needle** or **evacuated tube and needle collection system** (Fig. 3-9). The use of the evacuated (vacuum) tube system allows the blood to pass directly from the vein into the collection tube. Veins in the forearm are most commonly used when this system is used. The three main veins in the forearm are the cephalic, median cubital, and median basilic (Fig. 3-10). The **median cubital vein** is usually chosen for venipuncture. The median basilic might roll or move, and the skin over the cephalic might be tougher to penetrate. Other sites may be used when necessary.

The phlebotomy may be done and blood collected by either the syringe method or the evacuated (vacuum) tube method (see Procedure 3-3). An infusion or butterfly set can be used in combination with the evacuated tube method (see Procedure 3-4). (see Fig. 3-11). In the syringe method, a needle is attached to a syringe and inserted into the vein. The plunger of the syringe is drawn back, which creates suction, drawing the blood into the syringe. In the evacuated tube method, one end of a two-way needle is partially attached by means of a holder device to the rubber stopper of a specially prepared vacuum tube. The other end of the two-way needle is inserted into the vein. Once that end is in the vein, the

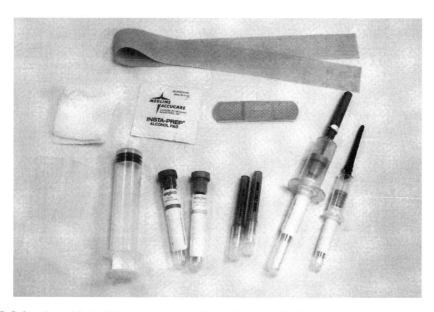

FIG 3-9. Assembled phlebotomy supplies. (From Powers LW: *Diagnostic Hematology.* St Louis, Mosby, 1989, p 423.)

end of the needle in the rubber stopper is pushed through the stopper to make a direct connection to the vacuum tube (Fig. 3-12). The vacuum tube creates suction, which draws the blood into the tube. One commercially available vacuum tube system is called VACUTAINER.* The NCCLS has published standards for the use of evacuated tubes for blood specimen collection.[5]

When doing a venipuncture, the phlebotomist should remain in a standing position, which gives the greatest freedom of movement. The patient should assume a comfortable position. A bed patient should remain lying down, and an **ambulatory patient** should be seated comfort-

---

*Becton Dickinson VACUTAINER Systems, Becton Dickinson & Co, Franklin Lakes, NJ.

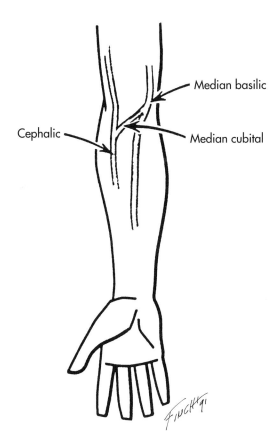

FIG 3-10. Major veins of the arms.

ably with the arm in an inclined position. The seated patient should put an arm on a table or other firm support and extend it for the phlebotomist.

Blood Collection Variables. The majority of clinical laboratory determinations are done on whole blood, plasma, or serum. Many of these analyses are done in the hematology or chemistry laboratories, but many other areas of the laboratory also require venous blood for testing.

Most venous blood specimens are drawn from fasting patients. Most fasting blood is drawn in the morning before breakfast. This means that the food from the previous meals has been completely digested and absorbed and any excess has been stored. Food intake, medication, activity, and time of day can all influence the laboratory results for blood specimens. Some of these facts are rarely taken into account by the persons interpreting the laboratory results. The fasting state is one fact that is carefully noted, however, especially for glucose, triglyceride, and phosphorus determinations. Through numerous studies it has been found that the average meal has no significant effect on the concentration of most blood constituents, with certain exceptions. Blood collected directly after a meal is described as a **postprandial specimen**. Food intake significantly affects blood glucose and triglycerides, giving a falsely high result, and phosphorus, giving a falsely low result. Because it is the most efficient time of day to draw specimens for the laboratory, most of the blood collecting is done early in the morning, and for this reason most of the patients are in the **fasting state** (having had no food or liquid other than water for 8 to 12 hours). Fasting specimens, however, are not necessary for most laboratory determinations. Blood should not be collected while intravenous solutions are being administered, if possible.

Other controllable biological variations in blood include posture (whether the patient is lying in bed or standing up), immobilization (resulting from prolonged bed rest, for example), exercise, circadian/diurnal variations (cyclical

Text continued on p. 63

PROCEDURE 3-3

Venipuncture Using the Evacuated Tube System[3,9]

1. Wash hands and put on gloves to comply with policies for standard precautions for blood collection.

2. Identify and reassure the patient. Ask the patient to state his or her full name. Always check the wrist identification to confirm the identity of the patient. This is especially important when blood specimens are being drawn from unconscious or mentally impaired patients.

3. Assemble necessary equipment and supplies (Fig. 3-9).
   a. Thread the short end of the double-pointed needle (called the hub of the needle) into the plastic holder and tighten securely, using the needle sheath as a wrench (see Fig. 3-12).
   b. Assemble sterile evacuated blood collection tubes as needed for the tests desired, ascertaining the proper order for collection. Before using, tap all tubes that contain additives to make certain that all the additive is dislodged from the stopper.
   c. Place the vacuum tube in the holder and push the stopper of the blood collection tube into the shorter shielded needle (within the holder) up to the recessed guideline on the needle holder. The needle will thus be embedded in the stopper without puncturing it and losing vacuum in the tube (see Fig. 3-12, *A*). Do not push the tube beyond the guideline, as a premature loss of vacuum may result. Because of this potential problem, some phlebotomists prefer not to attach the tube at this stage.
   d. Remove the needle shield, and inspect the tip of the longer needle visually to see if it is free of hooks at the end of the point and the opening is clear. Leave the needle covered loosely until the actual venipuncture can be performed. Do not contaminate it.

4. Position the patient. For ambulatory patients: a chair with side supports is used to prevent accidental falling. The patient should be seated comfortably in the chair, with the arm extended to form a straight line from the shoulder to the wrist and inclined in a downward position. The arm should rest across a narrow table or on a slanting armrest, which can be part of the chair. The arm and elbow should be supported firmly, and the arm should not be bent at the elbow. Add more support if needed.

   For patients in bed: make certain they are in a comfortable supine position. If additional support is needed, a pillow may be placed under the arm on which the venipuncture is to be done. The patient should extend the arm to form a straight line from the shoulder to the wrist.

5. Close the patient's hand (unnecessary if veins are prominent).

6. Select the vein site to be used. If possible, the site is selected without the tourniquet. However, on many patients the tourniquet is used at this point (Procedure 3-5). Observe both arms. Select the median cubital vein that appears fullest. These veins are usually easily palpable, fairly well anchored in place, and bruise less. If necessary, use the cephalic vein, in preference to the basilic vein. The cephalic vein does not roll and bruise as easily as the basilic, although the blood usually flows more slowly. Palpate and trace the vein several times with the tip of the index finger. Feel the "bounce" of a full vein. A vein feels much like an elastic tube and gives under pressure. Even if you can see the vein, palpate until you can be certain of its location and direction.

PROCEDURE 3-3

Venipuncture Using the Evacuated Tube System—cont'd

Unlike veins, arteries pulsate and have a thick wall. Thrombosed veins feel cordlike and roll.

Muscle tendons are usually apparent.

Blood can be forced into the vein by gently massaging the arm from wrist to elbow. Several sharp taps at the vein site with the index and second fingers may cause the vein to dilate. Application of heat to the site may have the same result. Lowering the arm over the chair will allow the veins to fill to capacity. If a vein is not readily apparent, use a tourniquet temporarily. Do not leave the tourniquet in place for more than one or two minutes for this examination process.

The best location to perform the venipuncture is at the bend of the elbow, but if these sites are not usable, the flexor surfaces of the forearm, the wrist area above the thumb, the volar area of the wrist, or the back of the hand can be used. Use of the foot or ankle is rarely necessary.

Collection of blood from a site on which the tourniquet has been used for more than 2 minutes can result in inaccurate laboratory analyses. A tourniquet prevents blood from flowing freely, and the balance of fluid and blood elements may be disrupted.

Do not use areas of obvious hematomas, where blood has been collected before, as some laboratory results may be erroneous. If no other veins are available, collect below (distal to) the hematoma.

Do not collect blood from scarred areas or from an arm where intravenous fluids are being given. Use the other arm. Special procedures must be followed if blood is collected from an arm where an intravenous solution is being administered.

Only experienced phlebotomists should draw blood specimens from intravascular devices—cannula, fistula, vascular graft, or heparin-locked catheter.

7. Apply the tourniquet so that it can be easily released (Fig. 3-13 and Procedure 3-5). The tourniquet increases venous filling with blood and makes the veins more prominent and easier to enter. Do not leave the tourniquet on for longer than 1 minute, if possible; apply just before venipuncture is to be performed. Never apply a tourniquet above an intravenous site, a fistula, a shunt, a cannula, or a heparin-locked catheter. Avoid pinching the skin. The tourniquet should remain "flat" around the patient's arm.

8. Clean the skin at the venipuncture site. Usually the vein site is cleaned with an isopropyl alcohol solution or medicated alcohol on a gauze pad, using a circular motion starting from the actual site of entry and working toward the periphery. This is done to prevent any chemical or microbiologic contamination of either patient or specimen. Allow the area to air-dry in order to prevent hemolysis of the blood sample and alcohol seepage into the puncture. For blood culture collection, a triple application of povidone-iodine solution is required.

   If the area is touched before the puncture, it should be recleaned.

9. Place the selected collection tubes and needle assembly within easy reach.

Continued

PROCEDURE 3-3

Venipuncture Using the Evacuated Tube System—cont'd

10. Grasp the patient's arm and anchor the vein. The patient's arm should be grasped firmly, with the palm of the hand under the elbow. The patient's arm should be fully extended. Use the thumb, placed 1 or 2 in. below the puncture site, to anchor the vein by drawing the skin taut. Ask the patient to open and close the hand.

11. Perform the venipuncture:
    a. Keep the patient's arm in a downward position and maintain the tube below the site throughout the procedure to prevent backflow from the tube into the patient's vein.
    b. Turn the needle so that the bevel side is up.
    c. Line up the needle with the vein.
    d. Puncture the vein. The puncture of the skin and vein should be done in two steps, if possible, the skin first and then the vein, at approximately a 15- to 30 degree angle and in a direct line with the vein. A sensation of resistance will be felt, followed by ease of penetration as the vein is entered.
    e. As soon as the needle is positioned sufficiently in the vein, insert the vacuum tube into the needle holder as far as it will go so that blood can flow into the vacuum tube (see Fig. 3-12, *B*). Do this by grasping the flange of the needle holder from the top, between the index and third fingers, and triggering the tube forward by pushing with the thumb until the hub end of the needle punctures the stopper. This will activate the vacuum action to draw the blood into the collection tube.
    f. Allow the tube to fill until the vacuum is exhausted and blood flow ceases, in order to ensure the correct ratio of anticoagulant to blood. The tube normally will not be filled completely. As the blood flow ceases, remove the tube from the needle holder, being careful not to change the position of the needle in the vein. If multiple samples are to be drawn, remove the tube as soon as the blood flow stops and insert the next tube into the holder. The shut-off device on the hub of the needle covers the point at which the tube is removed and stops the blood from flowing until the next tube is inserted. Adhere to the proper order for the draw: first, sterile tubes for culture, then nonadditive tubes, tubes for coagulation studies, and finally the tubes with additives.
    g. As the tube containing an additive is removed, mix immediately by gently inverting the tube five to ten times. To avoid hemolysis, do not shake or mix vigorously.
    h. To collect multiple samples, carefully insert the next tube into the holder, taking care not to change the position of the needle in the vein. Collect as many tubes as needed, using the same technique.

PROCEDURE 3-3

Venipuncture Using the Evacuated Tube System—cont'd

12. Open the patient's hand. Ask the patient to open his or her hand; this reduces the amount of venous pressure.

13. Release the tourniquet (preferably at 1 minute). Remove the tourniquet as soon as blood flow is established in the last tube to be drawn. If the tourniquet has been left on too long before blood is acquired, some test results are altered owing to stasis of cells and movement of fluid out of the vein into the tissue. The arm will become cyanotic. **The tourniquet must always be released before the needle is removed from the vein.**

14. Position a dry gauze pad. Lightly place a gauze pad over (covering) the venipuncture site.

15. Quickly, but gently, remove the needle. Then apply pressure on the gauze pad. Hold the dry gauze pad over the needle and puncture site. Quickly remove the needle while keeping the bevel in an upward position, exercising care not to scratch the patient's arm. Apply mild pressure to the site as soon as the needle is withdrawn. Continue to apply pressure on the gauze pad until bleeding is stopped. Special attention should be given to patients with prolonged bleeding.

16. Bandage the arm, if needed. If the patient continues to bleed, apply a pressure bandage over the venipuncture site. Tell the patient to leave the bandage on for 15 to 30 minutes. It is recommended that adhesive bandages not be placed on small children; they may remove, chew, or swallow them.

17. Dispose of the puncturing unit. Avoid puncturing your own skin. **NEVER attempt to reshield the needle.** Special sharps biohazard disposal systems are available, which allow for direct disposal of the needle. Dispose of all waste supplies immediately in the proper disposal containers.

18. Label tubes. Be sure to properly label all tubes with the patient's name, identification number, date of collection, and other necessary patient information, and mix the tubes adequately with their additive or anticoagulant. In the clinical laboratory, blood tube labels must exactly match the patient data on the test request forms.

19. Remove gloves and wash hands.

20. Leave the patient only after all signs of bleeding have stopped.

PROCEDURE 3-4

Venipuncture Using an Infusion Set and the Evacuated Tube System

1. Attach the tube holder and adapter to the end of the infusion/butterfly needle tubing (Fig. 3-15).

2. Hold the butterfly needle with the bevel up, at approximately 15 to 30 degrees to the patient's skin and in a direct line with the vein to be entered.

3. Apply tourniquet (Fig. 3-13 and Procedure 3-5).

4. Anchor the vein.

5. Insert the needle into the vein with one smooth aggressive motion. Some blood will appear in the tubing if the vein has been entered.

6. When using the evacuated tube system, as soon as the needle enters the vein, insert the collection tube into the holder as far as it will go.

7. If multiple tubes are needed, remove the tube as the blood flow stops and insert the next tube into the holder.

8. When the last tube has filled, remove the tourniquet and then the needle and tubing, positioning a dry gauze over the needle and puncture site Apply mild pressure to the site as soon as the needle is withdrawn.

9. Apply pressure on the venipuncture site until bleeding has stopped.

10. Bandage the arm, if needed. If the patient continues to bleed, apply a pressure bandage over the venipuncture site. Tell the patient to leave the bandage on for 15 to 30 minutes. It is recommended that adhesive bandages not be placed on small children; they may remove, chew, or swallow them.

11. Dispose of the puncturing unit. Avoid puncturing your own skin. Special sharps biohazard disposal systems are available, which allow for direct disposal of the infusion system. Dispose of all waste supplies immediately in tthe proper disposal containers.

12. Label tubes. Be sure to properly label all tubes with the patient's name, identification number, date of collection, and other necessary patient information, and mix the tubes adequately with their additives or anticoagulants. In the clinical laboratory, blood tube labels must exactly match the patient data on the test request forms.

13. Remove gloves and wash hands.

14. Leave the patient only after all signs of bleeding have stopped.

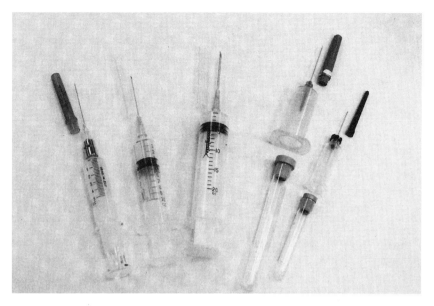

FIG 3-11. Phlebotomy equipment: syringe, needles, and evacuation system. *Left to right:* Syringe with Luer-Lok needle, disposable plastic syringes and needles, VACUTAINER evacuation systems. (From Powers LW: *Diagnostic Hematology.* St Louis, Mosby, 1989, p 418.)

variations throughout the day), recent food ingestion (caffeine effect, for example), smoking (nicotine effect), alcohol ingestion, and administration of drugs. The concentrations of certain plasma constituents are affected by some of these factors, and for some laboratory tests it is important to take into consideration the time of day, posture of the patient, dietary intake, and so forth, prior to collection of the blood specimen. Standardization of collection policies can minimize the effect of these variables on test values, but in most health care facilities, this is difficult to do. Specimen requirements for the various tests to be done should always be kept in mind by the person collecting the blood.

Application of the Tourniquet. The use of a **tourniquet** is desirable to enlarge the veins, so that they become more prominent. A strip of flat tubing (about 1 in. wide) can serve as a tourni-

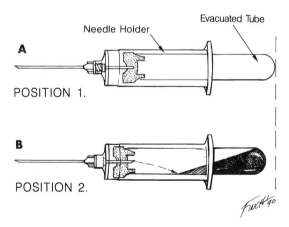

FIG 3-12. Standard double-ended blood collecting needle with holder using vacuum tube system. **A,** Preparation for venipuncture. **B,** Collection of specimen.

quet. It is applied around the arm just above the bend in the elbow and should be just tight enough to obstruct the venous blood flow (Fig. 3-13). The patient should also be instructed to close his or her hand to make the veins more prominent and easier to enter. The proper way to apply an elastic tubing tourniquet is described in Procedure 3-5.

General Venipuncture Considerations. The most prominent vein is usually chosen for venipuncture. If the veins are difficult to find, have the patient open and close the hand a few times; this will build up more pressure. Veins may be made more prominent by use of a tourniquet, by allowing the arm to hang down for 2 to 3 minutes, by massaging the vein toward the trunk of the body, or by sharply tapping the site of the puncture with the index and second fingers. If a tourniquet has been used to locate the vein site, release the tourniquet for a few minutes and then reapply to perform the venipuncture. The tourniquet should not be in place for more than one minute—or two at the maximum. Veins may be hardened or rubbery in elderly persons or in persons who have had repeated venipuncture. Rolling veins may be held in place by putting the thumb and index finger on the vein so that 2 to 5 cm of vein lies between them. As soon as the vein is entered, the thumb and finger are removed.

The veins can be felt by touching or palpating with the index finger. They reveal themselves as elastic tubes under the surface of the skin. By pressing up and down on the vein gently several times, the path of the vein can be felt.

Once the site for venipuncture has been chosen and the vein observed or palpated, the area is cleaned with an antiseptic solution. One suitable antiseptic is a solution of medicated alcohol (or isopropyl alcohol). The area of puncture is cleansed thoroughly with the antiseptic. After application of the antiseptic, the area must not be touched until after the actual puncture is made.

To insert the needle properly into the vein, the skin and vein are first fixed in place by grasping

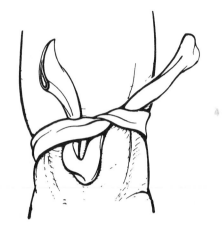

FIG 3-13.   Application of a tourniquet.

the patient's arm with the other hand and pulling the skin taut. This can be accomplished by placing the thumb about 1 or 2 in. below the puncture site (Fig. 3-14). The bevel of the needle should be facing up, and the needle should be positioned in the same direction as the vein. The syringe or evacuated tube assembly should be held so that the needle makes a 15- to 30-degree angle with the patient's arm. The tip of the needle is then placed on the vein and pushed deliberately forward. (See also Procedure 3-3.) A sensation of resistance is felt, followed by ease of penetration as the vein is entered. When the vein has been punctured and a suitable amount of blood collected into the tube or syringe, the patient releases the clenched hand, the tourniquet is released, a dry gauze is placed over the puncture site, and the needle is withdrawn. After the needle has been removed, pressure may be applied on the puncture site, using dry gauze, until bleeding has stopped. Special attention must be given to patients with prolonged bleeding times.

If difficulty is experienced in entering the vein (no blood appears in the tube or syringe) and especially if a **hematoma** (collection of blood under the skin) starts to form, release the tourniquet and promptly withdraw the needle; then apply pressure to the wound. It is best to select an alternative site for repeated venipunctures on the same patient.

PROCEDURE 3-5

Application of a Tourniquet

1. Place the tourniquet under the patient's arm, just above the bend in the elbow (see Fig. 3-11).

2. Grasping the ends of the tourniquet, pull up so that tension is applied to the tourniquet. This tension must be maintained throughout the procedure.

3. With the proper tension, cross the end of the tourniquet and tuck a loop in the tourniquet from the top down, leaving the ends up and away from the venipuncture site. Do not tie a bow or a knot. The loop must be made in such a way that the tourniquet can easily be released by pulling on a free end of the tourniquet when it is to be removed (see Fig. 3-11). Avoid pinching the skin, if possible. The tourniquet should remain flat around the patient's arm.

4. Do not leave the tourniquet on for long periods of time because this will cause stoppage of the circulation (stasis). Prolonged stasis results in gross alterations in the blood constituents. Leave the tourniquet in place for no longer than one minute, if possible.

It is most important that the tourniquet be released before the needle is removed from the skin. If this is not done, excessive bleeding will occur. If the venipuncture is poorly done (if there is trauma to the tissues), a hematoma may result. This should be avoided, if at all possible.

The evacuated tube system is an ideal means of collecting multiple samples with ease. The NCCLS has published standards for the use of evacuated tubes for blood specimen collection.[5] A multiple-sample needle is used (see Fig. 3-12 and Procedure 3-3). After blood has filled the first tube, the tube is removed from the needle holder, leaving the needle anchored in the vein, and a second tube is inserted into the tube holder. Blood will fill the second tube just as it did the first. Each tube must be thoroughly and immediately mixed with any additive or anticoagulant in the tube by inverting the tube gently 5 to 10 times to ensure proper mixing of the additive and blood. The multiple-sample needle has a special adaptation that prevents blood from leaking out during the exchange of tubes. Some vacuum tube collection systems can be purchased with an added guard closure, which helps to shield the laboratorian against exposure to blood specimens. All tubes must be immediately la-

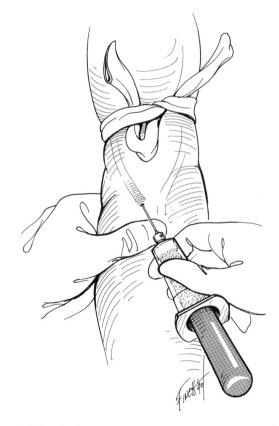

FIG 3-14. Venipuncture technique using evacuated tube system.

beled according to the labeling protocol established for the facility.

If blood must be drawn from a patient who has intravenous equipment attached to one arm, the blood sample should be drawn from a vein in the other arm. If neither arm is free, an ankle vein is the site of choice for the venipuncture.

In weak or elderly patients, the venous pressure may be so low that the pressure of the needle or the negative pressure of the vacuum tube may collapse the vein. In these cases it may be advisable to use a syringe, for then the negative pressure can be controlled.

If the patient's clothing is too tight above the venipuncture site, it will slow down the flow of blood and may cause a hematoma. If the tourniquet is too tight, it will cause the arterial flow to stop. The radial pulse should be felt with the tourniquet in place correctly. A tight tourniquet can cause cyanosis, and it pinches the skin, causing unnecessary discomfort to the patient. It may also cause the vein to disappear before the puncture is made. When this happens, the vein has collapsed, and the tourniquet should be released for a few minutes and the procedure repeated.

The placement of the needle—the angle of entry and the entry itself—is important (Fig. 3-14). The angle of entry of the needle with the skin should be 15 to 30 degrees. If the skin and the vein are penetrated at one time, the needle may go straight through the vein. It is best to make the penetration in two steps: the skin first and then the vein. The bevel of the needle must always be covered by skin before the vacuum tube is fully engaged; otherwise the vacuum in the tube is lost. If there is a poor flow of blood, the needle may be half into the vein or the bevel may be partly occluded. To correct this problem, gently turn the needle, push in, or press down to keep the vein wall off the bevel. The needle bevel must be in the lumen of the vein and the needle itself in line with the vein in order to have a good flow of blood.

Hemolysis, when destruction of red cells has occurred, causes erroneous results in some chemistry measurements using serum. Hemolytic serum will appear pink. For a summary of general considerations for venipuncture using the evacuated tube system, see Box 3-2.

Venipuncture Using Syringe and Needle. A syringe and needle are often used to collect blood from patients with difficult veins. With the use of the same preparation procedures as for the vacuum tube system, the syringe and needle system is assembled and the vein entered. When making preparations for doing the venipuncture, remove the syringe from its protective wrapper and the needle from the sterile package and assemble them, allowing the covering to remain over the needle when not in use. Attach the needle so that the bevel faces in the same direction as the graduation marks on the syringe. Check to make sure the needle is sharp, the syringe moves smoothly, and there is no air left in the syringe.

Blood will enter the syringe spontaneously if a clean entry into the vein has been made. In persons with low venous pressure, the plunger of the syringe is withdrawn slightly to make certain that the needle has entered the vein. Withdraw the blood by using the left hand to pull back the plunger while steadying the syringe with the right hand (do not push in the plunger, as air will be injected into the patient's vein).

When sufficient blood has been withdrawn, release the tourniquet and remove the needle and syringe from the vein. Place a dry gauze pad over the site of the venipuncture, and maintain gentle pressure for a few minutes. Do not leave the patient until the bleeding stops.

Remove the needle from the syringe, and gently expel the blood into a collection tube (place used collection supplies into the proper disposal container immediately). Avoid foaming or rupture of the cells by using gentle pressure on the plunger of the syringe. Stopper the tube, and gently invert it 5 to 10 times to mix blood with additive, if one is used.

If an evacuated collection tube is used to hold the blood, push the needle through the stopper and allow the blood to collect in the tube by using the vacuum in the tube.

BOX 3-2

General Considerations for Venipunctures Using the Evacuated Tube System

1. If a tube begins to fill and then stops, change the position of the needle, first in a forward direction, then slightly backward, or rotate the needle half a turn. Loosen the tourniquet. The bevel of the needle may not be fully in the lumen of the vein.

2. If a tube is not filling with blood but the needle is in the vein, try another vacuum tube; sometimes the vacuum tubes are defective and the vacuum has been lost.

3. Do not probe with the needle. It is painful for the patient.

4. If another venipuncture attempt is necessary, try the other arm in the cubital fossa, or another puncture in the same arm in a site below the first puncture.

5. Never attempt a venipuncture more than twice. Request that another phlebotomist or a physician draw the specimen.

6. Sometimes a capillary puncture may be used in place of the venipuncture.

7. Clothing may be too tight above the site of the venipuncture. This can slow the flow of blood and may cause a hematoma.

8. If the tourniquet is too tight (the radial pulse should be felt at all times), arterial flow of blood will stop and this may cause the vein to disappear before the puncture is done. A tight tourniquet may cause pinching of skin (an unnecessary discomfort), cyanosis, fluid shifts, and possible erroneous laboratory results.

9. Needle placement and angle of entry are important. The angle of the needle with the skin should be about 30 degrees. If the angle is greater than 30 degrees, the needle can pass straight through the vein. If skin and vein are penetrated at one time, blood may spurt from the puncture hole. The needle bevel should be well covered by skin before the vacuum tube is fully attached, or the vacuum will be lost. With small veins, the bevel may be rotated down to help increase blood flow.

10. If the vein disappears at puncture (some veins collapse when touched), the tourniquet pressure may be tightened slightly.

11. If the vacuum collapses the vein (the size and softness of veins vary), tighten the tourniquet, press the needle down gently, or rotate it so that the vein wall is not occluding the bevel.

12. Undue bleeding and hematoma formation can be prevented if the puncture is made only in the uppermost wall of the vein and by making certain that it is fully penetrated; by removing the tourniquet before removing the needle; by immediately applying pressure to the venipuncture site after removing the needle; by applying pressure on the gauze pad over the venipuncture site for several minutes until bleeding stops; or by covering the site with an adhesive dressing, except with small children. If bleeding appears to be excessive, a roll of gauze under an adhesive bandage may be effective. Patients with bleeding must be observed again at 5 minutes.

13. To prevent hemolysis in the blood specimen, avoid drawing blood from an area where there is a hematoma and, in general, do not mix blood in nonadditive tubes (except for serum separator tubes, which must be tipped two or three times to activate the clotting process). Allow blood to clot at room temperature for 30 minutes before centrifuging for serum separation. Mix anticoagulated specimens thoroughly but by gentle inversion five to ten times.

A syringe and needle or an **infusion set (Butterfly)** is often used for coagulation studies, for babies and small children with small veins, for very obese patients whose veins are hard to find, for patients receiving intravenous chemotherapy for cancer (whose veins have become scarred), for patients who have frequent venipunctures (leukemia patients), and for veins other than those in the antecubital fossa.

Venipuncture Using the Infusion Set (Butterfly Needle). The infusion set, or Butterfly Needle* is generally used for drawing a blood specimen from a patient with small, fragile, "rolly" veins or for drawing from veins in the wrist area, back of the hand, ankle, foot, or scalp. This system has generally replaced the syringe method of blood collection in many institutions. A 25-gauge needle is recommended for the smallest and most fragile veins. A syringe collection system, rather than an evacuated tube method, is recommended when the 25-gauge infusion set is used. The infusion set is often used for drawing blood specimens from pediatric patients (see Procedure 3-4).

An infusion set is used with an additional collection method—either by attaching it to a sterile syringe and manually filling the syringe or by attaching it to an adapter, which is in turn attached to an evacuated tube holder (Fig. 3-15). The specimen is eventually transferred to or collected directly into an evacuated tube.

Obtaining Blood From Existing Intravascular Devices or Indwelling Lines. When vascular access is needed over an extended period of time, for administration of therapeutic blood products or for infusion of fluids, medications, or parenteral nutrition solutions, without the necessity for multiple venipunctures, **vascular access devices (VAD)** are used. These devices are also called **indwelling lines** or **intravascular devices.** It is also possible, with skill and experience, to collect a venous or arterial blood sample from these devices. Because infection and sep-

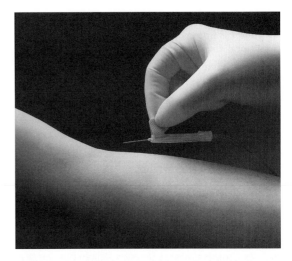

FIG 3-15.   Butterfly Needle (infusion set). (Courtesy Becton Dickinson & Co, Becton Dickinson VACU-TAINER Systems, Franklin Lakes, NJ.)

ticemia are serious consequences, especially in immunosuppressed patients, adherence to a strict asepsis control protocol for collection from intravascular devices is required. Each health care facility has its own policy and procedure for dealing with these devices, and this must be followed to prevent complications from infection due to improper use of the devices. For this reason, a special training program for phlebotomists drawing blood from intravascular devices is necessary.

An intravascular device consists of a silicone catheter and a self-sealing silicone septum encased in a metal or plastic port and may have other types of access ports. It is surgically implanted with the use of local or general anesthesia. The catheter is tunneled through the subcutaneous tissue to a major blood vessel, and the portal is secured to the fascia under the skin. The device is accessed by needle puncture through the skin into the port or through a diaphragm. For venous ports, catheters are placed in a vein. Several different intravascular devices are used.

The decision to use an intravascular device for obtaining a blood specimen is made by the attending physician.

---

*Becton Dickinson & Co, Franklin Lakes, NJ.

Obtaining Blood With Heparin Locks. A **heparin-lock system** consists of an indwelling winged Butterfly Needle and can be used in a vein for 36- to 48-hour periods to administer medication intravenously or as a source for venous blood samples. This device is used to "save" veins for patients and to lessen trauma to the veins. Repeated venipunctures can be painful to patients and can, after time, result in scarring of the vein lining, which makes the vein unusable.

The Butterfly system is carefully placed in the vein and must be maintained by careful adherence to infection control procedures, since the needle is a foreign body being placed directly into the patient's vein. These procedures include the use of antibiotic ointments and careful monitoring for signs of inflammation.

A dilute heparin solution is used in the line to keep the blood in it from clotting. This heparin flush is injected through the tubing, and a plug at the end of the butterfly line holds the solution in place. Before any blood is used for analysis, a waste specimen of 2 to 3 mL must be withdrawn and discarded to free the specimen of the heparin solution. There must be a special period of training and education before a phlebotomist draws specimens from a heparin lock.

Blood Collection for Culture. To ensure that the blood collected for culture is free from contamination (from the patient, the phlebotomist, or other personnel), extra precautions are taken for cleaning the skin and the collection tube prior to the actual collection. The skin is cleaned three times with a povidone-iodine solution or a chlorhexidine gluconate preparation. By use of a scrub applicator, the povidone-iodine solution must be applied to the puncture site in a concentric outward-moving circle, beginning at the site. This step is repeated three times. After the triple cleaning, the povidone-iodine may be removed with an alcohol pad if the color of the solution makes it difficult to locate the vein. If for any reason the vein must be touched prior to the actual venipuncture, the phlebotomist's gloved finger must be triple-cleaned with povidone-iodine. Perform the venipuncture using a sterile syringe and needle, or collect directly into culture bottles using an evacuated (vacuum) system.

Each culture bottle top must be cleaned with an alcohol pad prior to injection of the required amount of blood sample into the bottle. Culture bottles are labeled and brought to the laboratory.

Additives and Anticoagulants

Blood is a combination of formed elements (red cells, white cells, and platelets) in a liquid portion called plasma. In vivo (in the body) the blood is in a liquid form, but in vitro (outside the body) it will clot in a few minutes. Blood that is freshly drawn into a glass tube appears as a translucent, dark red fluid. In a matter of minutes it will start to clot, or coagulate, forming a semisolid jelly-like mass. If left undisturbed in the tube, this mass will begin to shrink, or retract, in about 1 hour. Complete retraction normally takes place within 24 hours. When coagulation occurs, a pale yellow fluid called serum separates from the clot and appears in the upper portion of the tube. During the process of coagulation, certain factors present in the original blood sample are depleted or used up. Fibrinogen is one important substance found in the circulating blood (in the plasma portion) that is necessary for coagulation to occur. Fibrinogen is converted to fibrin when clotting occurs, and the fibrin lends structure to the clot in the form of fine threads in which the red cells (erythrocytes) and the white cells (leukocytes) are embedded. To assist in obtaining serum, collection tubes with a separator gel additive in them are commonly used (Fig. 3-16). Serum is used extensively for chemical, serologic, and other laboratory testing, and can be obtained from the tube of clotted blood by centrifuging.

If coagulation is prevented by the addition of an **anticoagulant**, the formed elements of the blood— red cells, white cells, and platelets—can be separated from the plasma. If the anticoagulated blood is centrifuged, it separates into three main layers: the red cells, the buffy coat (consisting of white cells and platelets), and the plasma.

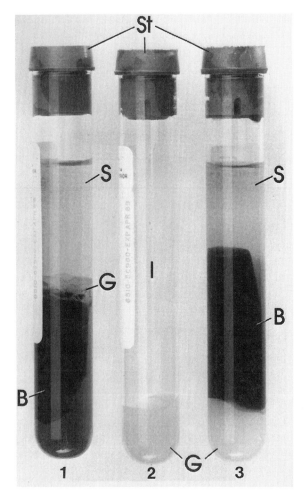

FIG 3-16. VACUTAINER phlebotomy tubes containing barrier gel (red-gray tops). *1,* Tube filled with blood and centrifuged. *2,* Unfilled tube. *3,* Tube filled with blood and not centrifuged. Note positions of gel before *(3)* and after centrifugation (*1*). *B,* Clotted blood; *St,* red-gray stoppers; *G,* barrier gel; *S,* serum. (From Kaplan LA, Pesce AJ: *Clinical Chemistry: Theory, Analysis, and Correlation,* ed 2. St Louis, Mosby, 1989, p 43.)

Hematologic studies are done primarily on whole anticoagulated venous blood or on fresh capillary blood. It is important that everyone involved in collecting blood specimens thoroughly understand the reason for using anticoagulants. Use of the appropriate **additive** is essential, and to do this the type of determination to be done

by the laboratory must be indicated on the request form.

Several anticoagulant additives are available for various purposes in the clinical laboratory. Some of the more commonly used anticoagulants are:

1. *Sodium fluoride:* This is a dry additive, a weak anticoagulant, used primarily for blood glucose specimens, since it is also an enzyme poison (preventing glycolysis, or destruction of glucose).

2. *Oxalates:* These dry additives are available as sodium, potassium, ammonium, or lithium oxalates. The oxalate in the anticoagulant forms an insoluble complex with the calcium in the blood, inhibiting the clotting mechanism. When calcium ions are combined with oxalate and are therefore not available to participate in clotting, the blood does not clot.

3. *Ammonium and potassium oxalate:* Also called balanced oxalate, or double oxalate, this combination is a dry additive. It is used for some hematology work. It is not used in chemistry, as a rule, because the presence of ammonium in the anticoagulant interferes with some of the chemistry determinations. Use of this anticoagulant has been replaced in most laboratories by the use of EDTA.

4. *EDTA (ethylenediaminetetraacetic acid):* EDTA is used as a disodium or dipotassium salt. It prevents coagulation by chelating (binding) calcium in the plasma. It is available as a dry (potassium or sodium EDTA) or liquid (potassium EDTA) additive and is used primarily in the hematology laboratory. It is the anticoagulant of choice for blood to be used in cell counts, hematocrit, hemoglobin, and cell differentials on stained blood films, to name but a few tests, because it preserves the morphologic structure of the blood cell elements.

5. *Sodium citrate:* This additive is widely used for coagulation procedures, including prothrombin times and partial thromboplastin

TABLE 3-1

Color Coding for Vacuum Tubes

Stopper Color	Use	Additive
Gray	Plasma or whole blood; glycolysis inhibition	Potassium oxalate and sodium fluoride
Yellow, pale	Sterile interior of tube; cultures	Sodium polyanetholesulfonate (SPS)
Yellow, bright	Blood bank	Acid citrate dextrose (ACD)
Green	Plasma or whole blood chemistries; viable lymphocytes or neutrophils	Lithium, ammonium, or sodium heparin
Red	Serum chemistries; serology; blood bank	No additive
Red and black	Serum chemistries	Inert serum separator gel
Light blue	Plasma or whole blood; coagulation assays	Sodium citrate
Dark blue	Tests for trace elements	Sodium heparin
Lavender	Plasma or whole blood; hematology, drug analyses	Sodium or potassium EDTA (dried); potassium EDTA (liquid)

tests. It prevents coagulation by inactivating calcium ions. The citrate helps to prevent the rapid deterioration of labile coagulation factors such as factor V and factor VII.

6. *Heparin:* This additive is theoretically the best anticoagulant, because it is a normal constituent of blood and introduces no foreign contaminants to the blood specimen. Heparin is available as sodium, lithium, and ammonium salts. It prevents coagulation for approximately 24 hours by neutralizing thrombin, thus preventing the formation of fibrin from fibrinogen. Only a small amount of heparin is needed, so that simply coating the insides of tubes or syringes is often enough to give a good anticoagulant effect.

Color Coding for Vacuum Tubes. Stopper color codes for additives have been generally accepted by manufacturers of vacuum (evacuated) tubes for blood collection and also for microcontainer systems. Table 3-1 explains the color coding system for vacuum tube stoppers.

Order for Drawing Blood into Collection Tubes. To avoid any possible cross-contamination of additives between tubes, it is recommended that blood collection tubes be drawn in a specific order. Each health care facility implements its own specific policy governing the order in which tubes for laboratory analyses are drawn. Policies on coagulation studies and blood cultures, for example, vary from place to place. In general, however, it is important to draw any sterile blood culture specimens first, then specimens that require no additives (plain tubes), followed by tubes needed for coagulation studies (usually sodium citrate or heparin), if they are drawn at the same time. Last, tubes with the various other additives are drawn, with gel separator tubes first, then EDTA, then oxalates and fluorides. It is possible that there can be additive contamination from tube to tube, especially if the blood drawing is slow and difficult. If, for example, the EDTA tube is collected prior to the heparin tube for electrolyte analysis, the potassium salt of EDTA may falsely elevate the potassium determination.

Adverse Effects of Additives. The additives chosen for specific determinations must be such that they do not alter the blood components and do not affect the laboratory tests to be done. The following are some adverse effects of using an improper additive or using the wrong amount of additive.

1. The additive may contain a substance that is the same, or reacts in the same way, as the substance being measured. An example would be the use of sodium oxalate as the anticoagulant for a sodium determination.

2. The additive may remove the constituent to be measured. An example would be the use of an oxalate anticoagulant for a calcium determination; oxalate removes calcium from the blood by forming an insoluble salt, calcium oxalate.

3. The additive may affect enzyme reactions. An example would be the use of sodium fluoride as an anticoagulant in an enzyme determination. Fluoride destroys many enzymes.

4. The additive may alter cellular constituents. An example would be the use of oxalate in cell morphology studies in hematology. Oxalate distorts the cell morphology; red cells become crenated, vacuoles appear in the granulocytes, and bizarre forms of lymphocytes and monocytes appear rapidly when oxalate is used as the anticoagulant. Another example is the use of heparin as an anticoagulant for blood to be used in the preparation of blood films that will be stained with Wright's stain. Unless the films are stained within 2 hours, heparin gives a blue background with Wright's stain.

5. If too little additive is used, partial clotting will occur. This interferes with cell counts.

6. If too much liquid anticoagulant is used, it dilutes the blood sample and thus interferes with certain quantitative measurements.

Laboratory Processing of Blood Specimens

Blood specimens must be properly handled after collection. The NCCLS has published standards for handling blood specimens after collection by venipuncture.[10] As discussed previously, if no anticoagulant is used, the blood will clot and serum is obtained. After being placed in a plain tube with no additives, the blood is allowed to clot. The serum is then removed from the clot by centrifugation. To prevent excessive handling of biological fluids, many laboratory instrumentation systems can now use the serum directly from the centrifuged tube, without another separation step and without removing the stopper. In the past, the serum was removed and placed in a clean, dry storage tube or vial prior to analysis.

Serum Separator Devices. To assist in the processing of clotted whole blood to obtain the serum, special **serum separator collection tubes** are available. An evacuated glass tube serves as the single system for both collection and processing of the blood. Serum separator tubes are of two major types, those used during centrifugation and those used after centrifugation.

The tubes used during centrifugation may be either integrated gel tube systems or devices inserted into the collection tube just before centrifugation. The integrated gel tubes contain a special silicone gel layer, which, because of its viscosity and density, moves to form a barrier between cells and serum during centrifugation (see Fig. 3-14). Blood is forced into the gel layer during centrifugation, causing a temporary change in viscosity. The gel starts out at the bottom of the collection tube. Blood is added to the tube and the clot allowed to form for a minimum of 30 minutes. After clot formation, the tubes are centrifuged. The gel rises and lodges between the packed red cells and the top layer of serum. The gel hardens and forms an inert barrier. These tubes do not have to be unstoppered before centrifugation, thus eliminating aerosol production and possible evaporation. The serum separator tubes also give a higher yield of serum as well as a shorter processing time because only a single centrifugation step is needed.

Processing Blood for Serum. Serum can be used in the chemistry laboratory for tests for sodium, potassium, calcium, phosphorus, acid and alkaline phosphatase, cholesterol, uric acid, and liver function, to mention but a few. Serum is also used for serology testing.

It is important to remove the plasma or serum from the remaining blood cells, or clot, as soon as possible. Since biological specimens are being handled, the need for certain safety precautions is stressed. The standard precautions policy should be used, since all blood specimens should be considered infectious (see Chapter 2). Blood specimens should be handled with protective gloves. The outsides of the tubes may be bloody, and initial laboratory handling of all specimens necessitates direct contact with the tubes. When stoppers must be removed from the tubes, they must be removed carefully and not popped off, as this could cause infection by inhalation or by contact of the infectious aerosol with mucous membranes. Stoppers should be twisted gently while being covered with protective gauze to minimize the risk from aerosol. This processing step can be done with the use of a protective plastic shield so that no direct splashes can take place. To separate the serum and plasma from the remaining blood cells, the tube must be centrifuged. It is generally best to test specimens as quickly as possible. If the specimen must be stored prior to analysis, remove the serum/plasma from the clot/red cells to prevent alterations from taking place in the sample to be tested. It is especially important to remove the plasma quickly from the cell layer when potassium oxalate has been used as the anticoagulant, because the salt (potassium oxalate) shrinks the red blood cells and the intracellular water diffuses into the plasma (fluid inside the red cell leaves the cell and thus causes shrinkage). Centrifuge covers should always be in place during centrifugation to protect the worker from the

specimens, and the centrifuge should be placed as far from laboratory personnel as possible. If the centrifuged serum or plasma must be removed into a separate tube or vial, the safest procedure for this step is pipetting instead of pouring. Pipette the serum or plasma by using mechanical suction and a disposable pipette; use a protective plastic shield so that no direct splashes can take place. All serum and plasma tubes, as well as the original blood tubes, should be discarded properly in biohazard containers when they are no longer needed for the determination.

Appearance of Processed Specimens

Persons working with specimens in the laboratory must be able to recognize the appearance of normal as opposed to abnormal plasma or serum. Normally, serum or plasma is straw colored, but various shades of yellow are also normally seen. Abnormal-appearing serum and plasma can be clinical indications of serious disorders. Also, the use of such abnormal specimens can interfere with some determinations, especially chemistry tests.

Hemolysis. Hemolysis in specimens is perhaps the most common cause of the abnormal appearances to be considered. A specimen that is hemolyzed appears red, usually clear red, because the red blood cells have been lysed and the hemoglobin has been released into the liquid portion of the blood. Often the cause of hemolysis in specimens is the technique used for venipuncture. A poor venipuncture, with excessive trauma to the blood vessel, can result in a hemolyzed specimen. Collecting the blood in dirty tubes or tubes that are not entirely dry can also result in hemolysis. In these cases, carefully repeating the venipuncture and using clean, dry equipment will produce a normal-appearing specimen that can be used for chemical determinations. Hemolysis of blood can also be caused by freezing, prolonged exposure to warmth, unnecessarily forceful spraying of blood from the needle of a syringe when the blood is transferred to a specimen tube, or allowing the serum or plasma to remain too long on the cells before testing or removal to another tube. **Hemolyzed serum** or plasma is unsuitable for several chemistry determinations because substances usually present within cells can be released into the serum or plasma. If serum is left on the cells for a prolonged period, potassium will move out of the red cells and into the serum, resulting in falsely elevated levels of serum potassium. The procedure to be done should always be checked first to see if abnormal-appearing specimens can be used.

Jaundice. Jaundiced serum or plasma is another specimen with an abnormal appearance. When serum or plasma takes on a brownish-yellow color, there has most likely been an increase in bile pigments, namely bilirubin. Excessive intravascular destruction of red blood cells, obstruction of the bile duct, or impairment of the liver leads to an accumulation of bile pigments in the blood, and the skin becomes yellow. When this occurs, the skin of the patient is said to be jaundiced. The serum or plasma can also be jaundiced, or yellow. Those performing clinical laboratory determinations should note any abnormal appearance of serum or plasma and record it on the report form. Another term for jaundiced is icteric. Jaundiced serum or plasma is seen in patients with hepatitis. Once again, it is important to be observant in all areas of laboratory work—to notice things such as the appearance of a jaundiced specimen can assist the physician in making a diagnosis.

Lipemia. When the blood, serum, or plasma takes on a milky appearance, the specimen is said to be lipemic. The presence of lipids, or fats, in the serum causes this abnormal lipemic appearance. A blood specimen drawn from a patient soon after a meal may often appear lipemic. Use of a **lipemic serum** specimen, does not, for the most part, interfere with chemical determinations, except for triglyceride tests.

Storage of Processed Specimens

The processing of individual serum or plasma tubes will depend on the analysis to be done and the time that will elapse before analysis. Serum or plasma may be kept at room temperature, refrigerated, frozen, or protected from light, depending on the circumstances and the determination to be done. Some specimens must be analyzed immediately after they reach the laboratory, such as specimens for blood gas and pH analyses. Blood specimens for hematology studies can be stored in the refrigerator for 2 hours before being used in testing. After storage, anticoagulated blood, serum, or plasma must be thoroughly mixed after it has reached room temperature.

Plasma and serum often can be frozen and preserved satisfactorily until a determination can be done. Whole blood cannot be frozen, because red blood cells rupture on freezing. Freezing preserves most chemical constituents in serum and plasma and provides a method of sample preservation for the laboratory. In general, refrigerating specimens retards alterations of many constituents. With all biological specimens, however, preservation should be the exception rather than the rule. A laboratory determination is best done on a fresh specimen.

Urine: General Collection Information

The urine specimen has been referred to as a liquid tissue biopsy of the urinary tract that is painlessly and easily obtained. Urine yields a great amount of valuable information quickly and economically, but, as for all other human specimens used in the laboratory, the specimen must be carefully collected, preserved, and processed prior to analysis in order for the results reported to be regarded as reliable. A routine urine analysis (urinalysis) is included with many hospital admissions and visits to physicians' offices or clinics.

Types of Urine Collection

The composition of urine in random samples collected at different times during the day is likely to vary considerably, because the work of the kidney is so variable. The NCCLS recommends that a specimen for routine urinalysis be from a well-mixed, **first morning specimen** (eight-hour concentrated), that it be uncentrifuged, and that it be tested at room temperature.[7] It is not practical to collect an entire day's specimen (24-hour specimen), as it would take too long for any results to be ready for the physician; also, as urine stands, many of the more important constituents found in it disappear or are altered. A 24-hour specimen, or other **timed urine collection,** is required only when it is necessary to know the entire day's volume of urine output, or for quantitative tests in which the exact amount of urine must be known so that the exact amount of substance present may be reported. The NCCLS describes several types of urine collection.[11] Some of these are random, first morning, timed, midstream, clean-catch, catheterized, and suprapubic.

Urine testing should be done within two hours of collection. If this is not possible, the specimen should be stored at 4° C as soon as possible after collection. Specimens can be stored under refrigeration for 6 to 8 hours with no gross alterations in constituents.

Since a 24-hour collection is not necessary for a routine urinalysis, any random specimen that is passed during the day may be used. A **voided midstream urine specimen** is suitable for most routine urine tests. As discussed above, the first urine voided in the morning is usually recommended. This is true primarily because the first morning urine specimen is the most concentrated one passed during the day. It is more concentrated because less fluid (or water) is excreted during the night, while the same amount of solid or dissolved substance must be excreted for the kidney to perform its function of maintaining the composition of the extracellular fluid. To test for the presence of urine sugar, the best specimen to use is one voided 2 to 3 hours after a meal. This is the one exception to the recommended use of the first morning specimen.

Containers for Urine Collection

It is of prime importance that the containers used to collect the urine specimen be clean and dry. Containers should not be reused. Several types of containers are suitable for this purpose. The NCCLS has made several recommendations regarding urine collection containers.[7] Disposable, inert, plastic containers with sealable or screw-top lids and plastic bags or jars are most often used. These are available in several sizes and are preferred for routine screening urinalysis. Containers for routine urine tests should have a capacity of 50 to 100 mL with a round opening at least 2 in. in diameter and should have screw caps. Sterile containers with lids for collecting urine for microbiologic studies (cultures) are available. There are also special pediatric urine-collecting bags made of clear polyethylene. If a 24-hour pediatric specimen is required, a special tube can be attached to the bag, which is in turn connected to a collection bottle.

Large plastic containers with wide mouths and screw caps are used to collect timed specimens (24-hour collections) from adults, usually with added preservatives. The collection bottles should be refrigerated between voidings. Any bedpans that are used to collect voided urine must be scrupulously clean and free of cleaning agents or bleach. Any collection containers used must be labeled with complete patient identification. Labels must remain fixed to the container under refrigeration and must be on the container, not on the lid.

Preservation of Urine Specimens

If a fresh specimen of urine is left at room temperature for a period of time, the urine rapidly undergoes changes. It is for this reason that a good routine urinalysis should include the use of a fresh specimen. Decomposition of urine begins within 30 minutes after collection. Specimens left at room temperature will soon begin to decompose, mainly owing to the action of bacteria in the urine. Urea-splitting bacteria produce ammonia, which on combination with hydrogen ions forms ammonium. This causes an increase in urine pH. The increase in pH will result in decomposition of casts and certain cells, if they are present in the urine. The various laboratory tests to be performed on a specimen of urine should be done within 30 minutes after collection, if possible; no longer than 1 or 2 hours should elapse before the tests are done, unless the urine is preserved in some way.

If it is impossible to examine the urine specimen when it is fresh or if a timed urine collection (2-, 12-, or 24-hour) is required, the urine must be preserved. Various methods of preserving urine are available, most of which inhibit the growth of bacteria, thus preventing many of the alterations from occurring.

The best method of preservation is immediate refrigeration during (for timed collection) and after collection. The specimen may be kept 6 to 8 hours under refrigeration, with no chemical preservative added, with no gross alterations. Several chemical preservatives are available as additives for routine urine specimens. Most of them interfere in some way with the testing procedures, however, and it is best if no chemical preservative is added.

Toluene is one chemical preservative that can be used. It is a liquid that is lighter than urine or water. It has its preservation effect by preventing the growth of bacteria by excluding contact of urine with air. A thin layer of toluene is added, just enough to cover the surface of the urine. The toluene should be skimmed off or the urine pipetted from beneath it when the urine is examined. Toluene (toluol) is the best all-around preservative, because it does not interfere with the various tests done in the routine urinalysis. Other common preservatives for urine specimens are formaldehyde (formalin), thymol, and boric acid. Thymol, a crystalline substance, works to prevent the growth of bacteria. However, thymol may interfere with tests for urine protein and bilirubin. Formalin, a liquid preservative, acts by fixing the formed elements in the urinary sediment, including bacteria. It may, however, interfere with the reduction tests

for urine sugar and may form a precipitate with urea that interferes with the microscopic examination of the sediment. Preservative tablets that produce formaldehyde are commercially available. The tablets are more convenient to use than the liquid formalin and do not interfere with the usual chemical and microscopic examination.

Various disposable collecting systems are available commercially for collecting, storing, transporting, and testing urine specimens. New systems are continually being introduced to the market.

In general, it should be remembered that a fresh urine specimen is best for urinalysis tests. It is usually easy to collect and will give the most satisfactory results.

Collecting Urine Specimens

As stated previously, the specimen for urinalysis should be collected in a clean, dry container, and the specimen should be fresh. For routine screening, a freshly voided, random, preferably midstream (freely flowing) urine specimen is usually suitable. For most routine urinalysis, including protein content and urinary sediment constituents, the concentrated first morning specimen is the most satisfactory one to use.

Occasionally it may be necessary to obtain a catheterized urine specimen, but this procedure is not encouraged because of the risk of patient infection. These urine specimens are obtained by introducing a catheter into the bladder, through the urethra, for the withdrawal of urine. This procedure should be avoided whenever possible, as there is always a risk of introducing bacteria into an otherwise sterile bladder—this could initiate a urinary tract infection. Catheterized specimens may be necessary in female patients when contamination by vaginal contents may alter the examination (especially during menstruation). Catheterization may also be necessary for obtaining urine specimens for bacteriologic examination when a sterile sample is needed. Under many conditions, however, a freely flowing voided specimen is satisfactory for bacteriologic cultures. Urine obtained by means of catheterization should be handled very carefully in the

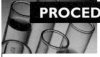

PROCEDURE 3-6

Clean-Catch, Midstream Urine Specimen For Culture (Patient Collection Instructions)[11]

1. Wash your hands thoroughly with soap and water.

2. Open the lid of the urine container provided. Be careful not to touch the inside.

3. Cleanse your genital area using the following procedure:

   Man
   a. If you are uncircumcised, draw back the foreskin before cleansing.

   b. Clean the tip of your penis using a sterile cleansing towelette, beginning at the tip and moving toward the base. Repeat the cleansing process using a second towelette.

   Woman
   a. Squat over the toilet, and use the fingers of one hand to separate and hold open the folds of the skin in your genital area.

   b. Clean the urinary opening and surrounding area with a sterile cleansing towelette, moving from front to back. Repeat the cleansing process using a second towelette.

4. Discard the towelettes in a trash receptacle (not in the toilet).

5. Begin urinating into the toilet bowl. After the urine has flowed for several seconds into the toilet, catch the midportion of the urine flow in the collection container. When sufficient urine has been collected (approximately one-half full), continue urinating into the toilet.

6. **Tightly** screw the cap on the specimen container.

7. Wash your hands thoroughly with soap and water.

8. Promptly give the specimen container to the nurse or laboratory personnel or leave in the place specified.

9. Ensure that the specimen label contains your proper identification.

---

laboratory. Remember that catheterization is an invasive procedure for the patient and does involve some degree of risk.

When both a bacteriologic culture and a routine urinalysis are needed on the same specimen, the culture should always be done first and then the routine tests, so as not to contaminate the culture. See Procedure 3-6 for collection of specimens suitable for culture.

Since on most days many urine specimens are sent to the laboratory, it is especially important that each container be properly labeled when it is collected from the patient. Each specimen must be accompanied by a request form.

When a 24-hour urine specimen is sent to the laboratory, it must be ascertained first that the specimen has been properly collected. A preservative must have been added at the beginning of the collection time, and the correct collection time must have been used (24 hours total time, for example). In the laboratory, the total volume of specimen is measured and recorded, the urine is thoroughly mixed, and an aliquot is withdrawn for analysis.

Collection of Timed Urine Specimens. The patient is carefully instructed about details of the collection process, if the collection will be done on an outpatient basis. The bladder is emptied at the starting time (8 A.M., for example), and this time is noted on the collection container. This urine is discarded and not put into the container. All subsequent voidings are collected and put into the container, up to and including that at 8 A.M. the following day. This urine specimen will complete the 24-hour collection. For timed collections of other than 24 hours, the sample collection principle applies. The first urine voided at the beginning of the collection is always discarded. These timed collection specimens are preserved by refrigeration between collections, with the appropriate chemical preservative being added to the container prior to the beginning of the collection process.

The total volume of the timed collection sample is measured and recorded, and the sample well mixed, before a measured aliquot is withdrawn for analysis.

Collection of Urine for Culture. A clean, voided midstream urine specimen (often referred to as a "clean catch") is desirable for culture (see Procedure 3-6). It is important that the glans penis in the male and the urethral orifice in the female be thoroughly cleaned with a mild antiseptic solution by means of sterile gauze or cotton balls. The patient should be instructed to urinate forcibly, and to allow the initial stream of urine to pass into the toilet or bedpan. Throughout the urination process for the female, the labia should be separated so that no contamination results. The midstream specimen should be collected in a sterile container, and no portion of the perineum (female) should come in contact with the collection container. After the specimen has been collected, the rest of the urine is passed into the toilet or bedpan.

Body Cavity Fluids (Extravascular)

When fluids normally found in small amounts in various cavities or spaces in the body—**body cavity fluids**—increase in amount and mechanically inhibit the action of certain key organs such as the heart or lungs, or when such a fluid is needed for diagnostic purposes, the fluid is aspirated. The procedure is done under sterile conditions by a physician. Fluids aspirated from the chest, abdomen, joints, cysts, or abscesses are often brought to the laboratory for various types of tests. The origin of the fluid and the tests to be done should be noted on the container and the request form, along with the usual label information required (patient name, hospital number, and so on.). Many different tests can be ordered on body cavity fluids, including chemistry determinations, cultures, cell counts and differentials, and examination for tumor cells.

The various types of extravascular fluids, or body cavity fluids, are examined in various departments of the clinical laboratory, depending on what test is to be done and what type of fluid is to be examined. Cell counts are done on most body fluid specimens. For this reason, in many institutions without a central specimen processing area, body cavity fluid specimens are brought first to the hematology laboratory, and are either examined there or sent on to a specific department for further analyses.

Most normal body cavity fluids are pale and straw colored. As the cell count and any abnormal debris and constituents increase, the fluid becomes more turbid.

Since cell counts are done on many body cavity fluid specimens, the specimen must be a fresh one. If it is not fresh, cell disintegration will occur. No cell counts may be done on a clotted specimen; anticoagulants must be used to prevent coagulation of the specimen when a cell count is needed. Specific gravity tests, when done, must also be done on a clot-free specimen. Tests for mucin and protein, however, can be done on clotted specimens. When a glucose determination is ordered, the specimen must be immediately preserved with sodium fluoride to prevent glycolysis. Generally, a blood glucose test is done simultaneously for comparison purposes. Body cavity fluid specimens to be cultured should be sent to the microbiology laboratory. Specimens to be tested for a chemical constituent should be sent to the chemistry laboratory as soon as possible. Sometimes only one specimen is sent to the laboratory, and several tests are required; except for culture, cell counts should always be done before other tests. For cell counts, the anticoagulant of choice is heparin or liquid EDTA. For examination for tumor cells, the fluid may be collected in EDTA or heparin. If the fluid is collected without any anticoagulant, clotting may be observed. The presence of clotting indicates a substantial inflammatory reaction. Sometimes so much fluid is aspirated that it must be collected in a gallon container instead of the usual tube. It is important to remember that the suitable anticoagulant must be placed in this large container just as in the tube. Many laboratory tests cannot be done on a clotted specimen of body fluid. With the standard precautions policy, all body cavity fluids should be considered contaminated, and all equipment must be decontaminated or discarded after being used.

Cerebrospinal Fluid

Cerebrospinal fluid (CSF) is the most frequently tested body cavity fluid other than blood or urine. It fills the ventricles of the brain, the central canal of the spinal cord, and the subarachnoid spaces of the brain and spinal cord; it is formed in the ventricles. It has many of the same characteristics as plasma, since most of its components are derived from the blood plasma. The only known function of the cerebrospinal fluid is mechanical—providing protection for the brain and spinal cord. Examination of the cerebrospinal fluid is important in the diagnosis of neurologic disorders, inflammatory diseases, and hemorrhage in the meninges.

The cerebrospinal fluid, or spinal fluid, is obtained by puncturing one of the spaces between the lumbar vertebrae with a needle. It is collected by lumbar puncture into the L3-4 lumbar interspace to avoid damaging the spinal cord. This procedure is done by a physician. The spinal fluid is usually collected into three or four sterile containers (numbered according to the order of collection), each containing between 1 and 3 mL of fluid. It is essential that the containers be properly labeled and handled with extreme care, as the procedure of collection cannot be easily repeated. There is a certain risk to the patient in this procedure, and for this reason the specimen is extremely precious and must be treated with the utmost care. Cerebrospinal fluid is considered infectious, and standard precautions must be used in connection with the specimen. A 5% phenol, concentrated bleach solution, alcohol solution, or other disinfectant solution can be used for decontamination of equipment that is not disposable. Specific decontamination protocol varies according to the laboratory facility. There is always the danger of spreading infectious pathogens if cerebrospinal fluid is not handled properly. Cell counts on a spinal fluid specimen must be done as soon as possible after the spinal tap has been completed, since the cells present will disintegrate within a short time. Tests for glucose in spinal fluid must also be performed immediately to prevent glycolysis. The use of sodium fluoride will slow down the glycolytic process. A blood specimen for a glucose assay should accompany a request for spinal fluid glucose for comparison purposes. For the chemical tests ordered, the specimen should be sent to the chemistry laboratory.

Normal cerebrospinal fluid appears clear and colorless. If the fluid is grossly bloody or blood tinged, the patient may have a serious brain or spinal injury. Sometimes, however, a drop of blood gets into the sample from the puncture needle. It is important for this reason to observe the collected tubes and to note the order in which they are collected. If blood has gotten into the tube from a **traumatic tap** (blood from the needle, skin, or muscle), the tubes will progressively clear. That is, the first tube collected will have more blood in it, and the succeeding tubes will have less. This is one reason why it is important to observe all the tubes collected, not just one. If all the tubes are bloody to the same degree, a hemorrhage in the brain or spinal cord is more likely. If the spinal fluid in the tubes appears cloudy, there is good reason to suspect an infection in the central nervous system. Most conditions for which spinal fluid testing is requested are very serious and require immediate diagnosis and treatment. This is why the laboratory tests are so important and why speed is essential.

Synovial Fluid

Synovial fluid is the fluid that is contained in the joint spaces. Normal synovial fluid resembles uncooked egg white; it is straw colored and viscous, and does not clot. Examination of this fluid from the joints provides information about joint diseases such as infections, gout, and rheumatoid arthritis.

Synovial fluid differs from other body cavity fluids because of the importance of finding crystals in the specimen and because it is normally very viscous. Ideally the specimen should be collected into three tubes: a sterile tube for culture; a tube with either sodium heparin or liquid EDTA anticoagulant, preferably heparin, for cell counts, crystal identification, and prepared smears; and a plain tube without additive anticoagulant (and not in a serum separator gel tube) to observe for gross appearance, crystal analysis, and fibrinogen clots and for chemistry or immunologic tests. Sodium heparin or liquid EDTA is the additive of choice because other anticoagulants are likely to have undissolved crystals present when the amount of specimen aspirated is small. Normal joints have very little synovial fluid. The additive crystals can cause confusion when the specimen is being examined for the presence of crystals. To test for clot formation, the fluid must be collected in a plain tube without anticoagulant.

Pericardial, Pleural, and Peritoneal Fluids

The fluids of the pericardial, pleural, and peritoneal cavities are called **serous fluids**. They normally are formed continuously in the body cavities and are reabsorbed, leaving only very small volumes. The normal appearance of these fluids is pale and straw colored. The fluid becomes more turbid as the cell count rises, an indication of inflammation. Increases in the amounts of these body cavity fluids formed are seen in inflammation and when the serum protein level

falls. Serous fluids are aspirated because they are mechanically inhibiting the function of the associated organs or for diagnostic purposes. These aspirations are done by the physician. The specimen is collected into various containers, depending on the laboratory testing to be done. An EDTA tube is used for cell counts and smear evaluation, sterile tubes for cultures, and oxalate or fluoride tubes for protein, glucose, or other chemistry tests. If a large volume of fluid is aspirated, it is collected in a gallon jar with an appropriate additive to prevent clotting. If the fluid clots, it is useless for many analyses.

Swabs for Culture

Swabs with samples of specimens from wounds, abscesses, throats, and so forth are brought to the laboratory in a sterile transport tube for culture. These swabs are potentially from infectious areas and should be treated very carefully in the laboratory. Again, the container with the swab in it must be properly labeled and the culture done immediately. Most bacteria will die if stored on a dry swab, so if the culture cannot be done immediately, a transport medium should be used— some means to keep the swab moist and cool. Most organisms can live for many hours if stored properly. Immediate culture is still best, however. Proper technique for disposal of contaminated material must be used.

Throat Culture Collection

Throat swab specimens are used for detection of group A β-hemolytic streptococci causing pharyngitis (see Procedure 3-7). The specimen collected can be used for the classic culture on sheep blood media or for one of the rapid direct tests utilizing extraction of the cell wall polysaccharide antigen and its recognition by antibody. These rapid tests have gained popularity, especially in physicians' offices, because results are available within minutes instead of hours.

Feces

Feces, or stool specimens, should be collected in a clean plastic container. The specimen should be collected and covered without being contami-

PROCEDURE 3-7

Throat Culture

1. Ask the patient to open his or her mouth.

2. Using a sterile tongue blade to hold the tongue down, and a sterile swab to collect the specimen, take the specimen directly from the back of the throat, being careful not to touch the teeth, cheeks, gums, or tongue when inserting or removing the swab (Fig. 3-17).

3. The tonsillar fauces and rear pharyngeal wall should be swabbed, not just gently touched, in order to remove organisms adhering to the membranes. White patches of exudate in the tonsillar area are especially productive for isolating the streptococcal organisms.

4. The swab containing the specimen can be placed in a special container with transport media. Commercial collection sets containing both swabs and transport media are available. Streptococci survive on dry swabs for up to 2 to 3 hours and on swabs in transport (holding) media at 4° C for 24 to 48 hours.

5. The specimen container must be labeled with the necessary patient identification.

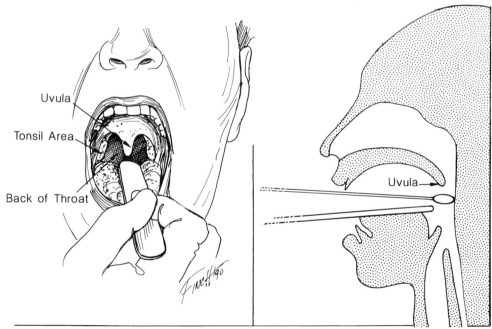

A. DEPRESS TONGUE FIRMLY   B. COLLECT THROAT CULTURE

FIG 3-17.   Obtaining a throat culture.

nated with urine. The amount collected depends on the test to be done. Most testing is done on a random specimen. The container should be labeled properly, including the time of collection (for a timed specimen) and the laboratory tests desired.

Small amounts of fecal material are frequently analyzed for the presence of occult, or hidden, blood. Occult blood is recognized as a most important sign of the presence of a bleeding ulcer or malignant disease in the gastrointestinal tract. The specimen is applied to commercially prepared filter paper slides that have been impregnated with reagent. These slides are then sent to the laboratory for analysis. Outpatients are often asked to recover small amounts of their own feces that have been excreted into the toilet and apply them directly to the slides, which have been supplied by the physician. These slides are then mailed back to the physician or laboratory for testing.

Feces from infants are usually recovered from the child's diaper for trypsin activity screening tests to detect cystic fibrosis. In adults, for certain metabolic balance studies and for measurement of fecal nitrogen and fat, 3-day (72-hour) fecal collections are needed.

Other Specimens

Other types of specimens, such as gallstones, kidney stones, sputum, seminal fluid, or tissue samples, may be sent to the laboratory for analysis. Each requires special collection and processing considerations.

CHAIN-OF-CUSTODY SPECIMEN INFORMATION

When specimens are involved in possible medicolegal situations, certain specimen handling policies are required. Medicolegal, or forensic, implications require that any data pertaining to the specimen in question be arrived at in such a way that they will be recognized by a court of law. Processing steps for such specimens, including the initial collection, transportation, storage, and analytic testing, must be documented

by careful record keeping. Documentation ensures that there has been no tampering with the specimen by any interested parties, that the specimen has been collected from the appropriate person, and that the results reported are accurate. Each step of the collection, handling, processing, testing, and reporting processes must be documented—this is called the chain of custody.

Chain-of-custody documentation must be signed by every person who has handled the specimens involved in the case in question. The actual process may vary in different health care facilities, but the general purpose of this process is to make certain that any data obtained by the clinical laboratory will be admissible in a court of law and that all steps have been taken to ensure the integrity of the information produced.

SPECIMEN TRANSPORTATION

Once the specimen has been collected and properly labeled, it must be transported to the laboratory for processing and analysis. In many institutions the specimen container is placed in a leak-proof plastic bag as a further protective measure to prevent pathogen transmission—the implementation of the standard precautions policy and the use of barriers. The request form must be placed on the outside of this bag. Many of these transport bags have a special pouch provided on the outside of the bag, into which the request form is placed.

Since some laboratory analyses require special handling of the specimens to be tested, beginning with the transporting of the specimen to the laboratory, specific requirements for specimens should be noted for each particular test to be done. For example, some tests require that the specimen be protected from light to prevent changes in the constituent to be measured. These specimens should be covered as soon as possible with a light-protective foil wrap and then transported to the laboratory for processing and testing. Some tests must be done on the specimen as soon after collection as possible. For other tests, the specimen can be processed and stored until testing is done at a later time. It is always the best rule to trans-

according to the requirements established by the receiving laboratory. Leak-proof and crush-proof primary containers and mailing containers should be used (Fig. 3-18).

All specimen containers to be shipped must be labeled with the necessary patient identification information, and the mailing package must include the properly completed request form for the tests to be done.

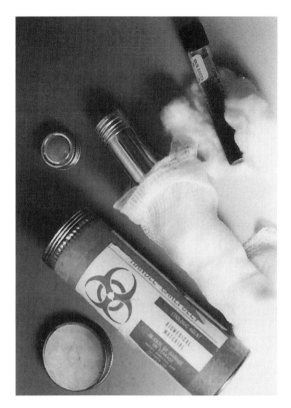

FIG 3-18. Proper containers for shipping biological specimens. (From Baron EJ, Finegold SM: *Bailey and Scott's Diagnostic Microbiology*, ed 8. St Louis, Mosby, 1990, p 15.)

port the specimen to the laboratory as quickly as possible, however, using the transport system implemented by the health care institution.

Shipping Specimens to Reference Laboratories

Sometimes it is necessary to ship a specimen to another laboratory, a large reference laboratory, for example, for testing. Tests infrequently performed, or those needing specialized technology, are sometimes more cost-effective if they are done in a central or reference laboratory setting where these special tests are performed. Such testing has become increasingly popular with the advent of the CLIA '88 regulations.

Since biological specimens are potentially infectious, care must be taken to ship them safely,

REFERENCES

1. *Ancillary (Bedside) Blood Glucose Testing in Acute and Chronic Care Facilities: Approved Guideline.* Villanova, Pa, National Committee for Clinical Laboratory Standards, 1994, NCCLS document C30-A.
2. *Blood Collection on Filter Paper for Neonatal Screening Programs: Approved Standard,* ed 3. Villanova, Pa, National Committee for Clinical Laboratory Standards, 1997, NCCLS document LA4-A3.
3. College of American Pathologists: *So You're Going to Collect a Blood Specimen: An Introduction to Phlebotomy,* ed 7. Northfield, Ill., College of American Pathologists, 1996.
4. *Devices for Collection of Skin Puncture Blood Specimens: Approved Guideline,* ed 2. Villanova, Pa, National Committee for Clinical Laboratory Standards, 1990, NCCLS document H14-A2.
5. *Evacuated Tubes for Blood Specimen Collection: Approved Standard,* ed 4. Villanova, Pa, National Committee for Clinical Laboratory Standards, 1996, NCCLS Document H1-A4.
6. *Guideline for Isolation Procedures in Hospitals.* Hospital Infection Control Practices Advisory Committee (HICPAC), Centers for Disease Control and Prevention (CDC), 1996.
7. *Physician's Office Laboratory Guidelines: Tentative Guideline,* ed 3. Villanova, Pa, National Committee for Clinical Laboratory Standards, 1995, NCCLS document POL1/2-T3.
8. *Procedures for the Collection of Diagnostic Blood Specimens by Skin Puncture: Approved Standard,* ed 3. Villanova, Pa, National Committee for Clinical Laboratory Standards, 1991, NCCLS document H4-A3.
9. *Procedures for the Collection of Diagnostic Blood Specimens by Venipuncture: Approved* Standard, ed 4. Villanova, Pa, National Committee for Clinical Laboratory Standards, 1998, NCCLS document H3-A3.

10. *Procedures for the Handling of Blood Specimens by Venipuncture: Approved Standard,* ed 3. Villanova, Pa, National Committee for Clinical Laboratory Standards, 1990, NCCLS document H18-A.
11. *Routine Urinalysis and Collection, Transportation, and Preservation of Urine Specimens: Approved Guideline.* Villanova, Pa, National Committee for Clinical Laboratory Standards, 1995, NCCLS document GP16-A.

BIBLIOGRAPHY

Burtis CA, Ashwood ER (eds): *Tietz Fundamentals of Clinical Chemistry,* ed 4. Philadelphia, WB Saunders Co, 1996.

Garza D, Becan-McBride, K: *Phlebotomy Handbook,* ed 3, Norwalk, Conn, Appleton & Lange, 1993.

Henry JB (ed): *Clinical Diagnosis and Management by Laboratory Methods,* ed 19. Philadelphia, WB Saunders Co, 1996.

NCCLS: *Procedures for the Handling and Transport of Diagnostic Specimens and Etiologic Agents: Approved Standard,* ed 3, Villanova, Pa, National Committee for Clinical Laboratory Standards, 1994; NCCLS Document H5-A3.

Protection of Laboratory Workers From Infectious Disease Transmitted by Blood, Body Fluids and Tissue: Tentative Standard, ed 2. Villanova, Pa, *National Committee for Clinical Laboratory Standards,* 1991, NCCLS document M29-T2.

Slockbower JM, Blumenfeld TA: *Collection and Handling of Laboratory Specimens.* Philadelphia, JB Lippincott Co, 1983.

STUDY QUESTIONS

1. An evacuated blood collection tube with a lavender-colored top is used for almost all tests relating to:

   A. Clinical chemistry
   B. Microbiologic cultures
   C. Coagulation studies
   D. Hematology

2. A red-topped or red-and-black-topped blood collection tube is used for:

   A. Plasma for coagulation tests
   B. Serum for chemistry tests
   C. Anticoagulated blood for hematologic tests
   D. Whole blood for glucose tests

3. Fasting blood is necessary for some chemistry tests because certain values increase substantially after eating. Which of the following assays does *not* require a fasting blood specimen?

   A. Glucose
   B. Cholesterol
   C. Triglyceride
   D. Phosphorus

4. Blood specimens are not acceptable for laboratory testing when which of the following is noted?

   A. There is no patient name or identification number on the label.
   B. The label on the request form and the label on the collection container do not match.
   C. The wrong collection tube has been used (i.e., anticoagulant additive instead of tube for serum).
   D. All of the above

5. If serum is allowed to remain on the clot for a prolonged period, which of the following effects will be noted?

   A. Elevated level of serum potassium
   B. Decreased level of serum potassium
   C. Elevated level of glucose
   D. Decreased level of glucose

6. Match each of the following abnormal serum appearances (1 to 3) with the likely cause for the color change (A to C).

   1. Red-pink
   2. Yellow
   3. Milky white
      _____ A. Elevated bilirubin (jaundice; icteric serum)
      _____ B. Lysis of red blood cells (hemolyzed serum)
      _____ C. Presence of lipids or fat (lipemic serum)

7. What is the preferred method for preserving a urine specimen if it cannot be tested within 2 hours of being voided?

8. What does the NCCLS recommend as a preferred specimen for routine urinalysis?

9. What instructions are necessary to convey to a patient about how a 24-hour urine collection should be done?

10. What would be the appearance of the cerebrospinal fluid in the series of tubes collected if there had been a traumatic tap?

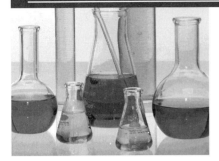

CHAPTER 4

Systems of Measurement and General Laboratory Equipment

Learning Objectives

From study of this chapter, the reader will be able to:

➤ Understand the metric units of measurement for weight, length, volume, and temperature, how the metric system is used in the laboratory, and the conversion of English units to metric units.

➤ Convert temperatures from degrees Celsius to degrees Fahrenheit and vice versa.

➤ Know how normal and molar solutions are prepared.

➤ Know how to prepare solutions and reagents of specific composition, about the various forms and grades of water used in the laboratory and how each is prepared, about the various grades of chemicals used in the laboratory, including their levels of quality and the purposes for which they are intended, and how to properly label a container used to store a laboratory reagent or solution.

➤ Describe the various types of and uses for laboratory volumetric glassware (pipettes, flasks, burets), the techniques for their use, and the various types of glass used to manufacture them.

➤ Describe and interpret how laboratory volumetric glassware is calibrated and how the calibration markings are indicated on the glassware.

➤ Solve a titration problem—that is, solve for *x* normality when the volume and normality of one solution are known and only the volume of the second solution is known.

➤ Know how to properly clean laboratory glassware and plastic ware.

➤ Describe the operation of and uses for laboratory balances—analytical, torsion, triple beam.

➤ Describe types and uses of laboratory centrifuges.

INTRODUCTION TO GENERAL LABORATORY MEASUREMENTS AND EQUIPMENT USED

If the results of laboratory analyses are to be useful to the physician in diagnosing and treating patients, the tests must be performed as accurately as possible. Many factors constitute the final laboratory result for a single determination. The use of high-quality analytic methods and instrumentation is of prime importance, but other basic principles and procedures also play a role.

In order to unify physical measurements worldwide, the International System of Units (SI units) has been adopted. Many of these units also relate to the metric system. A coherent system of measure units is vital to precise clinical laboratory analyses. The pertinent SI units of measure are discussed in this chapter, as well as the use of metric measurements in the laboratory.

A general discussion of laboratory glassware and plastic ware, including types used for measuring volume, is included. The importance of knowing the correct use of these various pieces of glassware must be thoroughly appreciated. The four basic pieces of volumetric glassware—volumetric flasks, graduated measuring cylinders, burets, and pipettes—are specialized,

with each having its own particular use in the laboratory.

The accuracy of laboratory analyses depends to a great extent on the accuracy of the reagents used. Traditional preparation of reagents makes use of balances and volumetric measuring devices such as pipettes and volumetric flasks—examples of fundamental laboratory apparatus. When reagents and standard solutions are being prepared, it is imperative that only the purest water supply be used in the procedure. For this reason, the various types of water are discussed. The careful preparation of reagents and standard solutions, along with the necessary knowledge about the chemicals used for these preparations, is basic to any analytic procedure in the clinical laboratory and therefore is discussed in this chapter.

Many and varied pieces of laboratory equipment are used in performing clinical determinations, and knowledge of the proper use and handling of this equipment is an important part of any laboratory work. Measurement of mass, using balances, and measurement of volume, using pipettes and burets, are important basic analytic procedures in the clinical laboratory. Centrifuges are also used in various ways in the laboratory.

The use of photometry, and spectrophotometers in particular, is covered in Chapter 6.

SYSTEMS OF MEASUREMENT

The ability to measure accurately is the keystone of the scientific method, and anyone engaged in performing clinical laboratory analyses must have a working knowledge of measurement systems and units of measurement. It is also necessary to understand how to convert units of one system to units of another system. Systems of measurement included here are the English, metric, and SI systems.

Metric System

Traditionally, measurements in the clinical laboratory have been made in metric units. The **metric system** is based on a decimal system, a system of divisions and multiples of tens. It has not been widely used in the United States, except in the scientific community. The meter (m) is the standard metric unit for measurement of length, the gram (g) is the unit of mass, and the liter (L) is the unit of volume. Multiples or divisions of these reference units constitute the various other metric units.

International System (SI System)

Another system of measurement, the **International System of Units** (from le Système International d'Unités, or **SI**) has been adopted by the worldwide scientific community as a coherent, standardized system, based on seven base units. There are also derived units and supplemental units, in addition to the base units. The SI base units describe seven fundamental, but independent, physical quantities. The derived units are calculated mathematically from two or more base units.

The SI system was established in 1960 by international agreement and is now the standard international language of measurement. The **International Bureau of Weights and Measures** is responsible for maintaining the standards on which the SI system of measurement is based.

The term *metric system* generally refers to the SI system and, for informational purposes, metric terms that remain in common usage are described where needed. Since the English system is common in everyday use, English system equivalents are also given in the discussion of units.

The National Committee for Clinical Laboratory Standards (NCCLS) recommends that an extensive educational effort be put forth to implement the SI system in clinical laboratories in the United States.[6] Any changes in units used to report laboratory findings should be done with great care, to avoid misunderstanding and confusion in interpretation of laboratory results.

Base Units of the SI System

In the SI system the base units of measurement are the metre (meter), kilogram, second, mole, ampere, kelvin, and candela. These seven base units and their accepted abbreviations are listed in Table 4-1.

All units in the SI system can be qualified by standard prefixes that serve to convert values to more convenient forms, depending on the size of the object being measured. These prefixes are listed in Table 4-2.

TABLE 4-1

Base Units of the SI System

Measurement	Unit Name	Abbreviation
Length	Metre*	m
Mass	Kilogram	kg
Time	Second	s
Amount of substance	Mole	mol
Electric current	Ampere	A
Temperature	Kelvin†	K
Luminous intensity	Candela	cd

*The spelling *meter* is more commonly used in the United States and is used in this book.

†Although the basic unit of temperature is the kelvin, the degree Celsius is regarded as an acceptable unit, since kelvins may be impractical in many instances. Celsius is more commonly used in the clinical laboratory.

TABLE 4-2

Prefixes of the SI System

Prefix Name	Symbol	Factor	Decimal
Tera	T	10^{12}	1 000 000 000 000
Giga	G	10^9	1 000 000 000
Mega	M	10^6	1 000 000
Kilo	k	10^3	1 000
Hecto	h	10^2	100
Deka	da	10^1	10
Deci	d	10^{-1}	0.1
Centi	c	10^{-2}	0.01
Milli	m	10^{-3}	0.001
Micro	μ	10^{-6}	0.000 001
Nano	n	10^{-9}	0.000 000 001
Pico	p	10^{-12}	0.000 000 000 001
Femto	f	10^{-15}	0.000 000 000 000 001
Atto	a	10^{-18}	0.000 000 000 000 000 001

Various rules should be kept in mind when one is combining these prefixes with their basic units and using the SI system; some of these rules follow. An *s* should not be added to form the plural of the abbreviation for a unit or for a prefix with a unit. For example, 25 millimeters should be abbreviated as 25 mm, not 25 mms. Do not use periods after abbreviations (use mm, not mm.). Do not use compound prefixes; instead, use the closest accepted prefix. For example, 24 x 10^{-9} gram (g) should be expressed as 24 nanograms (24 ng) rather than 24 millimicrograms (25 mμg). In the SI system, commas are not used as spacers in recording large numbers, since they are used in place of decimal points in some countries. Instead, groups of three digits are separated by spaces. When recording temperature on the Kelvin scale, omit the degree sign. Therefore, 295 kelvins should be recorded as 295 K, not 295° K. However, the symbol for degree Celsius is ° C, and 22 degrees Celsius should be recorded as 22° C. Multiples and submultiples should be used in steps of 10^3 or 10^{-3}. Only one solidus or slash (/) is used when indicating *per* or a denominator: thus meters per second

squared (m/s²), not meters per second per second (m/s/s), and millimoles per liter-hour (mmol/L · hour), not millimoles per liter per hour (mmol/L/hour). Finally, although the preferred SI spellings are *metre* and *litre,* the spellings *meter* and *liter* remain in common usage in the United States and are used in this book.

The base units of measurement that are used most often in the clinical laboratory are those for length, mass, and volume.

Length. The standard unit for the measurement of length or distance is the **meter (m)**. The meter is standardized as 1,650,763.73 wavelengths of a certain orange light in the spectrum of krypton 86. One meter equals 39.37 inches (in.), slightly more than a yard in the English system. There are 2.54 centimeters (cm) in 1 in.

Further common divisions and multiples of the meter, using the system of prefixes previously discussed, follow. One tenth of a meter is a decimeter (dm), one hundredth of a meter is a centimeter (cm), and one thousandth of a meter is a millimeter (mm). One thousand meters equals 1 kilometer (km). The following examples show equivalent measurements of length:

$$25 \text{ mm} = 0.025 \text{ m}$$
$$10 \text{ cm} = 100 \text{ mm}$$
$$1 \text{ m} = 100 \text{ cm}$$
$$0.1 \text{ m} = 100 \text{ mm}$$

Other units of length that were in common usage in the metric system but are no longer recommended in the SI system are the angstrom and the micron. The angstrom (Å) is equal to 10^{-10} m or 10^{-1} nanometer (nm). This unit is permitted but not encouraged. The micron (μ), which is equal to 10^{-6} m, has been replaced by the micrometer (μm).

Mass (and Weight). Mass denotes the quantity of matter, while weight takes into account the force of gravity and should not be used in the same sense as mass. However, they are commonly used interchangeably and may be so used in this book. The standard unit for the measurement of mass in the SI system is the **kilogram (kg).** This is the basis for all other mass measurements in the system. The standard kilogram is the mass of a block of platinum-iridium kept at the International Bureau of Weights and Measures. One kilogram weighs approximately 2.2 pounds (lb) in the English system. Conversely, 1 lb equals approximately 0.5 kg.

The kilogram is divided into thousandths, called grams (g). One thousand grams equals 1 kg. The gram is used much more often than the kilogram in the clinical laboratory. The gram is divided into thousandths, called milligrams (mg). Grams and milligrams are units commonly used in weighing substances in the clinical laboratory. One millionth of a gram, a microgram (μg), may also be encountered. Some examples of weight measurement equivalents follow:

$$10 \text{ mg} = 0.01 \text{ g}$$
$$0.055 \text{ g} = 55 \text{ mg}$$
$$25 \text{ g} = 25,000 \text{ mg}$$
$$1.5 \text{ kg} = 1,500 \text{ g}$$

Units that were once used to describe mass and that may still be encountered are the gamma and parts per million. The term gamma (γ) should not be used; instead, use microgram (μg). The term parts per million (ppm) should be replaced by micrograms per gram (μg/g).

Volume. In the clinical laboratory the standard unit of volume is the **liter (L).** It was not included in the list of base units of the SI system because the liter is a derived unit. The standard unit of volume in the SI system is the cubic meter (m^3). However, this unit is quite large, and the cubic decimeter (dm^3) is a more convenient size for use in the clinical laboratory. Thus in 1964 the Conférence Générale des Poids et Mésures (CGPM) accepted the litre (liter) as a special name for the cubic decimeter. Previously, the standard liter was the volume occupied by 1 kg of pure water at 4° C (the temperature at which a volume of water weighs the most) and at normal atmospheric pressure. On this basis, 1 L equals 1,000.027 cubic centimeters (cm^3), and the units milliliters and cubic centimeters were used interchangeably, although there is a slight difference between them. One liter is slightly more than 1 quart (qt) in the English system (1 L = 1.06 qt).

The liter is divided into thousandths, called milliliters (mL); millionths, called microliters (μL); and billionths, called nanoliters (nL). Some examples of volume equivalents are:

$$500 \text{ mL} = 0.5 \text{ L}$$
$$0.25 \text{ L} = 250 \text{ mL}$$
$$2 \text{ L} = 2,000 \text{ mL}$$
$$500 \text{ }\mu\text{L} = 0.5 \text{ mL}$$

Since the liter is derived from the meter (1 L = 1 dm^3), it follows that 1 cm^3 is equal to 1 mL and that 1 millimeter cubed (mm^3) is equal to 1 μL. The former abbreviation for cubic centimeter (cc) has been replaced by cm^3. Although this is a common means of expressing volume in the clinical laboratory, milliliter (mL) is preferred.

Amount of Substance. The standard unit of measurement for the amount of a (chemical) substance in the SI system is the mole (mol). The mole is defined as the quantity of a chemical equal to that present in 0.0120 kg of pure carbon 12. A mole of a chemical substance is the relative atomic or molecular mass unit of that substance. Formerly, the terms atomic and molecular weight were used to describe the mole. These are further defined and discussed below.

Temperature. Three scales are commonly used to measure temperature, namely, the Kelvin, Celsius, and Fahrenheit scales. The **Celsius scale** is sometimes referred to as the centigrade scale, which is an outdated term.

The basic unit of temperature in the SI system is the kelvin (K). However, as mentioned previously, the degree Celsius is regarded as an acceptable unit, since the kelvin may be impractical in many instances. The Celsius scale is the one used most often in the clinical laboratory. The Kelvin and Celsius scales are closely related, and conversion between them is simple since the units (degrees) are equal in magnitude. The difference between the Kelvin and Celsius scales is the zero point. The zero point on the Kelvin scale is the theoretical temperature of no further heat loss, which is absolute zero. The zero point on the Celsius scale is the freezing point of pure water. Remember, however, that the magnitude of the degree is equal in the two scales. Therefore, since water freezes at 273 kelvins (273 K), it follows that 0 degrees Celsius (0° C) equals 273 kelvins (273 K) and that 0 Kelvin (0 K) equals minus 273

degrees Celsius (–273° C). Thus, to convert from kelvins to degrees Celsius, add 273; to convert from degrees Celsius to kelvins, subtract 273.

$$K = °C + 273$$
$$°C = K - 273$$

Since the Celsius scale was devised so that 100° C is the boiling point of pure water, the boiling point on the Kelvin scale is 373 K.

Converting from Celsius to Fahrenheit is not as simple, since the degrees are not equal in magnitude on these two scales. The Fahrenheit scale was originally devised with the zero point at the lowest temperature attainable from a mixture of table salt and ice, while the body temperature of a small animal was used to set 100° F. Thus, on the Fahrenheit scale the freezing point of pure water is 32°, while the temperature at which pure water boils is 212°. It is rare that readings on one of these scales must be converted to the other, as almost without exception readings taken and used in the clinical laboratory will be on the Celsius scale.

Examples of comparative readings of the three scales with common reference points are given in Table 4-3.

It is possible, however, to convert from one scale to the other. The basic conversion formulas are:
1. $1° C = \frac{9}{5}° F$
   $1° F = \frac{5}{9}° C$
2. To convert Fahrenheit to Celsius:
   Method A: Add 40, multiply by $\frac{5}{9}$, and subtract 40 from the result.

TABLE 4-3

Common Reference Points on the Three Temperature Scales

	Kelvin	Degrees Celsius	Degrees Fahrenheit
Boiling point of water	373	100	212
Body temperature	310	37	98.6
Room temperature	293	20	68
Freezing point of water	273	0	32
Absolute zero (coldest possible temperature)	0	–273	–459

Method B: $^\circ C = \frac{5}{9}(^\circ F - 32)$

3. To convert Celsius to Fahrenheit:
   Method A: Add 40, multiply by $\frac{9}{5}$, and subtract 40 from the result.
   Method B: $^\circ F = \frac{9}{5}^\circ C + 32$

Non-SI Units

Several non-SI units are relevant to clinical laboratory analyses, such as minutes (min), hours (hr), and days (d). These units of time have such historic use in everyday life that it is unlikely that new SI units derived from the second (the base unit for time in the SI system) will be implemented. Another non-SI unit is the liter (L). This has already been discussed with the base SI units of volume. Pressure is expressed in millimeters of mercury (mm Hg) and enzyme activity in international units (IU) (1 IU is defined as the amount of enzyme that will catalyze the transformation of 1 mol/sec of substrate in an assay system).

Reporting Results in SI Units

In order to give a meaningful laboratory result, it is important to always report both the numbers and the units by which the result is measured. The unit expresses or defines the dimension of the measured substance—concentration, mass, or volume—and it is an important part of any laboratory result.

Laboratory results can be reported as a mass concentration unit—mass/liter (as g/dL)—or as a molar unit (moles/L). Commonly, laboratories in the United States have been using the mass per liter system in results reporting. Worldwide, moles per liter units are used. Implementation, or conversion, to SI units (moles/L) would mean that some previously reported units will change. With SI units, whenever the molecular weight of the measured analyte is known, its concentration is to be expressed in moles per liter (mol/L) or a subunit, rather than in mass per liter. If the molecular weight is not known, as in specific proteins, mixtures of proteins, or other complex molecules, the concentration should be expressed in mass per liter.

Conversion to the molar (mol/L) unit from a mass concentration unit (g/dL) first involves multiplication by 10 for volume conversion and then division by the molecular weight of the substance. If any conversion is made, no greater precision should be given than was present in the original measurement.

LABORATORY GLASSWARE AND PLASTIC WARE

The general laboratory supplies, or laboratory ware, described in this chapter are those used for storage, measurement, and containment. Laboratory glassware and plastic ware, as well as automatic pipetting and diluting devices, are included. Most laboratory glassware and other laboratory ware can be divided into two main categories according to the use to which they are put: containers and receivers and volumetric ware. Examples of containers and receivers are beakers, test tubes, Erlenmeyer flasks, and reagent bottles. Examples of volumetric ware are pipettes, automatic and manual; volumetric flasks; graduated cylinders; and burets.

Glassware

Clinical laboratories still use glassware for the greater part of the analytic work done, even with the advent of plastic ware. Glassware is used in all departments of the laboratory, and special types of glass apparatus have been devised for special uses. These special types of glassware are discussed where applicable. The chemistry department probably has the greatest variety and amount of glassware. Certain types of glass can be attacked by reagents to such an extent that the determinations done in them are not valid. It is therefore important to use the correct type of glass for the determinations being done.

Types of Glass

Clinical laboratory glassware can be divided into several types: glass with high thermal resistance, high-silica glass, glass with a high resistance to alkali, low-actinic glass, and standard flint glass.

Thermal-Resistant (Borosilicate) Glass. High-thermal-resistant glass is usually a borosilicate glass with a low alkali content. This type of glassware is resistant to heat, corrosion, and thermal shock and should be used whenever heating or sterilization by heat is employed. Borosilicate glass, known by the commercial name of Pyrex* or Kimax,[†] is used widely in the laboratory because of its high qualities of resistance. Laboratory apparatus such as beakers, flasks, and pipettes are usually made from borosilicate glass. Other brands of glassware are made from lower-grade borosilicate glass and may be used when a high-quality borosilicate glass is not necessary. If the various pieces of glassware found in the laboratory are examined, it will be seen that one or more of these brand names will be found on many different kinds of glassware. It is essential to choose glassware that has a reliable composition and that will be resistant to laboratory chemicals and conditions. In borosilicate glassware, mechanical strength and thermal and chemical resistance are well balanced.

Alumina-Silica Glass. Alumina-silica glass has a high silica content, which makes it comparable to fused quartz in its heat resistance, chemical stability, and electrical characteristics. It is strengthened chemically rather than thermally. Corex* brand is made from alumina-silica. This type of glassware is used for high-precision analytic work, is radiation resistant, and can also be used for optical reflectors and mirrors. It is not used for the general type of glassware found in the laboratory.

Alkali-Resistant Glass. Glass with high resistance to alkali was developed particularly for use with strong alkaline solutions. It is boron-free. It is often referred to as soft glass, as its thermal resistance is much less than that of borosilicate glass, and it must be heated and cooled very carefully. Its use should be limited to times when

solutions of, or digestions with, strong alkalis are made.

Low-Actinic Glass. Low-actinic glassware contains materials that usually impart an amber or red color to the glass and reduce the amount of light transmitted through to the substance in the glassware. It is used for substances that are particularly sensitive to light, such as bilirubin or vitamin A.

Standard Flint Glass. Standard flint glass, or soda-lime glass, is composed of a mixture of the oxides of silicon, calcium, and sodium. It is the most inexpensive glass and is readily made into a variety of types of glassware. This type of glass is much less resistant to high temperatures and sudden changes in temperature, and its resistance to chemical attack is only fair. Glassware made from soda-lime glass can release alkali into solutions and can therefore cause considerable errors in certain laboratory determinations. For example, manual pipettes made from soda-lime glass may release alkali into the pipetted liquid.

Disposable Glassware. The widespread use of relatively inexpensive disposable glassware has greatly reduced the need to clean glassware. Disposable glassware is made to be used and discarded, and no cleaning is necessary either before or after use, in most cases. Disposable glass and plastic are used to manufacture test tubes of all sizes, pipettes, slides, Petri dishes for microbiology, and specimen containers, to mention but a few.

Containers and Receivers

This category of glassware includes many of the most frequently used and most common pieces of glassware in the laboratory. Containers and receivers must be made of good-quality glass. They are not calibrated to hold a particular or exact volume, but rather are available for various volumes, depending on the use desired. Beakers, Erlenmeyer flasks, test tubes, and reagent bottles are made in many different sizes (Fig. 4-1). This glassware, like the volumetric glassware, has cer-

---

*Corning Glass Works, Corning, NY.
[†]Kimble Glass Co, Vineland, NJ.

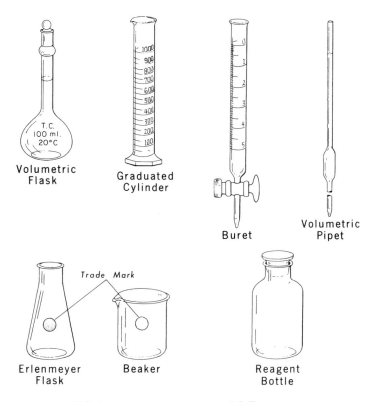

FIG 4-1. Laboratory glassware. *T.C.*, To contain.

tain information indicated directly on the vessel. The volume and the brand name, or trademark, are two pieces of information found on items such as beakers and test tubes. Containers and receivers are not as expensive as volumetric glassware, because the process of exact volume calibration is not necessary.

Beakers. Beakers are wide, straight-sided cylindrical vessels and are available in many sizes and in several forms. The most common form used in the clinical laboratory is known as the Griffin low form. Beakers should be made of glass that is resistant to the many chemicals used in them and also resistant to heat. Beakers are used along with flasks for general mixing and for reagent preparation.

Erlenmeyer Flasks. Erlenmeyer flasks are used commonly in the laboratory for preparing

reagents and for titration procedures. They, too, come in various sizes and must be made from a resistant form of glass.

Test Tubes. Test tubes come in many sizes, depending on the use for which they are intended. Test tubes without lips are the most satisfactory, because there is less chance of chipping and eventual breakage. Disposable test tubes are used for most laboratory purposes. Since chemical reactions occur in test tubes used in the chemistry laboratory, test tubes intended for such use should be made of borosilicate glass, which is resistant to thermal shock.

Reagent Bottles. All reagents should be stored in reagent bottles of some type. These can be made of glass or some other material; some of the more commonly purchased ones now are made of plastic. Reagent bottles come in various sizes; the size used should meet the needs of the particular situation.

Photometry Cuvettes. The special tubes used for photometry are called cuvettes or absorption cells. They may be round, square, or rectangular and may be made of glass, silica (quartz), or plastic. For most routine purposes in the clinical laboratory, a round cuvette made of good-quality glass is used. The amount of light transmitted by the cuvette varies significantly with the material used to make it. In order for cuvettes to be used interchangeably, they must be of uniform inside diameters so that the absorbance of a solution will be within a specified tolerance when measured in different cuvettes. To ensure this uniformity, only calibrated cuvettes must be used or plain tubes that have been optically matched (see also Chapter 6).

Volumetric Glassware

Volumetric glassware must go through a rigorous process of volume **calibration** to ensure the accuracy of the measurements required for laboratory determinations. In very precise work it is never safe to assume that the volume contained or delivered by any piece of equipment is exactly that indicated on the equipment. The calibration process is lengthy and time consuming; therefore the cost of volumetric glassware is relatively high compared with the cost of noncalibrated glassware (beakers, test tubes, and so on).

Volumetric Flasks. Volumetric flasks are flasks with a round bulb at the bottom. This tapers to a long neck, on which the calibration mark is found. The specifications set up by the National Bureau of Standards apply to all volumetric glassware and therefore to volumetric flasks (see Fig. 4-1).[4] Volumetric flasks are calibrated to contain a specific amount or volume of liquid, and therefore the letters TC are inscribed somewhere on the neck of the flask. There are many different sizes of volumetric flasks, for the different volumes of liquid that are used. The following are some of the sizes in which volumetric flasks can be purchased: 10, 25, 50, 100, and 500 mL, and 1 and 2 L.

Volumetric flasks have been calibrated individually to contain the specified volume at a specified temperature. They are not calibrated to deliver this volume. For each size of volumetric flask, there are certain allowable limits within which its volume must lie. These limits are called the tolerance of the flask. All volumetric glassware has a specific tolerance, the capacity tolerance, which is dependent on the size of the glassware. For example, if a 100-mL volumetric flask has a tolerance of ±0.08 mL, conditions are controlled during the calibration of a 100-mL volumetric flask to guarantee these limits. A tolerance of ±0.08 mL indicates that the allowable limits for the volume of a 100-mL volumetric flask are from 99.92 to 100.08 mL. A tolerance of ±0.05 mL for a 50-mL volumetric flask indicates allowable limits of 49.95 to 50.05 mL for the volume of the flask. Volumetric flasks are used in the preparation of specific volumes of reagents or laboratory solutions. They should be used with reagents or solutions at room temperature. Solutions diluted in volumetric flasks should be repeatedly mixed during the dilution so that the contents are homogeneous before they are made up to volume. In this way, errors due to the expansion or contraction of liquids during mixing are made negligible. An important factor in the use of any volumetric apparatus is an accurate reading of the meniscus level. For more information on reading a meniscus, see under Pipetting Technique Using Manual Pipettes later in this chapter.

Graduated Measuring Cylinders. A graduated measuring cylinder is a long straight-sided cylindrical piece of glassware with calibrated markings on it. Graduated cylinders are used to measure volumes of liquids when a high degree of accuracy is not essential. They can be made from plastic or polyethylene as well as from glass (see Fig. 4-1). Graduated cylinders come in various sizes according to the volumes they measure: 10, 25, 50, 100, 500, and 1000 mL. A 100-mL graduated cylinder can measure 100 mL or a fraction thereof, depending on the calibration, or graduation, marks on it. Most graduated cylinders are calibrated to deliver. This will be indicated directly on the glassware by the inscription TD. The letters TD can be found on many kinds of volumetric glassware, especially on the numerous kinds of pipettes used in the laboratory (see under Pipettes).

Graduated cylinders can be used to measure a specified volume of a liquid, such as water, in the preparation of laboratory re-agents. The calibration marks on the cylinder indicate its capacity at different points. If 450 mL of water is to be measured, the most satisfactory cylinder to use would be one with a capacity of 500 mL. Graduated cylinders are not calibrated as accurately as volumetric flasks. Therefore, the capacity tolerance for graduated cylinders allows a greater variation in volume. The capacity tolerance is greater for the larger graduated cylinders. A 100-mL graduated cylinder (TD) has a tolerance of ± 0.40 mL, meaning that the allowable limits are 99.60 to 100.40 mL.

Pipettes. Pipettes are another type of volumetric glassware used extensively in the laboratory. Many types of pipettes are available. It is important, however, to use only pipettes manufactured by reputable companies. Care and discretion should be used in selecting pipettes for clinical laboratory use, since their accuracy is one of the determining factors in the accuracy of the procedures carried out. A pipette is a cylindrical glass tube used in measuring fluids. Pipettes are calibrated to deliver, or transfer, a specified volume from one vessel to another (see Fig. 4-1). Manual and automatic pipettes are available.

Each manual pipette has at least one calibration or graduation mark on it, as does all volumetric glassware. A pipette is filled by using mechanical suction or an aspirator bulb. Mouth suction is never used. Strong acids, bases, solvents, or human specimens are much too potent or contaminated to risk pipetting them by mouth. Caustic liquids and some solvents are very dangerous; some destroy tissue immedi-

ately on contact. Some solvents have harmful vapors (see Chapter 2).

For most general laboratory use, there are two main types of manual pipettes: the **volumetric (or transfer) pipette** and the **graduated (or measuring) pipette**. They are classified according to whether they contain or deliver a specified amount; thus they may be called **to-contain pipettes** or **to-deliver pipettes**. A to-contain pipette is identified by the inscribed letters TC and a to-deliver one by the letters TD. The TD pipette is filled properly and allowed to drain completely into a receiving vessel. Portions of nonviscous samples, such as filtrates, serum, and standard solutions, are accurately measured by allowing the volumetric pipette to drain while it is held in the vertical position and by using only the force of gravity (see under Pipetting Technique Using Manual Pipettes). For most volumetric glassware the temperature of calibration is usually 20° C, and this is inscribed on the pipette (see under Calibration of Volumetric Glassware).

The opening (orifice) at the delivery tip of the pipette is of a certain size to give a specified length of time for drainage when the pipette is held vertically. A pipette must be held vertically to ensure proper drainage. It will not drain as fast when held at a 45-degree angle. The actual procedure is discussed further under Measurement of Volume: Pipetting and Titration.

Volumetric Pipettes. A pipette that has been calibrated to deliver a fixed volume of liquid by drainage is known as a volumetric pipette, or transfer pipette. These pipettes consist of a cylindrical bulb joined at both ends to narrow glass tubing. A **calibration mark** is etched around the upper suction tube, and the lower delivery tube is drawn out to a fine tip. Some important considerations concerning volumetric pipettes are that the calibration mark should not be too close to the top of the suction tube, the bulb should merge gradually into the lower delivery tube, and the delivery tip should have a gradual taper. To reduce drainage errors, the orifice should be of such a size that the flow out of the pipette is not too rapid. These pipettes should be made from a good-quality glass, such as Kimax or Pyrex (Fig. 4-2).

Volumetric pipettes are suitable for all accurate measurements of volumes of 1 mL or more. They are calibrated to deliver the amount inscribed on them. This volume is measured from the calibration mark to the tip. A 5-mL volumetric pipette will deliver a single measured volume of 5 mL, and a 2-mL volumetric pipette will deliver 2 mL. The **tolerance** of volumetric pipettes increases with the capacity of the pipette. A 10-mL volumetric pipette will have a greater tolerance than a 2-mL one. The tolerance of a 5-mL volumetric pipette is ±0.01 mL. When volumes of liquids are to be delivered with great accuracy, a volumetric pipette is used. Volumet-ric pipettes are used to measure standard solutions, unknown blood and plasma filtrates, serum, plasma, urine, cerebrospinal fluid, and some reagents.

Measurements with volumetric pipettes are done individually, and the volumes can be only whole milliliters, as determined by the pipette selected (e.g., 1, 2, 5, and 10 mL). To transfer 1 mL of a standard solution into a test tube volumetrically, a 1-mL volumetric pipette is used. To trans-

fer 5 mL of the same solution, a 5-mL volumetric pipette is used. After a volumetric pipette drains, a drop remains inside the delivery tip. The specific volume the pipette is calibrated to deliver is dependent on the fact that the drop is left in the tip of the pipette. Information inscribed on the pipette includes the temperature of calibration (usually 20° C), capacity, manufacturer, and use (TD). The technique involved in using volumetric pipettes correctly is very important, and a certain amount of skill is required (see under Pipetting Technique Using Manual Pipettes).

Graduated Pipettes. Another way to deliver a particular amount of liquid is to deliver the amount of liquid contained between two calibration marks on a cylindrical tube, or pipette. Such a pipette is called a graduated pipette, or measuring pipette. It has several graduation, or calibration, marks (see Fig. 4-2). Many measurements in the laboratory do not require the precision of the volumetric pipette. Graduated pipettes are used when great accuracy is not required. This does not mean that these pipettes may be used with less care than the volumetric pipettes. Graduated pipettes are used primarily in measuring reagents, but they are not calibrated with sufficient tolerance to use in mea-

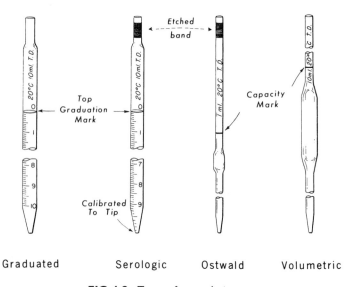

FIG 4-2. Types of manual pipettes.

suring standard or control solutions, unknown specimens, or filtrates.

A graduated pipette is a straight piece of glass tubing with a tapered end and graduation marks on the stem separating it into parts. Depending on the size used, graduated pipettes can be used to measure parts of a milliliter or many milliliters. These pipettes come in various sizes or capacities, including 0.1, 0.2, 1.0, 2.0, 5.0, 10, and 25 mL. If 4 mL of deionized water is to be measured into a test tube, a 5-mL graduated pipette would be the best choice. Since graduated pipettes require draining between two marks, they introduce one more source of error, compared with the volumetric pipettes, which have only one calibration mark. This makes measurements with the graduated pipette less precise. Because of this relatively poor precision, the graduated pipette is used when speed is more important than precision. It is used for measurements of reagents and is generally not considered accurate enough for measuring samples and standard solutions.

Two types of graduated pipettes are calibrated for delivery (see Fig. 4-2). One (called a Mohr pipette) is calibrated between two marks on the stem, and the other (a serologic pipette) has graduation marks down to the delivery tip. The serologic pipette has a larger orifice and therefore drains faster than the Mohr pipette (see under Serologic Pipettes).

The volume of the space between the last calibration mark and the delivery tip is not known in the Mohr pipette. In Mohr graduated pipettes, this space cannot be used for measuring fluids. Graduated pipettes are calibrated in much the same manner as volumetric pipettes; however, they are not constructed to as strict specifications, and they have larger tolerances. The allowable tolerance for a 5-mL graduated pipette is ±0.02 mL.

Micropipettes (To-Contain Pipettes). The **micropipette**, or to-contain pipette, when used properly, is one of the more precise pipettes used in the clinical laboratory. This type of pipette is calibrated to contain a specified amount of liquid. If a pipette contains only 10 μL (0.1 mL), and 10 μL of blood is needed for a laboratory de-

termination, then none of the blood can be left inside the pipette. The entire contents of the pipette must be emptied. If this pipette is rinsed well with a diluting solution, then all the blood or similar specimen will be removed from it. The correct way to use a to-contain pipette is to rinse it with a suitable diluent. Thus, a to-contain pipette cannot be used properly unless the receiving vessel contains a diluent; that is, a to-contain pipette should not be used to deliver a specimen into an empty receiving vessel. Since all the liquid in a to-contain pipette is rinsed out and used, there is only one graduation mark.

Micropipettes are used when small amounts of blood or specimen are needed. Many procedures require only a small amount of blood, and a micropipette is used for this measurement. Because even a minute volume remaining in the pipette can cause a significant error in micro work, most micropipettes are calibrated to contain the stated volume rather than to deliver it. They are generally available in small sizes, from 1 to 500 μL.

Unopette. A special disposable micropipette used in the hematology laboratory is a self-filling pipette accompanied by a polyethylene reagent reservoir. This unit is called a Unopette* and is used by many laboratories. A glass capillary pipette is fitted in a plastic holder and fills automatically with blood by means of capillary action. The plastic reagent bottle (called the reservoir) is squeezed slightly while the pipette is inserted. On release of pressure, the sample is drawn into the diluent in the reservoir. Intermittent squeezing fills and empties the pipette to rinse out the contents. This type of unit has been adapted for several chemical and hematologic determinations.

Capillary pipettes. An inexpensive, disposable micropipette is one made of capillary tubing with a calibration line marking a specified volume. This micropipette is filled to the line by capillary action, and the measured liquid is

---

*Becton, Dickinson & Co, Franklin Lakes, NJ.

delivered by positive pressure, as with a medicine dropper. These **capillary pipettes** are usually calibrated TC and require rinsing to obtain the stated accuracy.

Automatic micropipettors. These are **automatic pipetting devices**, which allow rapid, repetitive measurements and delivery of equivalent volumes of reagents or solutions. The most common type of micropipette used in many laboratories is one that is automatic or semiautomatic, called a micropipettor. These are piston-operated devices that allow repeated, accurate, reproducible delivery of specimens, reagents, and other liquids needing measurement in small amounts (see Fig. 4-10). Many pipettors are continuously adjustable so that variable volumes of liquids can be dispensed with the same device. Delivery volume is selected by adjusting the settings on the pipette device. Different types or models are available, which allow volume delivery ranging from 0.5 μL to 5,000 μL, for example. The calibration of these micropipettes should be checked periodically.

The piston, usually in the form of a thumb plunger, is depressed to a stop position on the pipetting device, the tip is placed in the liquid to be measured, and then slowly the plunger is allowed to rise back to the original position (see Fig. 4-10). This will fill the tip with the desired volume of liquid. The tips are usually drawn along the inside wall of the vessel from which the measured volume is drawn, so that any adhering liquid is removed from the end of the tip. These pipette tips are not usually wiped as is done with the manual pipettes, because the plastic surface is considered nonwettable. The tip of the pipette device is then placed against the inside wall of the receiving vessel, and the plunger is depressed. When the manufacturer's directions for the device being used are followed, sample delivery volume is judged to be extremely accurate.

The pipette tips are usually made of disposable plastic, so no cleaning is necessary. Various types of tips are available. Some pipetting devices automatically eject the tip after use. These

will also allow the user to insert a new tip as well as remove the used tip without touching it, minimizing infectious biohazard exposures. (See Pipetting Techniques Using Automatic Pipettes later in this chapter.)

Ostwald Pipettes. A special type of pipette designed for use in measuring viscous fluids such as whole blood is known as the Ostwald pipette (or the Ostwald-Folin pipette).

Serologic Pipettes. Another pipette used in the laboratory, but not often in the chemistry laboratory, is called a **serologic pipette**. It is much like the graduated pipette in appearance (see Fig. 4-2). The orifice, or tip opening, is larger in the serologic pipette than in other pipettes. The rate of fall of liquid is much too fast for great accuracy or precision. For use of the serologic pipette in chemistry, it would be necessary to retard the flow of liquid from the delivery tip. The serologic pipette is graduated to the end of the delivery tip and has an etched band on the suction piece. It is therefore designed to be blown out mechanically. The serologic pipette is less precise than any of the pipettes discussed above. It is designed for use in serology, in which relative values are sought. It is best not to use the serologic pipette for chemistry.

Burets. A **buret** is a long cylindrical tube of glassware with graduation divisions on it and a stopcock closing at one end (see Fig. 4-1). The stopcock on the delivery tip of the buret serves to control the flow of liquid. A buret is used to deliver measured quantities of fluids or solutions in the process of **titration**. Like all other volumetric glassware, burets are carefully calibrated according to the specifications set up by the National Bureau of Standards.

Burets also have a specific capacity tolerance depending on their size. Smaller burets are more accurate than larger ones (they have smaller tolerances). Burets with a maximum capacity of 2 mL or less are called microburets. They are usually calibrated with 0.01-mL or smaller divisions. Some common capacities for burets are 5, 10, and 25 mL. The capacity tolerances for burets are similar to those for graduated pipettes, which burets resemble very closely. For a 5-mL buret, the tolerance is ±0.02 mL. This means that the allowable limits for the volume of this particular buret are 4.98 to 5.02 mL. The chief difference between the buret and the graduated pipette is that the buret has a stopcock. The stopcock is made from either glass or Teflon. A glass stopcock requires the use of a lubricant, but a Teflon stopcock does not. Burets are used in titration, a means of quantitative measurement (see under Titration for more information on the use of the buret).

Calibration of Volumetric Glassware. Calibration is the means by which glassware or other apparatus used in quantitative measurements is checked to determine its exact volume. To calibrate is to divide the glassware or mark it with graduations (or other indices of quantity) for the purpose of measurement. Calibration marks will be seen on every piece of volumetric glassware used in the laboratory. Specifications for the calibration of glassware are established by the **National Bureau of Standards**.[4] High-quality volumetric glassware is calibrated by the manufacturer; this calibration can be checked by the laboratory using the glassware.

Each piece of volumetric glassware must be checked and must comply with these specifications before it can be accurately used in the clinical laboratory. Pipettes, burets, volumetric flasks, and other types of volumetric glassware are supposed to hold, deliver, or contain a specific amount of liquid. This specified amount, or volume, is known as the units of capacity and is indicated by the manufacturer directly on each piece of glassware.

Volumetric glassware is usually calibrated by weight, using distilled water. Water is commonly used as the liquid for calibration because it is readily available and because it is similar in viscosity and speed of drainage to the solutions and reagents ordinarily used in the clinical laboratory. The units of capacity determined will therefore be the volume of water contained in, or delivered by, the glassware at a particular temperature. The manufacturer knows what the weights of various amounts of distilled water are at specific temperatures. This information is used in the manual calibration of volumetric glassware. If a manufacturer wants a volumetric flask to contain 100 mL, a sensitive balance such as an analytical balance is used. Weights corresponding to what 100 mL of distilled water weighs at a specific temperature are placed on one side of the balance. The flask to be calibrated is placed on the other side of the balance, and distilled water is gradually added to it until equilibrium is achieved. The manufacturer then makes a permanent calibration mark on the neck of the flask at the bottom of the water meniscus level. This flask is then calibrated to contain 100 mL. Other sizes and types of volumetric glassware are similarly calibrated.

The volume of a particular piece of glassware varies with the temperature. For this reason it is necessary to specify the temperature at which the glassware was calibrated. Glass will swell or shrink with changes in temperature, and the volume of the glassware will therefore vary. Most volumetric glassware for routine clinical use is calibrated at 20° C. This means that the calibration process and checking took place at a controlled temperature of 20° C. On all volumetric glassware the inscription 20° C will be seen. Although 20° C has been almost universally adopted as the standard temperature for calibration of volumetric glassware, each piece of glassware will have the temperature of calibration inscribed on it. The volume of a volumetric flask is smaller at a low temperature than at a high temperature. A 50-mL volumetric flask that was calibrated at 20° C would contain less than 50 mL at 10° C.

Since the laboratory depends to such a great extent on the quality of its glassware in order to produce reliable results, it is necessary to be certain that the glassware is of the very best quality. The glass used for volumetric glassware must meet certain standards of quality. It must be transparent and free from striations and other surface irregularities. It should have no defects that would distort the appearance of the liquid surface or portion of the calibration line seen through the glass.

The design and workmanship for volumetric glassware are also specified by the National Bureau of Standards. The shape of the glassware must permit complete emptying and thorough cleaning, and it must stand solidly on a level surface.

Plastic Ware

The clinical laboratory has benefited greatly from the introduction of plastic ware. In many cases, plastic ware designed for laboratory use has replaced glassware. Much of the laboratory ware in general use, such as beakers, graduated cylinders, reagent bottles, capillary tubing for pipettes, and test tubes, can be manufactured from plastic as well as from glass. Plastic ware is cheaper and more durable, but glassware is frequently preferred because of its chemical stability and clarity. Plastic is unbreakable, which is its greatest advantage. Plastic is preferred for certain analyses in which glass can be damaged by chemicals used in the testing. Alkaline solutions must be stored in plastic.

The disadvantages of plastic are that there is some leaching of surface-bound constituents into solutions, some permeability to water vapor, some evaporation through breathing of the plastic, and some absorption of dyes, stains, or proteins. Because evaporation is a significant factor in using plastic ware, small volumes of reagent should never be stored in oversized plastic bottles for long periods of time.

Polymerized organic monomers are used to manufacture plastics for laboratory use. The most commonly used plastics include the polyolefins (polyethylene, polypropylene), polytetrafluoroethylene (Teflon, a fluorinated hydrocarbon), polystyrene, polycarbonate, and polyvinylchloride. These plastics are relatively chemically inert and as a group are unaffected by acids, alkalis, salt solutions, and most aqueous solutions. Most disposable plastic ware is made from polyethylene; it is very resistant to high temperatures, but can absorb some pigments and become discolored. Polyvinylchlorides are soft and flexible and are used to manufacture tubing. Some of the plastics can be autoclaved—Teflon, polycarbonate, and some of the polyolefin plastics. Polycarbonate plastic ware is clear and is ideal for graduated cylinders. Teflon is useful because it is almost totally chemically inert and is also resistant to a wide range of temperatures. Polyolefins are useful, in general, for their strength and their resistance to high temperatures. Specific physical properties for each type of plastic ware can be obtained from the manufacturer of the product. Materials used should be tested under the conditions present in the individual laboratory setting.

Automatic Measuring Devices
Automatic Pipettes

Automatic and semiautomatic pipettes are useful in many areas of laboratory work. Several different types are available, and each must be carefully calibrated before use. The problems encountered with automatic pipetting depend to a large degree on the nature of the solution to be pipetted. Some reagents cause more bubbles than others, and some are more viscous. Bubbles and viscous solutions can cause problems with measurement and delivery of samples and solutions.

Automatic pipetting devices permit rapid, repetitive measurement and delivery of predefined volumes of reagent or sample. With the use of these devices, efficient delivery of equal volumes of specific liquids is ensured. Specimens can be measured efficiently, followed by the addition of the necessary reagents or diluents. Some devices can measure the sample and then follow with a diluting reagent dispensed with the same apparatus. Other devices have tip-ejector capabilities, variable digital settings, or repetitive dispensing capabilities for added convenience. The capillary tips into which the sample is drawn can be made from glass or plastic. These are usually disposable. This eliminates cleaning and promotes proper discard techniques for infection control. Proper care, calibration, and maintenance are necessary to ensure precise, accurate sampling when these automatic pipetting devices are used. It is important to read and follow the manufacturer's instructions for each device (see also under Automatic Micropipettors in this chapter).

Automatic Dispensers or Syringes

Many types of automatic dispensers or syringes are used in the laboratory for repetitive adding of multiple doses of the same reagent or diluent. These devices are used for measuring serial amounts of relatively small volumes of the same liquid. The volume to be dispensed is determined by the pipettor setting. Dispensers are available with varieties of volume settings. Some are available as syringes and others as bottle top devices. Most of these dispensers can be cleaned by autoclaving.

Diluter-Dispensers

In automated instruments, diluter-dispensers are used to prepare a number of different samples for analysis. These devices pipette a selected aliquot of sample and diluent into the instrument or receiving vessel. These devices are mostly of the dual-piston type, one being used for the sample and the other for the diluent or reagent.

Cleaning Laboratory Glassware and Plastic Ware

Among the many factors that ensure accurate results in laboratory determinations is the use of clean, unbroken glassware. There is no point in exercising care in obtaining specimens, handling the specimens, and making the laboratory determination if the laboratory ware used is not extremely clean. Plastic ware must also be clean.

There are various methods of cleaning glassware, the one chosen depending on the glassware's use. In all cases, glassware for the clinical laboratory must be physically clean, in most cases it must be chemically clean, and in some cases it must be bacteriologically clean, or sterile.

Laboratory ware that cannot be cleaned immediately after use should be rinsed with tap water and left to soak in a basin or pail of water to which a small amount of detergent has been added. Never allow dirty glassware or plastic ware to dry out. Once dried out on the surface, it is difficult to remove most soil by ordinary means. For this reason it is important to have a soaking bucket available in the working area. Glassware that is new is often slightly alkaline and should be soaked for several hours in a dilute hydrochloric acid or nitric acid solution (about 1 mL/dL is satisfactory). This glassware should then be washed in the usual manner.

Glassware that is contaminated, as by use with patient specimens, must be decontaminated before it is washed. This can be done by presoaking in 5% bleach, or by boiling, autoclaving, or some similar procedure.

General cleaning methods involve the use of a soap, detergent, or cleaning powder. In most laboratories, detergents are used. If the dirty glassware has been soaking in a solution of the detergent water, the cleaning job will be much easier.

General Cleaning Procedure

There are various methods of cleaning laboratory ware. Most glassware and plastic ware (with the exception of pipettes) can be cleaned manually as described in Procedure 4-1.

Cleaning Plastic Ware

Most plastic ware can be cleaned in the same manner as glassware and using ordinary glassware washing machines, but the use of any abrasive cleaning materials should be avoided.

Plastic ware should be well cleaned and rinsed with deionized water prior to any necessary autoclaving, since some chemical reactions can occur at autoclaving temperatures that do not occur when the plastics are at room temperature. These reactions can cause deterioration of the plastic.

Some of the transparent plastics, such as polystyrene or polycarbonate, may absorb small quantities of water vapor during autoclaving and appear cloudy. This clouding effect will disappear as the plastic dries, and the plastic

---

PROCEDURE 4-1

Cleaning Glassware (Manual Method)

1. Put the specified amount of detergent into a dishpan or washing bucket containing moderately hot water. Allow the detergent to dissolve thoroughly.

2. Rinse glassware (or other items that can be washed) in tap water before placing it in the detergent solution. Never allow dirty glassware to dry out; always place it in a soaking bucket. Glassware should be completely submerged in the bucket or pan. Fill large pieces with detergent water and set aside to soak. Soaking glassware for at least 1 hour before washing makes the washing procedure much more efficient.

3. Using a cleaning brush, thoroughly scrub the glassware, being certain to clean all parts. Brushes of various sizes should be available to fit the different-sized test tubes, flasks, funnels, and bottles. Excessive brushing and improper use of brushes may cause scratching of the glassware. Avoid the use of abrasive cleaners on glassware.

4. Rinse glassware under running tap water; allow the water to run into each piece of glassware, pour it out, and repeat several times (seven to ten times is sufficient). Rinse the outside of the glassware, too. It is especially important to remove all the detergent from the glassware before use; if detergent remains, the alkali in it may interfere with laboratory determinations.

5. After thoroughly rinsing the glassware with tap water, rinse it with deionized water (type I or II) three to five times. Certain glassware used for microbiologic studies requires even longer rinsing with deionized water. Use deionized water (or distilled water in some instances) in the final rinsing of all laboratory glassware.

6. Glassware may be dried in a hot oven (no hotter than 100° C) or at room temperature. If a higher temperature is used, the glassware can become distorted. Always dry glassware or other equipment in an inverted position to ensure complete drainage of water as it dries. Never dry laboratory ware with a towel. Do not dry plastic ware or rubber items in an oven.

7. Check the glassware for cleanliness by observing the water drainage. Chemically clean glassware will drain uniformly; dirty glassware will leave water droplets adhering to the walls of the glass.

---

becomes transparent again. Drying the plastic ware in a 110° C oven can enhance the clearing effect.

Cleaning Pipettes

Nondisposable pipettes used in the laboratory are cleaned in a special way. Immediately after use, the pipettes should be placed in a special pipette container or cylinder containing water; the water should be high enough to completely cover the pipettes. Pipettes should be placed in the container carefully with the tip up to avoid breakage. When the pipettes are to be cleaned, they are removed from the cylinder and placed in another cylinder containing a cleaning solution. This cleaning solution can be a detergent or a commercial analytical cleaning product. The pipettes are allowed to soak in the cleaning solution for 30 minutes.

The next step involves thorough rinsing of the pipettes. This can be accomplished by hand, but more often it is done with the aid of an automatic pipette washer. The pipettes are rinsed with tap water, by use of the automatic pipette washer, for 1 to 2 hours. They are then rinsed in deionized or distilled water two or three times and dried in a hot oven.

Cleaning Photometry Cuvettes

Cuvettes must be scrupulously clean and free from grease smudges or scratches. If nondisposable cuvettes are used, they should be rinsed with tap water, filled with a mild detergent solution, and placed in a rubberized test tube rack as soon as possible after use. It is best not to put them into a regular dishwashing bucket, where they would rub against one another and be scratched. After standing with the detergent solution, the cuvettes are rinsed several times with tap water and two or three times with distilled or deionized water. When cuvettes are dried, high temperatures and unclean air should be avoided. A low to medium oven (not above 100° C) can be used for rapid drying. In some laboratories, there are special dishwashing machines that can adequately handle cuvettes.

Glass Breakage

It is important in the clinical laboratory to check all glassware periodically to determine its condition. No broken or chipped glassware should be used. Many laboratory accidents are caused by the use of broken glassware. Serious cuts may result, and infections may set in.

Each time a laboratory procedure is carried out, the glassware used should be checked; equipment such as beakers, pipettes, test tubes, and flasks should not have broken edges or cracks. To prevent breakage, glassware should be handled carefully; carrying too much glassware at one time from one place to another in the laboratory is to be avoided.

▌LABORATORY REAGENT WATER

The quality of water used in the laboratory is very important. Its use in reagent and solution preparation, reconstitution of lyophilized mate-

rials, and dilution of samples demands specific requirements for its level of purity. All water used in the clinical laboratory should be free from substances that could interfere with the tests being performed. It is important that the persons involved in doing the analyses understand the reasons for the special emphasis placed on the kinds of water used and the difficulties involved in obtaining and maintaining a pure reagent water supply. Significant error can be introduced into a laboratory assay if inorganic or organic impurities in the water supply have not been removed prior to analysis.

Levels of Water Purity

Three levels of laboratory water quality have been recommended by the National Committee for Clinical Laboratory Standards and the College of American Pathologists: type I, type II, and type III.[1,5]

Type I Reagent Water

This type of reagent water is the most pure and should be used for procedures that require maximum water purity. For preparation of standard solutions, buffers, and controls, in quantitative analytic procedures (especially when nanograms or subnanogram measurements are required), in electrophoresis, in toxicology screening tests, and in high-performance liquid chromatography, type I reagent water must be used.

Type II Reagent Water

For qualitative chemistry procedures and for most procedures carried out in hematology, immunology, microbiology, and other clinical test areas, type II water is suitable. Type II water can be used when the presence of bacteria can be tolerated.

Type III Reagent Water

This type of water can be used for some qualitative laboratory tests, such as those done in general urinalysis. Type III water can be used as a water source for preparation of type I or type II water and for washing and rinsing laboratory glassware. Any glassware should be given a final rinse with either type I or type II water, depending on the intended use for the glassware.

Criteria for Water Purity

The presence of ionizable contaminants in distilled or deionized water is most easily determined by measuring the conductance, or electrical resistance, of the water. This is the basis for having purity meters or conductivity warning lights on distillation and deionization apparatus.

There are several ways to test for water purity. With regard to the presence of inorganic ionized materials, as the purity of the water increases, the amount of dissolved ionized substances decreases and the ability of the water to conduct an electrical current decreases. This principle is used in commercially available resistance test analyzers for water purity. As the ability of the water to conduct an electrical current decreases, the resistance increases.

Water of the highest purity will vary with the method of preparation and may be referred to as nitrogen-free water, double-distilled water, or conductivity water, depending on the actual method used. However, a measure of conductance does not consider the presence of nonionized substances (organic contaminants) such as dissolved gases. Especially important in the clinical laboratory is dissolved carbon dioxide. Water free of such dissolved gases may be obtained by boiling it immediately before use and is often referred to as gas-free, or carbon dioxide–free, water. Such water may be necessary for the preparation of strongly alkaline solutions. Another contaminant of water may be substances dissolved from the storage container.

Accreditation or certification requirements for clinical laboratories, set up by state and federal agencies, have resulted in specific, well-defined criteria for water purity. The classification of and specifications for water purity are designed to enable laboratory personnel to specify the quality of the water needed for particular laboratory analyses and reagent preparation, for example. Each test performed in the laboratory must be

evaluated as to the type of water needed, to avoid potential interference with specificity, accuracy, and precision. It is well known, for example, that water contaminated with metal, when used in analyses of enzymes, can have a dramatic effect on the values obtained.

Storage of Reagent Water

It is important to store reagent water appropriately. Type I water must be used immediately after its production, to prevent carbon dioxide from being absorbed into it. There are no specified storage guidelines for Type I water, because it is not possible to maintain its high level of purity for any length of time. Types II and III water can be stored in borosilicate glass or polyethylene bottles but should be used as soon as possible to prevent contamination with airborne microbes. Containers should be tightly stoppered to prevent absorption of gases. It is also important to keep the delivery system for the water protected from chemical or microbiologic contamination.

Methods of Purifying Water

The original source of water varies greatly with the health care facility. Water originating from rivers, lakes, springs, or wells contains a variety of inorganic, organic, and microbiologic contaminants. No single purification system can remove all the contaminants. For this reason, a variety of methods, in differing combinations, are used to obtain the particular types of water used in a single laboratory facility. Two general methods are employed to prepare water for laboratory use: deionization and distillation. Sometimes it is necessary to further treat distilled water with a deionization process to obtain water with the degree of purity needed.

Deionized Water

In the process of **deionization**, water is passed through a resin column containing positively (+) and negatively (−) charged particles. These particles combine with ions present in the water to remove them—this water is known as **deionized** water. Therefore, only substances that can ionize will be removed in the process of deionization; organic substances and other substances that do not ionize are not removed. Further treatment with membrane filtration and activated charcoal is necessary to remove organic impurities, particulate matter, and microorganisms to produce Type I water from deionized water.

Distilled Water

In the process of distillation, water is boiled, and the resulting steam is cooled; condensed steam is distilled water. Many minerals are found in natural water. Among those commonly found are iron, magnesium, and calcium. Water from which these minerals and others have been removed by distillation is known as **distilled water**. The process of distillation also removes microbiologic organisms, but volatile impurities such as carbon dioxide, chlorine, and ammonia are not removed. Water that has been distilled meets the specifications for type II and type III water.

Double-Distilled Water. Distilled or deionized water is not necessarily pure water. There may be contamination by dissolved gases, by nonvolatile substances carried over by steam in the distillation process, or by dissolved substances from storage containers. For example, in tests for nitrogen compounds (such as urea nitrogen, a common clinical chemistry determination) it is important to use ammonia-free (nitrogen-free) water. This may be specially purchased by the laboratory for such determinations or prepared in the laboratory by a specific method, double distillation, to remove the contaminating ammonia.

Combinations of Deionization and Distillation

Water of higher purity is also produced by special distillation units in which the water is first deionized and then distilled; this eliminates the need for double distillation. Other systems may first distill the water, then deionize it.

Reverse Osmosis

The process of reverse osmosis passes water under pressure through a semipermeable membrane made of cellulose acetate, or other materials. This treatment removes approximately 90% of dissolved solids, 98% of organic impurities, insoluble matter, and microbiologic organisms. It does not remove dissolved gases and only about 10% of ionized particles.

Other Processes of Purification

Filtration of water through semipermeable membranes will remove insoluble matter, pyrogens, and microorganisms if the pore size of the membrane is small enough. Adsorption by activated charcoal, clays, silicates, or metal oxides can remove organic matter. Type I water can be processed through a combination of deionization, filtration, and adsorption.

Tap Water

Rarely is tap water used in the clinical laboratory, the exception being for the initial cleaning of laboratory glassware. Plain tap water is not used in any laboratory analyses or in the preparation of any reagents.

REAGENTS USED IN LABORATORY ASSAYS

The validity of the laboratory data obtained by analysis of patient specimens is dependent on the use of specific laboratory measuring apparatus and also on the use of specific reagents and materials or products devised for that apparatus. Analytic procedures require the use of properly prepared solutions or reagents. The accuracy of the determinations depends to a large extent on the accuracy of the reagents used.

A **reagent** is defined as any substance employed to produce a chemical reaction. In preparing reagents, instructions should be followed exactly. Often certain reagents will be purchased in a fully prepared state; in this case it is important that they be obtained only from reputable chemical companies. When preprepared reagents are used, manufacturers' instructions must always be followed. When a reagent is prepared, the set of instructions or directions provided for the preparation of the reagent must be followed explicitly.

Reagent Preparation

Instructions for preparing a reagent resemble a cooking recipe in that they tell what quantities of ingredients to mix together. They tell the names of the chemicals needed, the number of grams or milligrams needed, and the total volume to which the particular reagent should be diluted. The solvent most commonly used for dilution is deionized or distilled water.

Measurement of Mass and Volume

To prepare reagents, either measurement of mass by use of a balance for weighing or reconstitution of a freeze-dried or otherwise concentrated reagent product is necessary.

Preparation of reagents in the traditional way involves the use of a balance (the analytical, triple-beam, or torsion balance, for example) and other special volumetric measuring devices (such as volumetric flasks and graduated cylinders). The types of volumetric glassware available are discussed under Laboratory Glassware and Plastic Ware.

Since chemicals are used in the preparation of reagents and the accuracy of laboratory determinations depends on the quality of the reagents employed, it is essential that only chemicals from reliable manufacturers be used.

Concentrations of Solutions

Using solutions of the correct concentrations is of the greatest importance in attaining good results in the laboratory. Quantitative transfer, along with accurate initial measurement of a chemical, helps to ensure that a solution will be of the correct concentration.

The **concentration of a solution** may be expressed in different ways. With the use of SI units, traditional expression of concentration in terms of mass of solute per volume of solution

has been replaced by the use of moles of solute per volume of solution for analyte analyses whenever possible, and the use of the liter as the reference value.

In the clinical chemistry laboratory, where the vast majority of the total laboratory analyses are performed, most measurements are concerned with the concentrations of substances in solutions. The solution is usually blood, serum, urine, cerebrospinal fluid, or other body fluid, and the substance to be measured is dissolved in the solution. This substance is known as the **solute**. Therefore, the substances being measured in the analyses (whether they are organic or inorganic, or of high or low molecular weight) are solutes. The substance in which the solute is dissolved is known as the **solvent**.

When a reagent is being prepared, and the solution is being diluted with water, its volume is increased and its concentration decreased, but the amount of solute remains unchanged.

Laboratory Chemicals

A chemical is a substance that occurs naturally or is obtained through a chemical process; it is used to produce a chemical effect or reaction. Chemicals are produced in various purities or grades.

Standards of Purity. There are many **grades of chemicals** available, and it is essential to understand which grade or type should be used for which reagent.

When quantitative determinations are to be performed and accurate standard solutions prepared, it is necessary to use pure chemicals. In such cases, the more costly, reagent-grade chemicals are necessary for accuracy. Different companies have their own descriptions for the various degrees of purity, and there is no official designation. The label on the bottle and the supplier's catalog may give important information, such as the maximum limits of impurities or an actual analysis of the chemical. Directions for reagent preparation usually specify the grade, and in many instances state the particular brand of chemical. These directions must be followed to ensure reliable results.

The purity of organic chemicals is generally inferior to that of inorganic chemicals. This is due both to the manner in which they are prepared or synthesized and to changes that occur as they stand or are stored.

Grades of Chemicals. The following is a general description of the various grades of chemicals available for the clinical laboratory.

1. Reagent grade or analytic reagent (AR) grade. These chemicals are of a high degree of purity and are used often in the preparation of reagents in the clinical laboratory. The American Chemical Society has developed specifications for many reagent-grade or AR chemicals, and those that meet their standards are designated by the letters ACS.
2. Chemically pure (CP) grade. These chemicals are sufficiently pure to be used in many analyses in the clinical laboratory. However, the designation does not reveal the limits of impurities that are tolerated, and so they may not be acceptable for research and various clinical laboratory techniques unless they have been specifically analyzed for the desired procedure. It may be necessary to use this grade when higher-purity biochemicals are not available.
3. USP and NF grade. These reagents meet the specifications stated in the *United States Pharmacopeia (USP)* or the *National Formulary (NF)*. They are generally less pure than CP grade, as the tolerances specified are such that they are not injurious to health rather than chemically pure.
4. Purified, practical, or pure grade. These chemicals may be used as starting materials for synthesis of chemicals of greater purity but generally should not be used in the clinical laboratory.
5. Technical or commercial grade. These chemicals are used only for industrial purposes and are generally not used in the preparation of reagents for the clinical laboratory.
6. National Bureau of Standards, the College of American Pathologists (CAP), and the National Committee for Clinical Laboratory Standards (NCCLS).[3] These agencies or bureaus all supply certified clinical laboratory standards. The highest grade or purest chemicals are available from the National Bureau of Standards. However, very few such compounds are available to the clinical laboratory, and they are known as standards, clinical type.

Physical Forms of Chemicals. Chemicals used in the laboratory have various physical forms. Persons using these chemicals must know the various forms and which form should be used in the preparation of a specific reagent. Some of the common forms are lumps, sticks, pellets, granules, fine granules, crystalline powder, crystals, fine crystals, powder, and liquid. There are some special forms, such as chips, scales, and flakes, but these are not frequently used in reagent preparation.

Hazardous Chemicals Communication Policies. Information and training regarding hazardous chemicals must be provided to all persons working with them in the clinical laboratory. The Occupational Safety and Health Administration (OSHA) regulations ensure that all sites where hazardous chemicals are used comply with the necessary safety precautions. Any information about signs and symptoms associated with exposures to hazardous chemicals used in the laboratory must be communicated to all persons. Reference materials about the individual chemicals are provided by all chemical manufacturers and suppliers by means of the **material safety data sheet (MSDS)**. This information accompanies the shipment of all hazardous chemicals and should be available in the laboratory for anyone to review. The MSDS contains information about possible hazards, safe handling, storage, and disposal of the particular chemical it accompanies (see Chemical Hazards in Chapter 2).

Storage of Chemicals. It is important that chemicals kept in the laboratory be stored properly, as described in Chapter 2. Chemicals that require refrigeration should be refrigerated immediately. Solids should be kept in a cool, dry place. Acids and bases should be stored separately and in well-ventilated storage units. Flammable solvents (e.g., alcohol, chloroform) should be stored in specially constructed well-ventilated storage units with appropriate labeling in accordance with OSHA regulations. Flammable solvents such as acetone and ether should always be stored in special safety cans or other appropriate storage devices in appropriate storage units. Fuming and volatile chemicals, such as solvents, strong acids, and strong bases, should be opened, and reagent preparation resulting in fumes should be done, only under a fume hood so that the vapors will not escape into the room. Chemicals that absorb water should be weighed only after desiccation or drying in a hot oven; otherwise the weights will not be accurate.

It is very important that the label on a chemical be read for instructions about storage details. Most chemicals are stable at room temperature without desiccation. Some must be stored at refrigeration temperature, some must be frozen, and some that are light sensitive must be stored in brown bottles.

Chemicals Used to Prepare Standard Solutions. Chemicals used to prepare **standard solutions** are the most highly purified types of chemicals available. The group includes primary, reference, and certified standards. Primary standards meet specifications set by the Committee on Analytical Reagents of the American Chemical Society. Each lot of these chemicals is assayed, and the chemicals must be stable substances of definite composition. Reference standards are chemicals whose purity has been ensured by the National Bureau of Standards list of standard reference materials (SRM). Certified standards are also available.[3] For example, the CAP certifies bilirubin and cyanmethemoglobin standards, and the NCCLS certifies a standardized protein solution.

Quantitative Transfer and Dilution of Chemicals for Reagents

In preparing any solution in the clinical laboratory, it is necessary to utilize the practice known as quantitative transfer (Procedure 4-2). It is essential that the entire amount of the weighed or measured substance be used in preparing the solution. In **quantitative transfer**, the entire amount of the measured substance is transferred from one vessel to another for dilution. The usual practice in preparing most laboratory reagents is to weigh the chemical in a beaker (or other suitable vessel, such as a disposable weighing boat) and quantitatively transfer the chemical to a volumetric flask for dilution with deionized or distilled water. The volumetric flask chosen must be of the correct size; that is, it must hold the amount of solution that is desired for the total volume of the reagent being prepared.

The most common amount of solution prepared at one time is 1 L. If 1 L of reagent is needed, the measured chemical must be transferred quantitatively to a 1-L volumetric flask and diluted to the calibration mark with deionized water or the required solvent. The method of quantitative transfer requires a great deal of care and accuracy.

Dissolving the Chemical into Solution. There are several methods by which the dissolution of solid materials can be hastened. Heating usually increases the solubility of a chemical, and heat also causes the fluid to move (the currents help in dissolving). Even mild heat, however, will decompose some chemicals, and therefore heat must be used with caution. Agitation by a stirring rod or swirling by means of a mechanical shaker increases solubility by removing the saturated solution from contact with the chemical. Rapid addition of the solvent is another means

PROCEDURE 4-2

Quantitative Transfer

1. Place a clean, dry funnel in the mouth of the volumetric flask.

2. Carefully transfer the chemical in the measuring vessel into the funnel.

3. Wash the chemical into the flask with small amounts of deionized water or the required solvent for the reagent.

4. Rinse the measuring vessel (beaker) three to five times with small portions of deionized water or the required solvent until all of the chemical has been transferred from the vessel into the volumetric flask (add each rinsing to the flask).

5. Rinse the funnel with deionized water or the required solvent, and remove the funnel from the volumetric flask.

6. Dissolve the chemical in the flask by swirling or shaking it. Some chemicals are more difficult to dissolve than others. On occasion, more special attention must be given to the problem of dissolving the chemical.

7. Add deionized water or the required solvent to about 0.5 in. below the calibration line on the flask, allow a few seconds for drainage of fluid above the calibration line, and then carefully add deionized water or the required solvent to the calibration line (the bottom of the meniscus must be exactly on the calibration mark).

8. Stopper the flask with a ground-glass stopper, and mix well by inverting at least 20 times.

9. Rinse a properly labeled reagent bottle with a small amount of the mixed reagent in the volumetric flask. Transfer the prepared reagent to the labeled reagent bottle for storage.

---

of hastening the solution of solid materials. Some chemicals tend to cake and form aggregates as soon as the solvent is added. By adding the solvent quickly and keeping the solids in motion, aggregation may be prevented. Since the flask is calibrated at 20° C, the solution must be returned to room temperature before final volume adjustment is made.

Labeling the Reagent Container

Containers for storage of reagents (usually reagent bottles) should be labeled before the material is added. A reagent should never be placed in an unlabeled bottle or container. If an unlabeled container is found, the reagent in it must be discarded. Proper labeling of reagent bottles is of the greatest importance. All labels should include the name and concentration of the reagent,

Test Used For	✔O.K.
Name of Reagent	
Date Prepared	Initial of Maker

FIG 4-3. Sample label.

the date on which the reagent was prepared, and the initials of the person who made the reagent (Fig. 4-3).

Checking the Reagent Before Use

After the prepared reagent is in the reagent bottle, it must be checked by some means before it is put into actual use in any procedure. This can be done in one of several ways, depending on the reagent itself. After the reagent has been checked, this is noted on the label, and the solution can then be put into active use in the laboratory.

Ready-Made Reagents

In many laboratories, ready-made reagents are used, especially where large automated instruments are utilized. The manufacturers of these instruments usually provide the necessary specific reagents for use with their instruments. These reagents must be handled with extreme care and always must be used according to the manufacturers' directions.

Immunoreagents

Special commercial reagent kits are commonly used for clinical immunology and radioimmunoassay tests. A typical test kit will contain all necessary reagents, including standards, labeled antigen, and antibody, plus any other associated reagents needed. The laboratory must maintain strict evaluation policies for these kits, to ensure their reliability. The disadvantage of these kits is that the laboratory is dependent on the supplier to produce and maintain components, which must meet the necessary standards. Each new kit must be evaluated by the laboratory according to a strict protocol, and then a periodic monitoring program must be maintained to ensure the reliability of the results produced.

MEASUREMENT OF MASS: WEIGHING AND THE USE OF BALANCES

General Use of Balances

Probably some of the most important measurement devices are the various types of balances used in the **measurement of mass or weight** (**gravimetric analysis**) in preparing the reagents and standard solutions used in the laboratory. This is one method of **quantitative analysis** in the clinical laboratory. Almost every procedure performed in the laboratory depends to some extent on the use of a balance. Laboratory balances function by either mechanical or electronic means.

In the traditional clinical laboratory, gravimetric analysis (analysis by measurement of mass or weight) is used in the preparation of some reagents and standard solutions. Most procedures depend on the use of an accurately prepared standard solution. In many laboratories today, however, reagents, standard solutions, and control solutions are purchased ready to use, and the actual laboratory preparation of these reagents and solutions is not done. Since measurement of mass remains fundamental to all analyses, the technique of weighing should continue to be fundamental to the base of knowledge for all persons working in a clinical laboratory. Even with the use of purchased laboratory solutions, it is likely that a balance will be needed for preparing reagents or standards for certain laboratory determinations. Because of the added cost of purchasing prepared standards, some laboratories routinely prepare their own standard solutions. Another use for weighing is the calibration of volumetric equipment. The measurement of mass continues to be the quantitative means by which this equipment is calibrated.

Some solutions require more accurately weighed chemicals than others. The accuracy needed depends on what the solution is to be used for. One must decide what type of balance (or scale) is most appropriate for the precision or reproducibility required in weighing the chemicals to be used for a particular solution. The different kinds of balances are suited to particular needs. A balance that sacrifices precision for speed should not be used when precision is needed.

Types of Balances Used in the Laboratory

The balance considered to be the backbone of the clinical laboratory, especially clinical chemistry, is the analytical balance. This balance and other types—namely, the triple-beam balance, the Cent-O-Gram, and the torsion balance—are discussed in this section. A single laboratory is likely to have all of these types, and for this reason persons working in a laboratory should understand how the various balances are used.

Every laboratory should have some type of analytical balance and at least one other, less sensitive type of balance. These are the minimum requirements for weighing devices.

Analytical Balance

Many different types of analytical balances are made by different companies, and they have various degrees of automatic operation. In this discussion, analytical balances are divided into two types: manually operated (mechanical) analytical (Fig. 4-4) and automatic or electronic analytical (Fig. 4-5) balances. Each company that manufactures analytical balances has its own trade name for each of the analytical balances produced. Some of the fine analytical balances used in the clinical laboratory are the Ainsworth, Voland, Christian-Becker, Mettler, Ohaus, and Sartorius balances. Others are also available. It is important to investigate carefully several different analytical balances before deciding on one for use in a particular laboratory.

General Principles of Analytical Balances. The basic principle in the quantitative measurement of mass is to balance an unknown mass

(the substance being weighed) with a known mass. The **analytical balance** uses the basic concept of a simple lever or beam that pivots on a knife-edge fulcrum placed at the center of gravity of the lever. By use of this principle, balances are designed in different ways.

In the traditional mechanical analytical balance, two pans of equal mass are suspended from the ends of the lever or beam and calibrated weights are placed on one pan to counterbalance an object of unknown mass on the other pan. A rider or chain weight device is utilized for fractional weights.

The electronic analytical balance is a single-pan balance that uses an electromagnetic force to counterbalance the load placed on the pan. This pan is mechanically connected to a coil that is suspended in the field of a permanent cylindrical electromagnet. When a load is placed on the pan, a force is produced that displaces the coil within the magnetic field. A photoelectric cell scanning device changes position and generates a current just sufficient to return the coil to its original position; this is called electromagnetic force compensation. This current is proportional to the weight of the load on the pan and is dis-

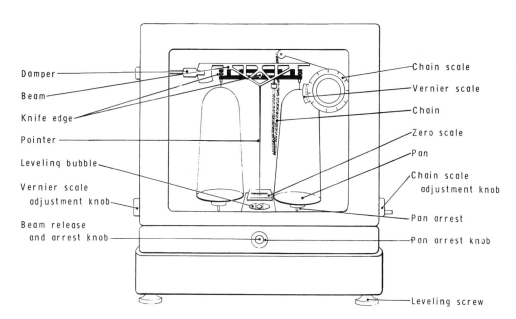

Damper — Beam — Knife edge — Pointer — Leveling bubble — Vernier scale adjustment knob — Beam release and arrest knob

Chain scale — Vernier scale — Chain — Zero scale — Pan — Chain scale adjustment knob — Pan arrest — Pan arrest knob

Leveling screw

FIG 4-4. Manual (mechanical) analytical balance.

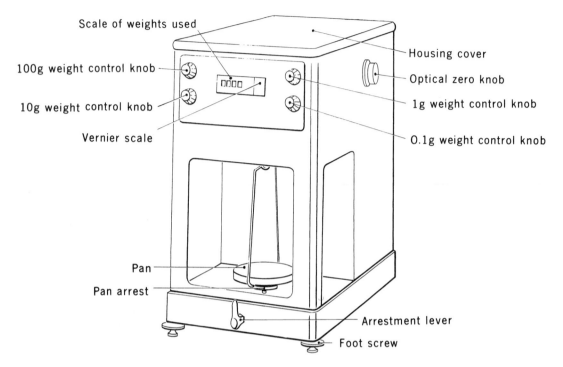

FIG 4-5. Electronic analytical balance.

played for the person using the balance to see visually, or it can be interfaced with a data output device. The greater the mass placed on the pan, the greater the deflecting force and the stronger the compensating current required to return the coil to its original position. There is a direct linear relationship between the compensation current and the force produced by the load placed on the pan. Electronic balances permit fast, accurate weighings, with a high degree of resolution. They are easy to use and have replaced the traditional mechanically operated analytical balance in most clinical laboratories.

Uses for the Analytical Balance. All analytical balances are used to weigh very small amounts of substances with a high degree of accuracy, but how this is accomplished differs slightly from one balance to another. Some require little or no manual operation, and some are more time consuming and require much more manipulation on the part of the operator.

Almost every procedure performed in the traditional clinical laboratory depends on the use of balances, the most important one being the analytical balance. Before any procedure is started, reagents and standard solutions are prepared. Standard solutions are always very accurately prepared, and the analytical balance is used to weigh the chemicals for these solutions. The analytical balance might be called the starting point of each method used in the laboratory. Its accuracy determines the accuracy of many clinical determinations. An instrument that is so sensitive and so essential must be made with great skill and treated very carefully by those using it.

The analytical balance should be cleaned and adjusted at least once a year to ensure its continued accuracy and sensitivity. Its accuracy is what makes this instrument so essential in the clinical laboratory. The accuracy to which most analytical balances used in the clinical laboratory should weigh chemicals is commonly 0.1 mg, or 0.0001 g. Whenever this accuracy is needed, the analytical balance must be used. Differences between electronic and manual analytical balances lie mainly in the manner in which the weights are added in the weighing procedure. With the manual balance the weights are physically placed on one of the balance pans by the user. With the electronic balance the weights are added by manipulating a series of dials.

General Rules for Weighing With an Analytical Balance. Weighing errors will occur if the balance is not properly positioned. It is therefore very important that the balance be located and mounted in an optimal position. The balance must be level. This is usually accomplished by adjusting the movable screws on the legs of the balance. The firmness of support is also important. The bench or table on which the balance rests must be rigid and free from vibrations. Preferably the room in which the balance is set up should have constant temperature and humidity. Ideally, the analytical balance should be in an air-conditioned room. The temperature factor is most important. The balance should not be placed near hot objects such as radiators, flames, stills, or electric ovens. Likewise, it should not be placed near cold objects, especially not near an open window. Sunlight or illumination from high-power lamps should be avoided in choosing a good location for the analytical balance.

The analytical balance is a delicate precision instrument, which will not function properly if abused. When learning to use an analytical balance, one should be responsible for knowing and adhering to the rules for the use of that particular balance. The following general rules apply:

1. Set up the balance where it will be free from vibration.
2. Load and unload the balance only when the pans are arrested; if the pans are not arrested, the delicate knife edges can be damaged.
3. Close the balance case before observing the reading; any air currents present will affect the weighing process.

4. Never weigh any chemical directly on the pan; a container of some type must be used for the chemical.
5. Never place a hot object on the balance pan. If an object is warm, the weight determined will be too little because of convection currents set up by the rising heated air.
6. Whenever the shape of the object to be weighed permits, handle it with tongs or forceps. Round objects such as weighing bottles may be handled with the fingers, but take care to prevent weight changes caused by moisture from the hand. Do not hold any object longer than necessary.
7. On completion of weighing, remove all objects and clean up any chemical spilled on the pans or within the balance area. Close the balance case.
8. Weighed materials should be transferred to labeled containers or made into solutions immediately.

Speed in weighing is obtained only through practice (Procedure 4-3).

Basic Parts of the Analytical Balance. It is essential that the parts of the analytical balance be thoroughly understood, so that the weighing process can be carried out to the degree of accuracy necessary. Once the correct use of an analytical balance has been mastered, one should be able to use any of the available types, as they all have the same basic parts. Each manufacturer supplies a complete manual of operating directions, as well as information on the general use and care of the balance, with each balance purchased. These directions should be followed. The following parts are common to most analytical balances, electronic or mechanical (manually operated):

1. *Glass enclosure.* The analytical balance is enclosed in glass to prevent currents of air and collection of dust from disturbing the process of weighing.
2. *Balancing screws.* Before any weighing is done on the balance, it must be properly leveled. This is done by observing the lev-

PROCEDURE 4-3

Weighing With an Electronic Analytical Balance

1. Before doing any weighing, make certain that the balance is properly leveled. Observe the spirit level (leveling bubble), and adjust the leveling screws on the legs of the balance if necessary.

2. To check the zero point adjustment, fully release the balance and turn the adjustment knob clockwise as far as it will go. The optical scale zero should indicate three divisions below zero on the vernier scale. Using the same adjustment knob, adjust the optical scale zero so that it aligns exactly with the zero line on the vernier scale. Arrest the balance.

3. With the balance arrested, place the weighing vessel on the pan, using tongs if possible, so that no humidity or heat is brought into the weighing chamber by the hands. Close the balance window.

4. Weigh the vessel in the following manner: Partially release the balance and turn the 100-g weight control knob clockwise. When the scale moves up, turn the knob back one step. Repeat this operation with the 10-g, 1.0-g, and 0.1-g knobs, in that order. Arrest the balance. After a short pause, release the balance, and allow the scale to come to rest. Read the result and arrest the balance. With the balance arrested, unload the pan and bring all knobs back to zero.

5. Add the weight of the sample desired to the weight of the vessel just weighed to get the total to be weighed. Set the knobs (100, 10, 1.0, and 0.1 g) to the correct total weight needed. When the 0.1-g knob has been set at its proper reading, the balance should be placed in partial release. Slowly add the chemical to the vessel until the optical scale begins to move downward. When the optical scale starts downward, fully release the beam, and continue to add the chemical until the optical scale registers the exact position desired. To obtain the reading to the nearest 0.1 mg (the sensitivity of most analytical balances), the vernier scale must be used in conjunction with the chain scale.

6. With the balance arrested, unload the pan, and bring all the knobs back to zero. Clean up any spilled chemical in the balance area.

eling bubbles, or spirit level, located near the bottom of the balance. If necessary, adjust the balancing screws located on the bottom of the balance case (usually found on each leg of the balance).

3. *Beam.* This is the structure from which the pans are suspended.

4. *Knife edges.* These support the beam at the fulcrum during weighing and give sensitivity to the balance. Knife edges are vital parts and are constructed of hard metals to give a minimum amount of friction.

5. *Pans for weighing.* In the manually operated analytical balance, there are two pans: the

weights are placed on the right-hand pan, and the object to be weighed is placed on the left-hand pan. In the electronic analytical balance, there is only one pan. The object to be weighed is placed on this pan. The pans are suspended from the ends of the beam.

6. *Weights.* In the manual balance, the weights are found in a separate weight box. These weights are never handled with the fingers but are removed from the box and placed on the balance pan by using special forceps. Mishandling of weights, either by using the fingers or by dropping, can result in an alteration of the

actual and true mass of the weight. Weights come in units ranging from 50 g to 100 mg. The values of the weights are stamped directly on top of them. In the electronic analytical balance, the weights are inside the instrument and are not seen by the operator unless there is a need to remove the casing for repair or adjustment. With the electronic analytical balance, the weights are added by manipulating specific dials calibrated for the weighing process. The built-in weights are on the same end of the beam as the sample pan and are counterbalanced by a fixed weight at the opposite end. There is always a constant load on the beam, and the projected scale has the same weight regardless of the load. The total weight of an object is registered automatically by a digital counter or in conjunction with an optical scale.

7. *Pan arrest.* This is a means of arresting the pan so that sudden movement or addition of weights or chemical will not injure the delicate knife edges. The pan arrests (usually found under the pans) can absorb any shock due to weight inequalities, so that the knife edges are not subjected to this shock. The pan must be released to swing freely during actual weighing. In the electronic analytical balance, the arresting mechanism for both the pan and the beam is operated by a single lever. Partial release or full release can be obtained, depending on how the lever is moved.

8. *Damping device.* This is necessary to arrest the swing of the beam in the shortest practical time, thus cutting down the time consumed in the weighing process.

9. *Vernier scale.* This is the small scale used to obtain precise readings to the nearest 0.1 mg. It is used in conjunction with the large reading scale to obtain the necessary readings (Fig. 4-6).

10. *Reading scale.* In the manual analytical balance, this scale is actually the reading

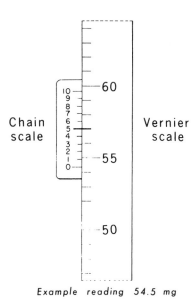

Example reading 54.5 mg

FIG 4-6. Reading obtained with a vernier scale.

scale for the chain that is used for weighing 100 mg or less. It is used in conjunction with the vernier scale to obtain readings to the nearest 0.1 mg. In the electronic analytical balance, this is usually a lighted optical scale, giving a high magnification and sharp definition for easier reading. The total weight of the object in question is registered automatically on this viewing scale.

Torsion Balance

Torsion balances are mechanical and are used mainly for weighing chemicals in the laboratory. They are sensitive, responsive instruments with an exceptionally long service life, during which there is no significant deterioration in performance. In normal use, they require very little maintenance. The unique attribute of the torsion balance movement, which is assembled as a single flexible structure by means of highly tensed torsion bands of watch-spring alloy, is that the use of knife edges, bearings, and other loose parts that would become dull, misaligned, and soiled is eliminated. Having no knife edges to dull or other loose parts to be adjusted accounts

PROCEDURE 4-4

Weighing With a Torsion Balance

1. Check to be sure that the balance is level, and adjust the leveling screws if necessary.

2. Check the zero adjustment. The optical reading scale should read zero with the pan empty and clean; adjust the optical zero with the small control knob if necessary.

3. Place the weighing vessel on the pan. Turn the weight control knob until the optical reading scale reads zero.

4. Add the chemical to the vessel until the desired weight registers on the optical scale. A vernier scale is present on most models so that the weight may be read to the accuracy needed.

5. Remove the vessel with the weighed chemical from the pan. Turn the control knob to zero, and wipe up any spilled chemical immediately.

for the popularity of the torsion balance. Little or no adjustment is required, and this is important in a laboratory, where time is important (Procedure 4-4). Most balances currently in use are a type of torsion balance.

Use and Basic Parts. The torsion balance has high sensitivity under a heavy load, permits fast weighing, and is relatively inexpensive. Care must be taken to avoid overloading these balances. Some models have a dial-controlled torque spring to eliminate the use of smaller loose weights. Other models are offered with dial-controlled built-in weights, which may further reduce the number of loose weights required. Many weighing determinations can be completed in about one-fifth the time formerly required. A sliding tare weight is provided to counterbalance the weighing vessel used. The beam is operated by a lever on the balance case. Some torsion balances are enclosed completely in glass or metal cases. Several of these balances have a damping feature, which brings the balance to equilibrium quickly. One such damping device is an oil dashpot, which is filled at the factory with silicone oil. Weighing can be done more rapidly on torsion balances with damping devices than on those lacking them.

There is usually a means by which the torsion balance can be arrested. This needs to be done only when the balance is to be moved to a new location or otherwise transported.

The sensitivity of the torsion balance varies with the model chosen. For most clinical laboratories, however, balances with a sensitivity of readings to the nearest 0.01 g are satisfactory. The manufacturer supplies a complete manual with directions for setting up, proper use, and care of the particular torsion balance. These directions should be followed closely.

Top-Loading Balance

A single-pan top-loading balance is one of the most commonly used balances in the laboratory. It is usually electronic and is self-balancing. It is much faster and easier to use than some of the balances described above. A substance can be weighed in just a few seconds. These balances are usually modified torsion or substitution balances. Top-loading balances are used when the substance being weighed does not require as much analytic precision, as when reagents of a large volume are being prepared.

Triple-Beam Balance

Another piece of laboratory apparatus used for weighing is the **triple-beam** or "trip" **balance** (Fig. 4-7). This mechanical balance is less sensitive, with an accuracy to the nearest 0.1 g. Whenever reagents are to be prepared with an

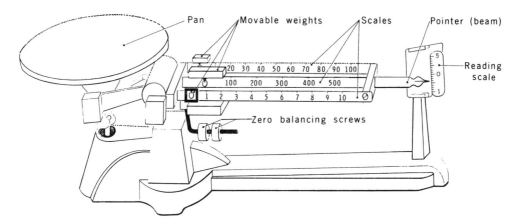

Pan   Movable weights   Scales   Pointer (beam)

Reading scale

Zero balancing screws

FIG 4-7. Triple-beam balance.

accuracy of 0.1 g or less, the triple-beam balance can be used. As the words triple-beam and trip suggest, three beams are present on the balance. Each beam provides a different weighing scale. Scales reading from 0 to 100 g, 0 to 500 g, and 0 to 10 g are usually provided on the triple-beam balance. These scales are provided with movable weights. The two larger scales have weights that lock into accurately milled notches at each calibration to ensure absolute accuracy at each position.

Some models of the triple-beam balance (called the Harvard triple-beam balance) have two pans, and some have a single pan. The principle of the weighing process is the same whether there are two pans or only one. Two-pan balances are used when two objects must be balanced against each other, as in balancing tubes for use in a centrifuge. One-pan balances are used a great deal in the laboratory for preparing reagents and chemical solutions.

On any type of triple-beam balance, the balance position of an object on the pan can be determined by observing the swing of the pointer. A swing of an equal number of divisions on either side of the zero mark on the dial indicates that the scale is balanced. It is not necessary to wait for the oscillation to stop to determine the correct weight. This observation enables the weighing process to be simple and rapid (Procedure 4-5).

Use and Basic Parts. Some type of less sensitive balance, such as the triple-beam or torsion balance, is an essential piece of equipment for every clinical laboratory, as many reagents are prepared that do not need the accuracy of the analytical balance. When an accuracy of 0.1 g or less is acceptable, the triple-beam balance can be used. It can be operated simply and rapidly and gives accurate weighings when used properly. However, even a balance with less sensitivity must be used carefully and according to the directions provided with the particular model.

The triple-beam balance should be placed on a reasonably flat and level surface. The beam should be near zero balance, with all the movable weights at their zero points. A final zero balance is attained by adjusting the balancing screws. It is advisable to check the zero balance periodically, especially if the balance has been moved. If an object is to be weighed, the balance must be set at zero before the weighing is begun. If a vessel is weighed in preparation for the addition of a chemical, it is not necessary to set the balance at the exact zero reading.

Parts basic to triple-beam balances are as follows:

1. *Pan:* where the object or weighing vessel holding the substance to be weighed is placed.

PROCEDURE 4-5

Weighing With a Triple-Beam Balance

1. Place the weighing vessel on the balance pan without previously bringing the balance to zero.

2. With the weighing vessel on the pan, bring the balance to zero by adjusting the movable weights on the three scales. Record the sum of the weights required for balance.

3. To the recorded weight add the amount of chemical to be weighed. For example, if the reagent to be prepared requires 10.5 g of NaCl and the weighing vessel weighs 35.5 g, the total weight is 46.0 g. Move the movable weights on the scales to give this total weight.

4. Gradually add the chemical until the pointer of the balance rests exactly at the zero mark on the vertical reading scale. Remove the weighing vessel, and return the movable weights to their zero positions. Transfer the chemical quantitatively to the flask for dilution.

5. Wipe up any spilled chemical immediately from the balance area.

2. *Beam:* a lever supported by a knife plane bearing at the center post. The length of beam to the right of the knife plane is graduated for placement of a sliding weight and ends in a pointer. The other end of the beam is attached to the pan guide with a knife-edge contact.

3. *Movable weights or poises:* sliding weights attached to the beam, which are moved to bring the balance into equilibrium. The trip balance has three beams, and various weight increments are added as the poises are advanced toward the pointer ends of the beams.

4. *Reading scale:* a scale located at the end of the beam pointer that shows when the balance is in equilibrium.

5. *Balancing screws or spindle:* a pair of threaded weights that are used to bring the empty balance into equilibrium.

MEASUREMENT OF VOLUME: PIPETTING AND TITRATION

Pipetting
Pipettes: An Overview and Uses

Pipettes are a type of volumetric glassware used extensively in the laboratory. Many kinds are available. Care and discretion should be used in selecting pipettes for clinical laboratory use, since their accuracy is one of the determining factors in the accuracy of the procedures carried out. A pipette is a cylindrical glass tube used in measuring fluids. It is calibrated to deliver, or transfer, a specified volume from one vessel to another.

Pipettes used in volumetric measurement in the laboratory must be free from all grease and dirt. For that reason, a special analytic cleaning solution is used. For a description of cleaning solutions, see Cleaning Laboratory Glassware and Plastic Ware.

Since the accuracy of laboratory determinations depends to such a large extent on the equipment used and since pipetting is a principal means of volume measurement, it is imperative that any pipettes used in the clinical laboratory be of the finest quality and be manufactured and calibrated by a reputable company. Care and discretion should be used in the selection of laboratory pipettes, whether manual or automatic.

Several types of pipettes are used commonly in the laboratory. It is necessary that their uses be understood and experience in how to handle them in clinical determinations be gained (see Pipettes, under Laboratory Glassware and Plas-

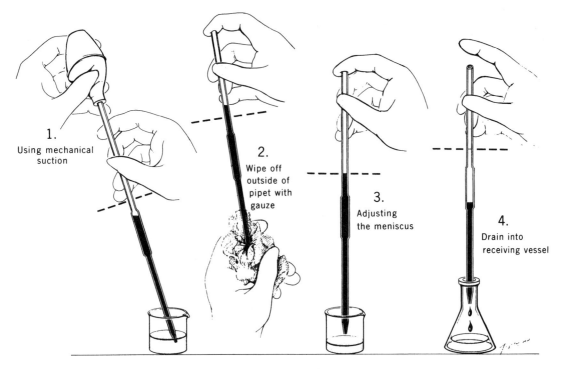

1.
Using mechanical suction

2.
Wipe off outside of pipet with gauze

3.
Adjusting the meniscus

4.
Drain into receiving vessel

FIG 4-8. Pipetting technique.

tic ware). Practice, again, is the key to success in the use of laboratory pipettes; only through practice will anyone become proficient in pipetting.

There are two categories of manual pipettes: to-contain (TC) and to-deliver (TD). TC pipettes are calibrated to contain a specified amount of liquid but are not necessarily calibrated to deliver that exact amount. A small amount of fluid will cling to the inside wall of the TC pipette, and when these pipettes are used, they should be rinsed out with a diluting fluid to ensure that the entire contents has been emptied. TD pipettes are calibrated to deliver the amount of fluid designated on the pipette; this volume will flow out of the pipette by gravity when the pipette is held in a vertical position with its tip against the inside wall of the receiving vessel. A small amount of fluid will remain in the tip of the pipette; this amount is to be left in the tip, as the calibrated portion has been delivered into the receiving vessel. There is another category of pipette, called

blowout. The calibration of these pipettes is similar to that of TD pipettes, except that the drop remaining in the tip of the pipette must be blown out into the receiving vessel. If a pipette is to be blown out, an etched ring will be seen near the suction opening (see discussions of serologic and Ostwald pipettes above). A mechanical device must be used to blow out the entire contents of the pipette.

Pipetting Technique Using Manual Pipettes

It is important to develop a good technique for handling pipettes (Fig. 4-8). It is only through practice that this is accomplished, however (Procedure 4-6). With few exceptions, the same general steps apply to pipetting with any of the manual pipettes described under Laboratory Glassware and Plastic Ware.

Laboratory accidents frequently result from improper pipetting techniques. The greatest potential hazard is when mouth pipetting is done

PROCEDURE 4-6

Pipetting With Manual Pipettes

1. Check the pipette to ascertain its correct size, being careful also to check for broken delivery or suction tips.

2. Wearing protective gloves, hold the pipette lightly between the thumb and the last three fingers, leaving the index finger free.

3. Place the tip of the pipette well below the surface of the liquid to be pipetted.

4. Using mechanical suction or an aspirator bulb, carefully draw the liquid up into the pipette until the level of liquid is well above the calibration mark.

5. Quickly cover the suction opening at the top of the pipette with the index finger.

6. Wipe the outside of the pipette dry with a piece of gauze or tissue to remove excess fluid.

7. Hold the pipette in a vertical position with the delivery tip against the inside of the original vessel. Carefully allow the liquid in the pipette to drain by gravity until the bottom of the meniscus is exactly at the calibration mark. (The meniscus is the concave or convex surface of a column of liquid as seen in a laboratory pipette, buret, or other measuring device.) To do this, do not entirely remove the index finger from the suction-hole end of the pipette, but, by rolling the finger slightly over the opening, allow a slow drainage to take place.

8. While still holding the pipette in a vertical position, touch the tip of the pipette to the inside wall of the receiving vessel. Remove the index finger from the top of the pipette to permit free drainage. Remember to keep the pipette in a vertical position for correct drainage. In TD pipettes, a small amount of fluid will remain in the delivery tip.

9. To be certain that the drainage is as complete as possible, touch the delivery tip of the pipette to another area on the inside wall of the receiving vessel.

10. Remove the pipette from the receiving vessel, and place it in the appropriate place for washing (see under Cleaning Laboratory Glassware and Plastic Ware).

instead of mechanical suction. Mouth pipetting is never acceptable in the clinical laboratory. Caustic reagents, contaminated specimens, and poisonous solutions are all pipetted at one time or another in the laboratory, and every precaution must be taken to ensure the safety of the person doing the work (see Chapter 2).

After the pipette has been filled above the top graduation mark, removed from the vessel, and held in a vertical position, the meniscus must be adjusted (Fig. 4-9). The **meniscus** is the curvature in the top surface of a liquid. The pipette should be held in such a way that the calibration mark is at eye level. The delivery tip is touched to the inside wall of the original vessel, not the liquid, and the meniscus of the liquid in the pipette is eased, or adjusted, down to the calibration mark.

When clear solutions are used, the bottom of the meniscus is read. For colored or viscous solutions, the top of the meniscus is read. All readings must be made with the eye at the level of the meniscus (Fig. 4-9).

Before the measured liquid in the pipette is allowed to drain into the receiving vessel, any liq-

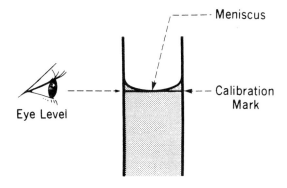

FIG 4-9. Reading the meniscus.

uid adhering to the outside of the pipette must be wiped off with a clean piece of gauze or tissue. If this is not done, any drops present on the outside of the pipette might drain into the receiving vessel along with the measured volume. This would make the volume greater than that specified, and an error would result.

Pipetting Technique Using Automatic Pipettes

Automatic pipettes allow fast, repetitive measurement and delivery of solutions of equal volumes. There are several commercially available types of automatic pipettes, either of the sampling type or of the sampling-diluting type (see Automatic Measuring Devices, under Laboratory Glassware and Plastic Ware). The sampling type measures the substance in question; the sampling-diluting type measures the substance and the adds the desired diluent. The sampling type of automatic pipette is mechanically operated and uses a piston-operated plunger. These are adjustable so that varying amounts of reagent or sample can be delivered with the same device. Disposable and exchangeable tips are available for these pipettes. Automatic pipettes or micropipettors must be calibrated before use.

Micropipettors. Micropipettors contain or deliver from 1 to 500 μL. It is important to follow the manufacturer's instructions for the device be-

ing used, as each one may be slightly different. In general, the following steps apply for use of a micropipettor (Fig. 4-10):

1. Attach the proper tip to the pipettor, and set the delivery volume.
2. Depress the piston to a stop position on the pipettor.
3. Place the tip into the solution, and allow the piston to slowly rise back to its original position (this fills the pipettor tip with the desired volume of solution).
4. Some tips are wiped with a dry gauze at this step, and some are not. Follow the manufacturer's directions.
5. Place the tip on the wall of the receiving vessel and depress the piston, first to a stop position where the liquid is allowed to drain, and then to a second stop position where the full dispensing of the liquid takes place.
6. Dispose of the tip in the waste disposal receptacle. Some pipettors automatically eject the used tips, thus minimizing biohazard exposure.

Repipettors. Several types of repipettors or dispensers are available; they allow repeated volumes of a specific reagent to be delivered to a solution or receiving vessel. These devices are useful for serial dispensing of relatively small volumes of the same liquid (reagent). The volume to be delivered is adjusted on the pipettor dispensing device, which generally is attached by tubing to a reagent bottle containing the reagent to be dispensed. The dispensing device consists of a plunger, a valve system, and the dispensing tip. Once the dispensing device has been primed with liquid, pressing on the plunger allows the selected volume of liquid to be dispensed into the receiving vessel. When the plunger returns to the original position, usually by means of a spring-activated device, the dispenser chamber is refilled with the liquid being measured.

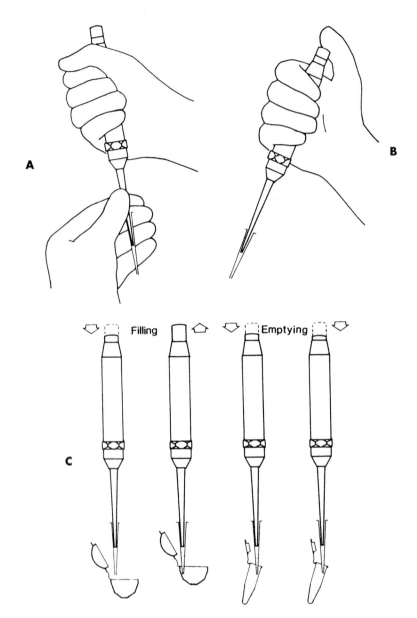

FIG 4-10. Steps in using piston-type automatic micropipette. **A,** Attaching proper tip size for range of pipette volume and twisting tip as it is pushed onto pipette to give an airtight, continuous seal. **B,** Holding pipette before use. **C,** Detailed instructions for filling and emptying pipette tip. (From Kaplan LA, Pesce A: *Clinical Chemistry: Theory, Analysis, and Correlation*, ed 3. St Louis, Mosby, 1996, p 16.)

Titration

Titration is a method of quantitative analysis, a volumetric technique in which the concentration of one solution is determined by comparing it with a measured volume of a solution whose concentration is known. If the concentration of a solution is unknown, it can be found by measuring the volume of the unknown solution that will react with a measured amount of the solution of known concentration (called a standard solution). This process is known as titration.

Use

In the clinical laboratory, titration is used to determine the concentrations of acids and bases, as the analytic tool for certain laboratory procedures, and in the preparation of some reagents.

This technique is often used to determine the concentration of an unknown acid or an unknown base by means of comparison with a known base or a known acid. In this case the quantity of hydronium ions that react with hydroxyl ions to form water is measured. However, numerous reactions, other than the neutralization reaction between an acid and a base, are used in titrations to determine the concentration of a solution.

The titration technique has numerous other uses in the clinical laboratory. It is the means of checking the concentrations of new reagents before they are used in the clinical laboratory. When weaker acids or bases are prepared from more concentrated solutions, the actual normality of the new solution must be determined by titration (Procedure 4-7).

Expression of Normality or Equivalents

When titration is used to determine concentration, the concentration is traditionally expressed in terms of normality or equivalents. Normality is employed because it provides a basis for direct comparison of strength for all solutions. Normality is the number of gram-equivalents per liter of solution. A gram-equivalent is the amount of a compound that will liberate, combine with, or replace one gram-atom of hydrogen. Therefore, 1 equivalent of any compound will react with exactly 1 equivalent of any other compound. For example, 1 equivalent of any acid will exactly neutralize 1 equivalent of any base. It is very convenient to have laboratory solutions of such concentrations that any chosen volume of one reagent reacts with an equal volume of another reagent. The system of equivalents or equivalent weights provides this useful tool. The equivalent weight of a substance is calculated by dividing the gram-molecular weight of the substance by the sum of the positive valences. A solution that contains 1 gram-equivalent weight of substance in 1 L of solution is called a normal (1N) solution (see also Chapter 7).

Essential Components for Titration

In any titration procedure, certain components must always be present:

1. A standard solution of known concentration
2. An accurately measured volume of the standard solution or unknown
3. An indicator to show when the reaction has reached completion
4. A buret (or similar device) to measure the volume of solution required to reach the end point

Standard Solutions. Standard solutions of a desired normality may be prepared by weighing on the analytical balance the exact amount of substance calculated to give that normality, dissolving it in a small amount of deionized water, and then diluting the solution to the number of liters required in the original calculation. Standard solutions prepared in this way (by direct weighing on the analytical balance) are known as primary standards. The chemical substances used in the preparation of standard solutions must be pure, must have a high molecular weight, and must not take up or give off moisture. Oxalic acid meets these

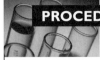

PROCEDURE 4-7

Titration

1. Use the buret clamp to fasten the buret, which must be clean and free from chips or cracks, to the buret stand, which will support it during the titration procedure. Fasten the clamp to the stand about halfway up the rod.

2. Grease the buret stopcock lightly. The stopcock should turn easily and smoothly, but an excess of lubricant will plug the stopcock capillary bore and prevent emptying of the buret. To grease a clean stopcock properly, apply a bit of grease with the fingertip down the two sides of the stopcock away from the capillary bore. Then insert the stopcock in the buret and rotate it until a smooth covering of the whole stopcock is obtained. If the buret is equipped with a Teflon plug, the stopcock need not be lubricated.

3. Rinse the buret with the titrant. In the case of an acid-base titration with phenolphthalein as the indicator, the titrant (or solution to be added and measured by means of the buret) will always be the base. In rinsing the buret, fill it completely with the titrant, and then let it drain. Discard the rinse solution. Fill the buret slowly and carefully to prevent air bubbles from forming in the narrow buret tube. It is essential that the buret be absolutely clean if the results are to be accurate. A clean buret will drain without any solution clinging to its sides; if the buret is dirty, there will be droplets of liquid clinging to the sides. After rinsing the buret several times with the titrant solution, fill it past the zero mark, and then bring the meniscus exactly to the zero mark by draining, using the stopcock to control the flow (see Fig. 4-11).

4. Into an Erlenmeyer flask, pipette the stated amount of the second solution to be employed in the titration. Pipette this solution with a volumetric pipette, using great care to ensure maximal accuracy.

5. Add the required amount of the indicator solution employed to show when the titration reaction has reached completion. (At this point, approximately 5 to 10 mL of water is often added to the Erlenmeyer flask to dilute the indicator and make the end point more visible. The volume of this diluent is not critical, since it does not enter into the reaction or affect the volumes of the solutions that are being titrated.)

6. Titrate each flask in the following manner:

   a. Inspect the buret to be sure that there are no air bubbles trapped in the capillary tube or tip. Air bubbles will add to the apparent volume required to reach the end point, leading to erroneous results. If bubbles are present, drain the buret and refill it with the titrant until there are no bubbles.

   b. Inspect to see that the meniscus is exactly at zero, or record the actual buret reading immediately before beginning the titration.

PROCEDURE 4-7

Titration—cont'd

c. Add the solution in the buret to the flask by rotating the stopcock carefully. A right-handed person encircles the buret stopcock with the left hand, using the right hand to swirl the flask during the titration (see Fig. 4-11). This will be awkward at first, but when mastered it will become natural.

d. With the buret tip well within the titration flask, the titrant may be added fairly rapidly at first, but as the reaction nears completion, the titrant is added drop by drop and finally by only portions of drops (split drops). Clues that the reaction is nearing completion depend on the particular reaction and indicator being employed. In the case of an acid-base titration with phenolphthalein as the indicator, there is a change from a colorless to a red solution. The phenolphthalein is colorless in acid solutions and red in alkaline solutions. In the neutralization reaction itself, hydronium ions react with hydroxyl ions to form water. The reaction begins with an excess of hydronium ions in the Erlenmeyer flask, and the titration is performed until all the hydronium ions have been neutralized by the hydroxyl ions added from the buret. The titration should be stopped at the actual point of neutralization, or as close to it as possible.

In practice, a pink color will appear when the alkali is added to the acid. This color will disappear on shaking. As the titration nears completion, the pink color will remain for a longer time. The base is then added slowly, by split drops, until a faint pink color remains. When the pink color no longer disappears but remains for more than 30 seconds, the end point (or neutralization) has been achieved. It is essential that any titration, using any indicator, be stopped at the actual end point, which is the first faint but permanent color change, or the results will be inaccurate.

e. Immediately on reaching the end point, record the buret reading. Be sure to record a figure that is significant, considering the tolerance of the particular buret being used.

7. Clean the buret by rinsing thoroughly with tap water and then with deionized water. Remove any grease from the stopcock. The titrant should not be left standing in the buret. Alkali will "freeze" the stopcock to the buret, and the concentration of the titrant will increase because of evaporation. When the buret is clean, it can be stored either in an inverted position on the buret clamp or in an upright position filled with deionized water.

8. Use the buret readings obtained in the titration procedure to determine the concentration of the unknown solution.

requirements and is often used as a primary standard. A solution of hydrochloric acid prepared from constant-boiling HCl is also often used as a primary standard. Bases are not often used as primary standards because they take up moisture when exposed to the air, which makes the measurement inaccurate.

Indicator for Reaction. The point at which equal concentrations of the standard and the unknown are present is called the end point of the titration. In the case of acid-base titrations, the end point is where neutralization occurs. Various means of detecting the end point are used, depending on the procedure. Sometimes the formation of a precipitate indicates that the end point has been reached. A change in color of one of the reacting solutions can also indicate the end point. The most common method of detecting the end point is through the use of an indicator solution. An indicator solution is a third solution added in the titration procedure (in addition to the standard solution and the unknown solution). The indicator solution is added in measured amounts to the titration flask. Most indicators are solids dissolved in water or alcohol. Phenolphthalein (0.1%) is commonly used as the indicator in acid-base titrations. Phenolphthalein is made up in a solution of alcohol. It is generally best to arrange the titration procedure so that one titrates from a colorless solution to the first sign of a permanent color rather than from a colored to a colorless solution. Phenolphthalein is colorless in an acid solution and red in an alkaline solution. When one is near the end point, the addition of a single drop from the buret may overrun the true end point considerably. This can cause significant error in the titration of small amounts of solutions. To avoid this drop error, the titrating solution should be added in split drops as the end point approaches. It is possible to control the flow from the buret with careful manipulation of the stopcock so that only part of a drop goes into the titration flask.

Burets. The device that is most often employed to measure the volume required to reach completion of the reaction in a particular titration procedure is the buret. The buret is basically a graduated pipette with a stopcock near the delivery tip to facilitate better control and delivery of the solution (see Figs. 4-1 and 4-11). Burets may be obtained in many capacities and tolerances. The particular buret capacity and tolerance used in a particular procedure are determined by the degree of accuracy that is desired. To ensure that the buret used is employed with maximum accuracy, a very specific technique or procedure must be followed. Mastery of this technique will come only with practice. It is essential that chemically clean, well-calibrated volumetric equipment be used throughout the procedure to ensure reliable results (see Burets, under Laboratory Glassware and Plastic Ware).

Calculations

To find the concentration of a solution, the following must be available: a standard solution of known concentration, the volume of the standard solution, and the volume of the undetermined solution required to reach completion in the particular reaction. As mentioned previously, the concentration is usually expressed in terms of normality, which permits direct comparison of solutions. Normality is the number of gram-equivalents per liter of solution, or milliequivalents per milliliter of solution. However, in practice, 1 L of a solution is rarely used; instead, parts of 1 L are used. Therefore, the number of equivalents is actually the normality of the solution times the volume that is used in the titration. All the ingredients required for the equation to determine the concentration of a solution in any titration are now present. If the equivalents of solution 1 are equal to the equivalents of solution 2, and if the number of equivalents of a particular solution is actually the normality of the solution times the volume, it follows that the normality of solution 1 times the volume of solution 1 is equal

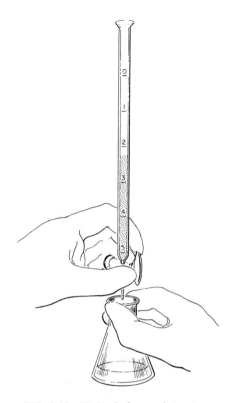

FIG 4-11. Method of manual titration.

to the normality of solution 2 times the volume of solution 2. Or in equation form:

Equivalents of solution 1 = Equivalents of solution 2

or

$$N_1 \times V_1 = N_2 \times V_2$$

In the case of a typical acid-base titration, assume that 2 mL of a standard 0.1000N HCl solution required 1.50 mL of NaOH, added from a buret, to reach the first permanent pink color. What is the normality of the NaOH?

$$N_{acid} \times V_{acid} = N_{base} \times V_{base}$$
$$0.1000N \times 2\ mL = N_{base} \times 1.50\ mL$$
$$N_{base} = \frac{0.1000N \times 2\ mL}{1.50\ mL} = 0.1333$$

That is, the normality of the sodium hydroxide is 0.1333.

General Considerations for Titration

Chemically clean, well-calibrated volumetric equipment, including flasks, pipettes, and burets, must be used in every titration procedure. Accurately prepared standard solutions are essential for accurate results. These are weighed analytically and diluted volumetrically. Indicators must be employed to show when the particular reaction has reached completion. These are often color indicators, which change from colorless to a faint permanent color when the reaction has reached completion. However, such instruments as pH meters may also be employed, in which case the end point is a particular hydronium ion concentration as recorded on the pH meter.

Acid-Base Titration

In acid-base titrations in the clinical laboratory, the most commonly used alkali is 0.1N sodium hydroxide (NaOH). This is relatively stable and can be used to determine the concentration of an acid. However, NaOH is not absolutely stable, and it should be checked daily against a standard acid to be considered reliable.

LABORATORY CENTRIFUGES

Centrifugation is used in the separation of a solid material from a liquid by application of increased gravitational force by rapid rotating or spinning. It is also used in recovering solid materials from suspensions, as in the microscopic examination of urine. The solid material or sediment packed at the bottom of the centrifuge tube is sometimes called the precipitate, and the liquid or top portion is called the supernatant. Another important use for the centrifuge is in the separation of serum or plasma from cells in blood specimens. The suspended particles, solid material, or blood cells usually collect at the bottom of the centrifuge tube because the particles are heavier than the liquid. Occasionally the particles are lighter than the liquid and will collect on the surface of the liquid when it is centrifuged. Centrifugation is employed in many areas of the clinical laboratory—in chemistry, urinalysis, hematology, and blood banking, among others. Proper use of the centrifuge is important for anyone engaged in laboratory work.

Types of Centrifuges

Centrifuges facilitate the separation of particles in suspension by the application of centrifugal force. Several types of centrifuges will usually be found in the same laboratory; each is designed for special uses. There are table-model and floor-model centrifuges, some small and others very large; there are refrigerated centrifuges, ultra-centrifuges, cytocentrifuges, and other centrifuges adapted for special procedures.

Two traditional types of centrifuges are used in routine laboratory determinations. One is a conventional **horizontal-head centrifuge** with swinging buckets, and the other is a **fixed angle-head centrifuge.**

With the horizontal-head centrifuge, the cups holding the tubes of material to be centrifuged occupy a vertical position when the centrifuge is at rest, but assume a horizontal position when the centrifuge revolves (Fig. 4-12). The horizontal-head, or swinging-bucket, centrifuge rotors hold the tubes being centrifuged in a vertical position when the centrifuge is at rest. When the rotor is in motion, the tubes move and remain in a horizontal position. During the process of centrifugation, when the tube is in the horizontal position, the particles being centrifuged constantly move along the tube and any sediment is distributed evenly against the bottom of the tube. When centrifugation is complete and the rotor is no longer turning, the surface of the sediment is flat with the column of liquid resting above it.

For the fixed angle-head centrifuge, the cups are held in a rigid position at a fixed angle. This position makes the process of centrifuging more rapid than it is with the horizontal-head centrifuge. There is also less chance that the sediment will be disturbed when the centrifuge stops. During centrifugation, particles travel along the side of the tube to form a sediment that packs against the bottom and side of the tube. Fixed angle-head centrifuges are used when rapid centrifugation of solutions containing small particles is needed—an example is the microhematocrit centrifuge. The microhematocrit centrifuge used in many hematology laboratories for packing red blood cells attains a speed of about 10,000 to 15,000 rpm with an RCF of up to 14,000 g.

A **cytocentrifuge** utilizes a very-high-torque and low-inertia motor to rapidly spread monolayers of cells across a special slide for critical morphologic studies. This type of preparation can be used for blood, urine, body fluid, or any other liquid specimen that can be spread on a slide. An advantage of this technology is that only a small amount of sample is used, producing evenly distributed cells that can then be stained for microscopic study. The slide produced can be saved and examined at a later time—in contrast to "wet" preparations, which must be examined immediately.

Refrigerated centrifuges are available, with internal refrigeration temperatures ranging from −15 to −25° C during centrifugation. This permits centrifugation at higher speeds, because the specimens are protected from the heat that is generated by the rotors of the centrifuge. The temperature of any refrigerated centrifuge should be checked regularly, and the thermometers should be checked periodically for accuracy.

Centrifuge Speed

Directions for use of a centrifuge are most frequently given in terms of speed, or revolutions per minute. The number of revolutions per minute (rpm) and the centrifugal force generated are expressed as **relative centrifugal force (RCF)**. The number of revolutions per minute is related to the relative centrifugal force by the following formula:

$$RCF = 1.12 \times 10^{-5} \times r \times (rpm)^2$$

where r is the radius of the centrifuge expressed in centimeters. This is equal to the distance from

Balanced Load

Top view of
Partially-Filled Rotor

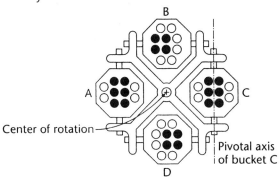

Center of rotation

Pivotal axis
of bucket C

A

Side View of Bucket A or C

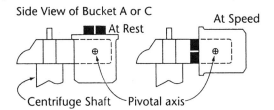

Centrifuge Shaft   Pivotal axis

Unbalanced Load

Top view of
Partially-Filled Rotor

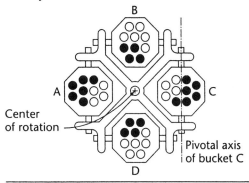

Center
of rotation

Pivotal axis
of bucket C

B

Side View of Bucket A or C

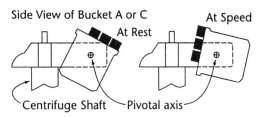

Centrifuge Shaft   Pivotal axis

Side View of Bucket B or D

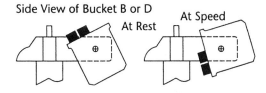

FIG 4-12. Examples of balanced and unbalanced loads in a horizontal-head centrifuge. **A,** Assuming all tubes have been filled with an equal amount of liquid, this rotor load is balanced. The opposing bucket sets A-C and B-D are loaded with equal numbers of tubes and are balanced across the center of rotation. Each bucket is also balanced with respect to its pivotal axis. **B,** Even if all the tubes are filled equally, this rotor is improperly loaded. None of the bucket loads are balanced with respect to their pivotal axes. At operating speed, buckets A and C will not reach the horizontal position. Buckets B and D will pivot past the horizontal. Also note that the tube arrangement in the opposing buckets B and D is not symmetrical across the center of rotation. (From *A Centrifuge Primer.* Palo Alto, Calif, Spinco Division of Beckman Instruments, 1980.)

the center of the centrifuge head to the bottom of the tube holder in the centrifuge bucket.

General laboratory centrifuges operate at speeds of up to 6,000 rpm, generating RCF up to 7,300 times the force of gravity (g). The top speed of most conventional centrifuges is about 3,000 rpm. Conventional laboratory centrifuges of the horizontal type attain speeds of up to 3,000

rpm—about 1,700 g—without excessive heat production caused by friction between the head of the centrifuge and the air. Angle-head centrifuges produce less heat and may attain speeds of 7,000 rpm (about 9,000 g).

Ultracentrifuges are high-speed centrifuges generally used for research projects, but for certain clinical uses, a small air-driven ultracentrifuge is available that operates at 90,000 to 100,000 rpm and generates a maximum RCF of 178,000 g. Ultracentrifuges are often refrigerated.

A rheostat is used to set the desired speed; the setting on the rheostat dial does not necessarily correspond directly to revolutions per minute. The setting speeds on the rheostat can also change with variations in weight load and general aging of the centrifuge.

The College of American Pathologists recommends that the number of revolutions per minute for a centrifuge used in chemistry laboratories be checked every 3 months. This periodic check can be done most easily by using a photoelectric tachometer or strobe tachometer. Timers and speed controls must also be checked on a periodic basis, with any corrections posted near the controls for the centrifuge.

Uses for Centrifuges

A primary use for centrifuges in clinical laboratories is to process blood specimens. Separation of cells or clotted blood from plasma or serum is done on an ongoing basis in the handling and processing of the many specimens needed for the various divisions of the clinical laboratory. The relative centrifugal force is not critical for the separation of serum from clot for most laboratory determinations; a force of at least 1,000 g for 10 minutes will usually give a good separation. When serum separator collection tubes are used that contain a silicone gel needing displacement up the side of the tube, a greater centrifugal force is needed to displace this gel— 1,000 to 1,300 g for 10 minutes. An RCF less than 1,000 g may result in an incomplete displacement of the gel. It is always important to follow the manufacturer's directions when special collection tubes or serum separator devices are being used. These may require different conditions for centrifugation (see Serum Separator Devices under Laboratory Processing of Blood Specimen, in Chapter 3).

In the hematology laboratory, a table-top version of the centrifuge has been specially adapted for determination of microhematocrit values.

This centrifuge accelerates rapidly and can be stopped in seconds. Centrifugation is needed to prepare urinary sediment for microscopic examination. The urine specimen is centrifuged, the supernatant decanted, and the remaining sediment examined. Refrigerated centrifuges are utilized in the blood bank and for other temperature-sensitive laboratory procedures. Ultracentrifuges, which can generate G forces in the hundreds of thousands, are used in laboratories where tissue receptor assays and other assays requiring high-speed centrifugation are needed.

Technical Factors in Using Centrifuges

The most important rule to remember in using any centrifuge is: always balance the tubes placed in the centrifuge. To **balance the centrifuge**, in the centrifuge cup opposite the material to be centrifuged, a container of equivalent size and shape with an equal volume of liquid of the same specific gravity as the load must be placed. (To see examples of a properly balanced centrifuge and one that is unbalanced, see Fig. 4-12.) For most laboratory determinations, water may be placed in the balance load.

Tubes being centrifuged must be capped. Open tubes of blood should never be centrifuged, because of the risk of aerosol spread of infection (see under Protection from Aerosols, in Chapter 2). Aerosols produced from the heat and vibration generated during the centrifugation process can increase the risk of infection to the laboratory personnel. Some evaporation of the sample can occur during centrifugation in uncapped specimen tubes.

Special centrifuge tubes can be used. These tubes are constructed to withstand the force exerted by the centrifuge. They have thicker glass walls or are made of a stronger, more resistant glass or plastic. Some of these tubes are conical, and some have round bottoms.

Before placing the centrifuge tubes in the cups or holders, check the cups to make certain that the rubber cushions are in place. If some cushions are missing, the centrifuge will not be properly balanced. In addition, without the cushions, the tubes are more likely to break.

Whenever a tube breaks in the centrifuge cup, it is most important that both the cup and the rubber cushion in the cup be cleaned well to prevent further breakage by glass particles left behind.

Covers specially made for the centrifuge should be used, except in certain specified instances. Using the cover prevents possible danger from aerosol spread and from flying glass should tubes break in the centrifuge. Keep the centrifuge cover closed at all times, even when not using the machine. In addition to the danger from broken glass, using the centrifuge without the cover in place may cause the revolving parts of the centrifuge to vibrate, which causes excessive wear of the machine.

Do not try to stop the centrifuge with your hands. It is generally best to let the machine stop by itself. A brake may be applied if the centrifuge is equipped with one. The brake should be used with caution, as braking may cause some resuspension of the sediment. Many laboratories discourage use of the brake except when it is evident that a tube or tubes have broken in the centrifuge.

Centrifuges should be checked, cleaned, and lubricated regularly to ensure proper operation. Centrifuges that are used routinely must be checked periodically with a photoelectric or strobe tachometer to comply with quality assurance guidelines set by the CAP.

REFERENCES

1. *Commission on Laboratory Inspection and Accreditation: Reagent Water Specifications.* Chicago, College of American Pathologists, 1985.
2. *International System of Units.* Washington, DC, National Bureau of Standards, 1972, special publication No. 330.
3. National Bureau of Standards: *Standard Reference Materials: Summary of the Clinical Laboratory Standards.* Washington, DC, US Department of Commerce, 1981, NBS special publication.
4. National Bureau of Standards: *Testing of Glass Volumetric Apparatus.* Washington, DC, US Department of Commerce, 1959, NBS circ 602.
5. *Preparation and Testing of Reagent Water in the Clinical Laboratory: Approved Guideline,* ed 2. Villanova, Pa, National Committee for Clinical Laboratory Standards, 1997, NCCLS document C3-A3.
6. *Quantities and Units (SI): Committee Report.* Villanova, Pa, National Committee for Clinical Laboratory Standards, 1983, NCCLS document C11-CR.

BIBLIOGRAPHY

Burtis CA, Ashwood ER (eds): *Tietz Fundamentals of Clinical Chemistry,* ed 4. Philadelphia, WB Saunders Co, 1996.

Campbell JM, Campbell JB: *Laboratory Mathematics: Medical and Biological Applications,* ed 4. St Louis, Mosby, 1997.

Henry JB (ed): *Clinical Diagnosis and Management by Laboratory Methods,* ed 19. Philadelphia, WB Saunders Co, 1996.

Kaplan LA, Pesce AJ: *Clinical Chemistry: Theory, Analysis, and Correlation,* ed 3. St Louis, Mosby, 1996.

STUDY QUESTIONS

1. Match the following measurements (1 to 3) with their standard metric units (A to C) and complete the metric units by filling in their accepted abbreviations:

   1. Volume
   2. Length
   3. Mass
      _____ A. Meter _____ (abbreviation)
      _____ B. Gram _____ (abbreviation)
      _____ C. Liter _____ (abbreviation)

2. Convert the following measurements of length from units listed to units requested:

   Example: 50 mm = _____ m (answer = 0.050 m)

   A. 100 mm = _____ m
   B. 20 cm = _____ mm
   C. 0.5 m = _____ cm
   D. 200 mm = _____ cm
   E. 10 mm = _____ m

3. Convert the following measurements of mass from units listed to units requested:

   A. 25 mg   = _____ g
   B. 500 mg = _____ g
   C. 100 g   = _____ kg
   D. 2.0 kg = _____ g
   E. 10 g   = _____ mg

4. Convert the following measurements of volume from units listed to units requested:

   A. 200 mL = _____ L
   B. 0.2 L   = _____ mL
   C. 500 μL = _____ mL
   D. 600 mL = _____ L
   E. 5 mL   = _____ μL

5. Convert 25° C to degrees Fahrenheit.

6. Convert 40° F to degrees Celsius.

7. If a 100-mL volumetric flask has a capacity tolerance of ±0.05 mL, what is the allowable range of volume for this flask?

8. Match each of the following types of volumetric glassware (1 to 3) with its primary use (A to C):

   1. 1-mL volumetric pipette
   2. 10-mL graduated pipette
   3. 100-mL volumetric flask
      _____ A. To prepare a reagent of specific total volume
      _____ B. To measure an unknown serum sample
      _____ C. To add a reagent to a reaction tube

9. In what form is the manufacturer's information about a chemical provided to the purchaser of the chemical?

10. What is meant by "quantitative transfer" in the preparation of a reagent?

11. Match each of the following types of balances (1 to 3) with its appropriate use (A to C):

    1. Analytical balance
    2. Torsion balance
    3. Triple-beam balance
       _____ A. To weigh chemicals to accuracy of 0.1 g or less
       _____ B. To weigh very small amounts of a substance to a high degree of accuracy
       _____ C. To weigh chemicals to accuracy of 0.01 g or less

12. Answer the following titration problem. What is the normality of an NaOH solution if 1.0 mL of a standard HCl solution (0.1000N) requires titration using 0.50 mL of the NaOH to reach the end point?

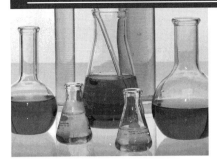

Use of the Microscope

Learning Objectives

From study of this chapter, the reader will be able to:

➢ Identify the parts of the microscope.
➢ Explain the difference between magnification and resolution.
➢ Explain what is meant by the term parfocal and how it
   is used in microscopy.
➢ Define alignment and describe the process of aligning
   a microscope.
➢ Describe the procedure for correct light adjustment to
   obtain maximum resolution with sufficient contrast.
➢ Describe the components of a phase-contrast microscope and tell how they differ from those of a brightfield microscope.
➢ Define the components of the compensated polarizing
   microscope and describe their locations and functions.

The microscope is probably the piece of equipment that receives the most use (and misuse) in the clinical laboratory. Microscopy is a basic part of the work in many areas of the laboratory—hematology, urinalysis, and microbiology, to name a few. Because the microscope is such an important piece of equipment and is a precision instrument, it must be kept in excellent condition, optically and mechanically. It must be kept clean, and it must be kept aligned.

DESCRIPTION

In simple terms, a microscope is a magnifying glass. The compound light microscope (or the **brightfield microscope,** the type used in most clinical laboratories) consists of two magnifying lenses, the objective and the eyepiece (ocular). It is used to magnify an object to a point where it can be seen with the human eye.

The total magnification observed is the product of the magnifications of these two lenses. In other words, the magnification of the objective times the magnification of the ocular equals the total magnification. For example, the total magnification of an object seen with a 10× ocular and a 10× objective is 100 times (100×). These magnification units are in terms of diameters; thus, 10× means that the diameter of an object is magnified to ten times its original size. (The object itself or its area is not magnified ten times; only the diameter of the object is magnified.) The magnification is inscribed on each lens as a number.

Because of the manner in which light travels through the compound microscope, the image that is seen is upside down and reversed. The right side appears as the left, the top as the bottom, and vice versa. This should be kept in mind when one is moving the slide (or object) being observed.

Besides magnification, resolution is a term that is basic in microscopy. **Resolution** tells how small and how close individual objects (dots) can be and still be recognizable. Practically, the resolving power is the limit of usable magnifica-

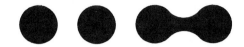

FIG 5-1. Resolution versus empty magnification.

tion. Further magnification of two dots that are no longer resolvable would be "empty magnification" and would result in a dumbbell appearance, as shown in Fig. 5-1.

The relative resolving powers of the human eye, the light microscope, and the electron microscope are shown below.

Human eye	0.25 mm	0.25×10^3 m	0.00025 m
Light microscope	0.25 μm	0.25×10^6 m	0.00000025 m
Electron microscope	0.5 nm	0.5×10^9 m	0.0000000005 m

Another term encountered in microscopy is **numerical aperture (NA).** The NA of a lens can be thought of as an index or measurement of the resolving power. As the numerical aperture increases, the closer objects can be positioned and still be distinguished from each other. Or, the greater the numerical aperture, the greater the resolving power of a lens. The numerical aperture can also be thought of as an index of the light-gathering power of a lens—a means of describing the amount of light entering the objective. Any particular lens has a constant rated numerical aperture, and this value is dependent on the radius of the lens and its focal length (the distance from the object being viewed to the lens or the objective); however, decreasing the amount of light passing through a lens will decrease the actual numerical aperture. The importance of this will become apparent when we discuss proper light adjustments with the microscope. The rated numerical aperture is inscribed on each objective lens.

The structures basic to all types of compound microscopes fall into four main categories: (1) the framework, (2) the illumination system, (3) the

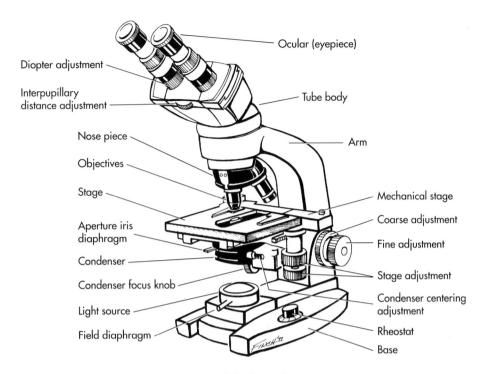

Diopter adjustment

Interpupillary
distance adjustment

Nose piece

Objectives

Stage

Aperture iris
diaphragm

Condenser

Condenser focus knob

Light source

Field diaphragm

Ocular (eyepiece)

Tube body

Arm

Mechanical stage

Coarse adjustment

Fine adjustment

Stage adjustment

Condenser centering
adjustment

Rheostat

Base

FIG 5-2.   Parts of the binocular microscope.

magnification system, and (4) the focusing system (Fig. 5-2).

PARTS OF THE MICROSCOPE

The framework of the microscope consists of several units. The base is a firm, horseshoe-shaped foot on which the microscope rests. The arm is the structure that supports the magnifying and adjusting systems. It is also the handle by which the microscope can be carried without damaging the delicate parts. The stage is the horizontal platform, or shelf, on which the object being observed is placed. Most microscopes have a mechanical stage, which makes it much easier to manipulate the object being observed.

Good microscope work cannot be accomplished without proper illumination. The illumination system is an important part of the compound light microscope. Different illumination techniques or systems that are useful in the clin-

ical laboratory include: (1) brightfield, (2) phase contrast, (3) interference contrast, (4) polarized and compensated polarized, (5) fluorescence, and (6) darkfield. The electron microscope is also useful but requires a more specialized laboratory than the routine clinical laboratory.

BRIGHTFIELD MICROSCOPE: GENERAL DESCRIPTION

The brightfield microscope is the type of illumination system most commonly employed in the clinical laboratory. It consists of an illumination system, a magnifying system, and a focusing system.

Illumination System
Light Source and Intensity Control

The illumination system begins with a source of light. The clinical microscope most often has a built-in light source (or bulb). The bulb is turned on with an on-off switch (or in some cases by a rheostat, which turns on the bulb and adjusts the intensity of light). The light intensity is controlled by a rheostat, dimmer switch or slide, ensuring both adequate illumination and comfort for the microscopist. When there is a separate on-off switch, the light intensity should be lowered before the bulb is turned off, to lengthen the life of the bulb. The light source is located at the base of the microscope, and the light is directed up through the condenser system. It is important that the bulb be positioned correctly for proper alignment of the microscope. (Proper alignment means that the parts of the microscope are adjusted so that the light path from the source of light through the microscope and the ocular is physically correct.) Microscopes are designed so that the light bulb filament will be centered if the bulb is installed properly. Many styles or types of bulbs are available (generally tungsten or tungsten-halogen), and it is important that the bulb designed for a particular microscope be used.

Condenser

Another part of the illumination system is the **condenser.** Microscopes generally use a substage Abbé-type condenser. The condenser directs and focuses the beam of light from the bulb onto the material under examination. The Abbé condenser is a conical lens system (actually consisting of two lenses) with the point planed off (Fig. 5-3). The condenser position is adjustable; it can be raised and lowered beneath the stage by means of an adjustment knob. It must be correctly positioned to correctly focus the light on the material being viewed. When it is correctly positioned, the image field is evenly lighted. The condenser body must be positioned, because, containing lenses, it has a fixed rated NA. When the microscope is properly used, the apparent NA of the condenser should be equal to or slightly less than the rated NA of the objective being used. The apparent or actual NA of the condenser can be varied by changing its position; as it is lowered, the apparent NA is reduced. Thus the condenser position must be adjusted

with each objective used in order to maximize the light focus and the resolving power of the microscope. When the apparent NA of the condenser is decreased below that of the rated NA of the objective, contrast and depth of field are gained and resolution is lost. This manipulation is often necessary in the clinical laboratory when wet, unstained preparations are being observed, such as urinary sediment. In this case, when a specimen is being scanned, in order to gain contrast, the condenser is lowered (or the aperture iris diaphragm partially closed), thus reducing the apparent NA of the condenser. Preferably, the condenser should be left in a generally uppermost position, at most only 1 or 2 mm below the specimen, and the light adjusted primarily by opening or closing the aperture iris diaphragm located in the condenser. The old procedure of "racking down" the condenser when one is looking at wet preparations is not acceptable.

Some microscopes are equipped with a condenser element, which is used in place for low-power work and swings out for high power. Others employ an element that swings out for low-power work and is used in place for higher magnification. This changes the apparent NA of the condenser, matching it with that of the objective. Other illumination systems employ different types of condensers, such as phase-contrast, differential interference-contrast, and darkfield condensers.

Aperture Iris Diaphragm

The **aperture iris diaphragm** also controls the amount of light passing through the material under observation. It is located at the bottom of the condenser, under the lenses but within the condenser body as shown in Fig. 5-3. This aperture diaphragm consists of a series of horizontally arranged interlocking plates with a central aperture (Fig. 5-4). It can be opened or closed as necessary, to adjust the intensity of the light, by means of a lever or dial. The size of the aperture, and consequently the amount of light permitted to pass, is regulated by the microscopist. Such regulation of the light affects the apparent NA of

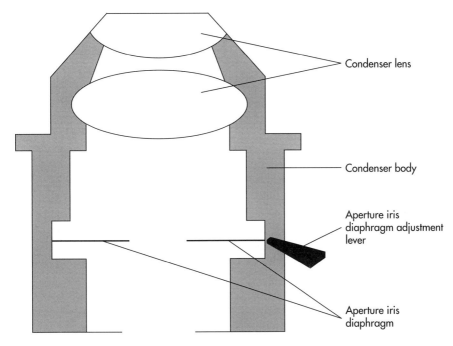

FIG 5-3. Abbé-type substage condenser with aperture iris diaphragm.

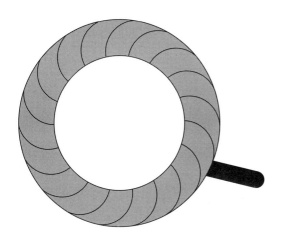

FIG 5-4. Aperture iris diaphragm.

the condenser; decreasing the size of the field under observation with the iris diaphragm decreases the apparent NA of the condenser. Thus, proper illumination techniques involve a combination of proper light intensity regulation, condenser position, and field size regulation.

Field Diaphragm

Better microscopes have a field iris diaphragm, located in the light port in the base of the microscope, through which light passes up to the condenser. The **field diaphragm** controls the area of the circle of light in the field of view when the specimen and condenser have been properly focused. It is also used in the alignment of the microscope.

Magnification System

The magnification system contains several important parts. It plays an extremely important role in the use of the microscope.

Ocular (Eyepiece)

The **ocular**, or **eyepiece**, is a lens that magnifies the image formed by the objective. The usual magnification of the ocular is 10 (10×); however, 5× and 20× oculars are also generally available. Most microscopes have two oculars and are called binocular microscopes. Some microscopes have only one ocular, and these are called monocular microscopes. The magnification produced by the ocular, when multiplied by the magnification produced by the objective, gives the total magnification of the object being viewed. The distance between the two oculars **(interpupillary distance)** is adjustable, as is the focus on one of the oculars **(diopter adjustment).**

Objectives

The **objectives** are the major part of the magnification system. There are usually three objectives on each microscope, with magnifying powers of $10\times$, $40\times$, and $100\times$. The objectives are mounted on the **nosepiece,** which is a pivot that enables a quick change of objectives. Objectives are also described or rated according to **focal length,** which is inscribed on the outside of the objective. Microscopes used in the clinical laboratory most commonly have 16-mm, 4-mm, and 1.8-mm objectives. The focal length is a physical property of the objective lens and is slightly less than the distance from the object being examined to the center of the objective lens. Practically speaking, then, the focal length of a lens is very close in value to the **working distance**—the distance from the bottom of the objective to the material being studied. The greater the magnifying power of a lens, the smaller the focal length and hence the working distance. This becomes very important when the microscope is being used, as the working distance is very short for the $40\times$ (4-mm) and $100\times$ (1.8-mm) objectives. For this reason, correct focusing habits are necessary to prevent damaging the objectives against the slide on the stage.

There are generally two types of objectives available in clinical microscopes: achromats and planachromats. Standard lenses in most microscopes are achromats, which correct for color (chromatic) aberrations. Although achromats are adequate for most laboratory work, the center of the field of view will be in sharp focus, while the edges appear out of focus and the field does not

appear to be flat. Planachromat objectives, while more expensive, are more appropriate for high-magnification work using a $40\times$ or $100\times$ objective, as the field of view is in focus and flat throughout. Apochromatic objectives are also available, which correct for chromatic and spherical aberrations. These are the finest lenses available, and may be necessary for photomicroscopy, but they are significantly more expensive and are not necessary for routine clinical work.

Objective lenses are inscribed with certain information, including type of lens, magnification, rated numerical aperture (NA), body tube length, and cover glass thickness or requirement for immersion oil.

Other terms that are commonly used to describe microscope objectives are *low power, high power* (also *high dry*), and *oil immersion.*

Low-Power Objective. The **low-power objective** is usually a $10\times$ magnification, 16-mm objective. This objective is used for the initial scanning and observation in most microscope work. For example, blood films and urinary sediment are routinely examined by using the low-power objective first. This is also the lens employed for the initial focusing and light adjustment of the microscope. Some routine microscopes also have a very low-power $4\times$ magnification lens. This is used in the initial scanning in the morphologic examination of histologic sections.

Often the term *parfocal* is used in speaking about a microscope. It means that if one objective is in focus and a change is made to another objective, the focus will not be lost. Thus the microscope can be focused under low power and then changed to the high-power or oil-immersion objective (by rotating the nosepiece), and it will still be in focus except for fine adjustment.

The rated NA of the low-power objective is significantly less than that of the condenser on most microscopes (for the $10\times$ objective the NA is approximately 0.25; for the condenser it is approximately 0.9). Therefore, to achieve focus, the

NAs must be more closely matched by reducing the light to the specimen; this is done by focusing or lowering the condenser slightly (1 or 2 mm below the specimen) and then reducing the size of the field of light, with the aperture iris diaphragm, to about 70% to 80%.

High-Power Objective. The **high-power objective,** or high-dry objective, is usually a 40× magnification lens with a 4-mm working distance. This objective is used for more detailed study, as the total magnification with a 10× eyepiece is 400× rather than the 100× magnification of the low-power system. The high-power objective is used to study histology sections, and to study wet preparations such as urinary sediment in more detail. The working distance of the 4-mm lens is quite short; therefore, care must be taken in focusing. The NA of the high-power lens is fairly close to (although slightly less than) that of most commonly used condensers (for most high-power objectives, NA = 0.85; for the condenser, NA = 0.9). Therefore, the condenser should generally be all the way up (or very slightly lowered) and the light field slightly closed with the aperture iris diaphragm for maximum focus.

Oil-Immersion Objective. The **oil-immersion objective** is generally a 100× lens with a 1.8-mm working distance. This is a very short focal length and working distance. In fact, the objective lens almost rests on the microscope slide when the microscope is in use. An oil-immersion lens requires that a special grade of oil, called immersion oil, be placed between the objective and the slide or coverglass. Oil is used to increase the NA and thus the resolving power of the objective. Since the focal length of this lens is so small, there is a problem in getting enough light from the microscope field to the objective. Light travels through air at a greater speed than through glass, and it travels through immersion oil at the same speed as through glass. Thus, to increase the effective NA of the

objective, oil is used to slow down the speed at which light travels, increasing the gathering power of the lens.*

Since the NA of the oil-immersion objective is greater than that of the condenser in most systems (for the 100× objective, NA = 1.2; for the condenser, NA = 0.9), the condenser should be used in the uppermost position and the aperture iris diaphragm should generally be open; practically speaking, however, partial closing of the iris diaphragm may be necessary. The oil-immersion lens, with a total magnification of 1,000× when used with a 10× eyepiece, is generally the limit of magnification with the light microscope.

The oil-immersion lens is routinely used for morphologic examination of blood films and microbes. The short working distance requires dry films, so wet preparations such as urinary sediment cannot be examined under an oil-immersion lens.

The high-power lens is also referred to as a high-dry lens because it does not require the use of immersion oil. Other objectives that might be present on a microscope in the clinical laboratory are a lower-power 4× scanning lens and a 50× or 63× low oil-immersion lens.

Focusing System

The **body tube** is the part of the microscope through which the light passes to the ocular. The tube length from the eyepiece to the objective lens is generally 160 mm. This is the tube that actually conducts the image. The required body tube length is also inscribed on each objective.

The adjustment system enables the body tube to move up or down for focusing the objectives. This usually consists of two adjustments, one coarse and the other fine. The coarse adjustment gives rapid movement over a wide range and is

---

*The speed at which light travels through a substance is measured in terms of the refractive index. The refractive index is calculated as the speed at which light travels through air divided by the speed at which it travels through the substance. The refractive index of air is therefore 1.00. The refractive index of glass is 1.515; immersion oil, 1.515; and water, 1.33.

used to obtain an approximate focus. The fine adjustment gives very slow movement over a limited range and is used to obtain exact focus after coarse adjustment.

CARE AND CLEANING OF THE MICROSCOPE

The microscope is a precision instrument and must be handled with great care. When it is necessary to transport the microscope, it should always be carried with both hands; it should be carried by the arm and supported under the base with the other hand. When not in use, the microscope should be covered and put away in a microscope case, or in a desk or cupboard. It should be left with the low-power (10×) objective in place, and the body tube barrel adjusted to the lowest possible position.

Cleaning the Microscope Exterior

The surface of most microscopes is finished with a black or gray enamel and metal plating that is resistant to most laboratory chemicals. It may be kept clean by washing with a neutral soap and water. To clean the metal and enamel, a gauze or soft cloth should be moistened with the cleaning agent and rubbed over the surface with a circular motion. The surface should be dried immediately with a clean, dry piece of gauze or cloth. Gauze should never be used to clean any of the optical parts of the microscope.

Cleaning Optical Lenses: General Comments

The glass surfaces of the ocular, the objectives, and the condenser are hand-ground optical lenses. These lenses must be kept meticulously clean. Optical glass is softer than ordinary glass and should never be cleaned with paper tissue or gauze. These materials will scratch the lens. To clean the lenses of the microscope, use lens paper. Before polishing with lens paper, take care that nothing is present that will scratch the optical glass in the polishing process. Such potentially abrasive dirt, dust, or lint can easily be blown away before polishing. Cans of compressed air are commercially available, or an air syringe can be made simply by fitting a plastic eyedropper or a 1-mL plastic tuberculin syringe with the tip cut off into a rubber bulb of the type used for pipetting (Fig. 5-5). This air syringe is used to blow away dust or lint that might otherwise scratch the optical glass in the polishing process.

Cleaning the Objectives

Oil must be removed from the oil-immersion (100×) objective immediately after use, by wiping with clean lens paper. If not removed, oil may seep inside the lens, or dry on the outside surface of the objective. The high-dry (40×) objective should never be used with oil; however, if this or any other objective or microscope part comes into contact with oil, it should be cleaned immediately. If a lens is especially dirty, it may be cleaned with a small amount of commercial lens cleaner, methanol, or a solution recommended by the manufacturer, applied to lens paper. Xylene should not be used, because it can damage the lens mounting if it is allowed to get beyond the front seal and because its fumes are toxic.

To properly clean the oil-immersion lens, first lower the stage; then rotate the objective to the front and wipe gently with clean lens paper. Then clean off the immersion oil with lens paper dampened with special lens cleaner or methanol. Alternatively, the cleaning agent may be applied to a wooden applicator stick wrapped with cotton or lens paper and moistened with the cleaning agent. Do not use a plastic applicator stick, as it will be dissolved by the solvent, ruining the objective. Apply the cleaning agent by blotting

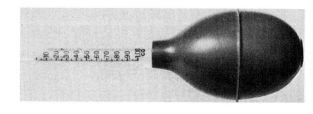

FIG 5-5. Air syringe.

and in a circular motion, beginning at the center and moving outward. Repeat with new dampened lens paper as necessary. Finally, blot dry with clean lens paper. Do not rub, as this may scratch the surface of the lens.

Lenses should never be touched with the fingers. Objectives must not be taken apart, as even a slight alteration of the lens setting may ruin the objective. Merely clean the outer surface of the lens as described. An especially dirty objective may be removed (unscrewed) from the nosepiece, then held upside down and checked for cleanliness by using the ocular (removed from the body tube) as a magnifying glass. Dust or lint can also be removed from the rear lens of the objective by blowing it away with an air syringe. Such removal of the objective from the nosepiece is not a routine cleaning procedure. The final step after using the microscope should always be to wipe off all objectives with clean lens paper.

Cleaning the Ocular

The ocular or eyepiece is especially vulnerable to dirt because of its location on the microscope and contact with the observer's eye. Mascara presents a constant cleaning problem. Dust can be removed from the lens of the ocular with an air syringe (or camel's hair brush). Air is probably easier to use and more efficient. The lens should then be polished with lens paper. The ocular can be checked for additional dirt by holding it up to a light and looking through it. When one is looking into the microscope, dirt on any part of the ocular will rotate with the ocular when it is turned. The ocular should not be removed for more than a few minutes, as dust can collect in the body tube and settle on the rear lens of an objective.

Cleaning the Condenser

The light source and condenser should also be free of dust, lint, and dirt. First blow away the dust with an air syringe or camel's hair brush; then polish the light source and condenser with lens paper. It may be necessary to clean them further with lens paper moistened with a commercial lens cleaner or methanol before polishing them with lens paper.

Cleaning the Stage; Coarse and Fine Adjustments

The stage of the microscope should be cleaned after each use by wiping with gauze or a tissue. After it has been cleaned thoroughly, the stage should be wiped dry.

The coarse and fine adjustments occasionally need attention, as does the mechanical stage adjustment mechanism. When there is unusual resistance to any manipulation of these knobs, force must not be used to overcome the resistance. Such force might damage the screw or rack-and-pinion mechanism. Instead, the cause of the problem must be found. A small drop of oil may be needed. It is best to call in a specialist to repair the microscope when a serious problem occurs. In addition, the microscope should be cleaned at least once a year by a professional microscope service company.

USE OF THE MICROSCOPE

When a microscope is being used, two conditions must be met: (1) the microscope must be clean, and (2) it must be aligned. The cleaning procedure has been described; alignment will now be discussed.

Alignment

When properly aligned, the microscope is adjusted in such a way that the light path through the microscope, from the light source to the eye of the observer, is correct. This is referred to as Kohler illumination. If a microscope is misaligned, the field of view will seem to swing—a very uncomfortable situation, often described as making the observer feel seasick. This can be corrected by properly aligning or adjusting the light path through the microscope. Many microscopes that are produced for student use are aligned by the manufacturer, and realignment requires special knowledge and experience, as the field diaphragm, condenser-centering adjustment screws, and removable eyepieces are not present. In such microscopes, realignment should be done by a professional microscope service company.

If the microscope has a field diaphragm, it is utilized in the alignment procedure. A field diaphragm is an iris diaphragm that is part of the built-in illuminator. With the low-power objective in place, close down the field diaphragm to a minimum. Then focus the condenser by adjusting the condenser height with the condenser focus knob, until the image of the field diaphragm is sharply visible in the field of view (Fig. 5-6, *A*). Next bring the image of the field diaphragm into the center of the field by means of the centering screws located on the condenser (Fig. 5-6, *B*). Now open the field diaphragm until it is just contained within the field of view (Fig. 5-6, *C*). At this point, it may be necessary to repeat the centering procedure. Finally, open the diaphragm until the leaves are just out of view.

Light Adjustment

With the low-power objective in position, the object to be examined, usually on a glass microscope slide, is placed on the stage and secured. Care must be taken to avoid damaging the objective when the specimen is placed on the stage. The slide is positioned so that the portion of the slide containing the specimen to be examined is in the light path, directly over the condenser lens.

The biggest concern in learning how to use a microscope for the first time is the lighting and fine adjustment maneuvers. One must be certain that the light source, condenser, and aperture iris diaphragm are in correct adjustment. Light adjustment is made before any focusing is done. The power supply is turned on and the light intensity adjusted to a bright but comfortable level. Light adjustment will be further accomplished by raising and lowering the condenser and opening and closing the aperture iris diaphragm. At the start of this initial light adjustment, the low-power (10×) objective should be in place. The condenser should be near its highest position, no more than 1 to 2 mm below the slide, with the aperture and field diaphragms open all the way and the body tube down so that the lens is approximately 16 mm from the slide (the working distance for the low-power lens). If the microscope is equipped with a field diaphragm, the condenser height should be adjusted so as to bring the field diaphragm into sharp focus, as described in the alignment procedure.

To adjust the aperture iris diaphragm, while looking through the ocular, close the diaphragm until the light just begins to be reduced. Or, if possible, remove the eyepiece and darken out approximately 20% to 30% of the light by closing the iris diaphragm while looking down the body tube (Fig. 5-7). Further closing of the iris diaphragm (or lowering of the condenser), while it

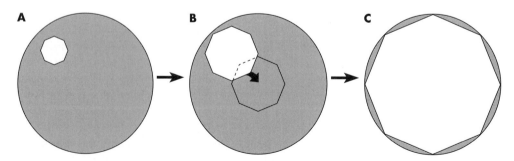

FIG 5-6. Microscope alignment; condenser centration. **A,** Stopped down field diaphragm image, off center or misaligned. **B,** Field diaphragm image widened and moved toward center by means of condenser adjustment knobs. **C,** Field diaphragm image diameter widened and centered.

may increase contrast and depth of focus, will reduce resolution.

Focusing

Focusing is the next technique to be mastered. If using a binocular microscope, adjust the interpupillary distance between the oculars so that the left and right fields merge into one. With the object to be examined on the stage, and while watching from the side, bring the low-power (10×) objective down as far as it will go, so that it almost meets the top of the specimen. Use the coarse adjustment for this procedure. The objective must not be in direct contact with the specimen. Watch from the side to avoid damaging the objective. Once the objective is just at the top of the specimen, slowly focus upward, using the coarse adjustment knob and looking through the ocular. When the object is nearly in focus, bring it into clear focus by use of the fine adjustment knob. Do this procedure with the right eye; then set the ocular diopter to the left eye, by rotating until the left eye is in clear focus, so that the object will be in focus with both eyes.

Further light adjustment should now be made to ensure maximum focus and resolution. Adjust

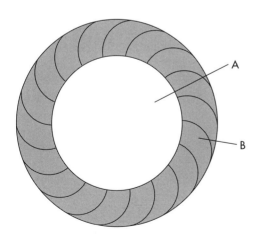

FIG 5-7. Adjusting the aperture iris diaphragm. **A,** 70% to 80% of light presented to objective. **B,** 20% to 30% of light restricted by stopping down the aperture iris diaphragm.

the light intensity with the brightness control so that the background light is sufficiently bright (white) but comfortable. Next adjust the iris diaphragm by opening it completely and then slowly closing it until the light intensity just begins to be reduced. Alternatively, remove the eyepiece and close the aperture iris diaphragm until about 80% of the body tube is filled with light.

When one is changing to another objective, the barrel distance need not be changed. As stated previously, most microscopes are parfocal. The only adjustment necessary should be made with the fine adjustment knob. It is essential to remember that fine adjustment is used continuously during microscopic examination, especially when wet preparations such as urine sediment are being examined.

When greater magnification is needed, more light is necessary. It is obtained by repositioning the condenser and aperture iris diaphragm in the manner previously described. In general, the condenser will be raised and the aperture iris diaphragm opened as the objective magnification increases. When the oil-immersion lens is used, the condenser should be raised to its maximum position.

Additional light is provided by the use of immersion oil, which is placed on the viewing slide when the oil-immersion (100×) objective is used. The oil directs the light rays to a finer point, reducing spherical aberration. When the oil-immersion lens is to be used, first find the desired area on the slide by using the low-power (10×) objective. Once this area is located, pivot the objective out of position, place a drop of immersion oil on the slide, and pivot the oil-immersion lens into the oil while observing it from the side. Next, move the objective from side to side to ensure contact with the oil and avoid the presence of air bubbles. The nosepiece, rather than the objective itself, should be grasped when lenses are being changed, to prevent damage to the objective. The ocular should not be looked through during this adjustment procedure. After the initial adjustment has been made, adjust the fine focus while looking through the ocular. After the study has been completed, clean off the oil remaining on the objective with lens paper as described previously.

OTHER TYPES OF MICROSCOPES (ILLUMINATION SYSTEMS)

Until recently, brightfield illumination has, with few exceptions, been the primary type of microscope illumination system used in the routine clinical laboratory. Now other illumination systems are becoming increasingly popular as refinements in microscope design have made them more reliable and easier to use in a clinical situation. These other types of illumination systems—phase contrast, interference contrast, polarizing, darkfield, fluorescence, and electron—will now be briefly described. The basic principles of microscopy and rules for usage apply with all of these variations; the primary difference is the character of light delivered to the specimen and illuminating the microscope.

Phase-Contrast Microscope

Another extremely useful illumination system is the phase-contrast microscope. A disadvantage of brightfield illumination is that it is necessary to stain (or dye) many objects to give sufficient contrast and detail. **Phase contrast** facilitates the study of unstained structures, which can even be alive, since wet preparations of cells or organisms are observed without prior dehydration and staining. As the name of the technique implies, the structures observed with this system show added contrast compared with the brightfield microscope. The phase-contrast microscope is basically a brightfield microscope with changes in the objective and the condenser. An annular diaphragm, or ring, is put into (or below) the condenser. This condenser annulus is designed to let a hollow cone or "doughnut" of light pass through the condenser to the specimen. A corresponding absorption ring is fitted into the objective. Each phase objective must have a corresponding condenser annulus (Fig. 5-8). In microscopes with multiple phase objectives, the annular diaphragms are usually placed in a rotating condenser arrangement (Fig. 5-9). Use of each phase objective requires an adjustment of the condenser to "match" the annular diaphragm and the phase absorption ring. The phase microscope may also be used as a brightfield microscope by setting the condenser to a standard brightfield (or open) position,

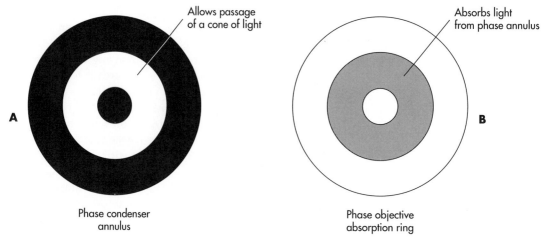

FIG 5-8. Phase annulus and absorption ring. **A,** Phase condenser annulus. **B,** Phase objective absorption ring.

which contains no annulus. However, since the phase objective blocks out a ring of light, the resolution or detail that can be achieved when phase objectives are used for brightfield examination is compromised. For more exact work, an additional brightfield objective should be employed in the microscope.

The annulus and the absorption ring must be perfectly aligned or adjusted so that they are concentric and superimposed. Therefore, a problem with the phase-contrast microscope is the necessity for perfect alignment. First the microscope must be aligned for brightfield work. To align the phase annulus, match the phase objective to the corresponding phase annulus in the condenser by rotating the phase turret. Insert the aperture viewing unit, either by insertion into the body tube or by inserting a phase telescope into an ocular tube. Focus the viewing apparatus until

the phase annulus (seen as a white ring of light) is in focus. There will be a bright (white) ring and a dark ring, which should be superimposed (Fig. 5-10). If not perfectly superimposed, the phase annulus can be repositioned by means of the annulus-centering knobs, located on the condenser. Each microscope will have a slightly different means of adjustment, and the operation directions for that microscope should be followed. However, all phase microscopes require alignment as for brightfield plus alignment of the phase annulus to the matching phase objective.

The net effect of phase contrast is to slow down the speed of light by one fourth of a wavelength. This diminution of the speed of light makes the system very sensitive to differences in refractive index. Objects with differences in refractive index, shape, and absorption characteristics show added differences in the intensity and

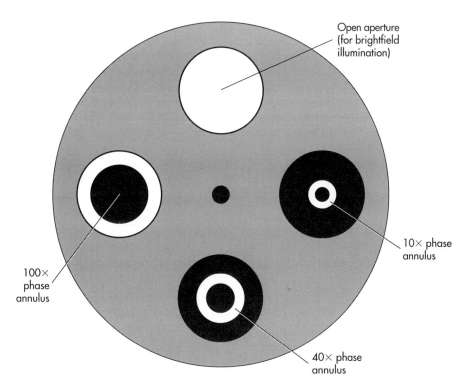

FIG 5-9. Rotating phase condenser with settings for brightfield, low power, high power, and oil immersion.

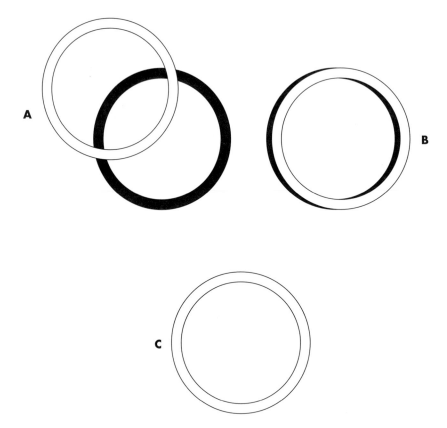

FIG 5-10. Alignment of phase annulus to phase absorption ring. **A,** Before alignment: phase annulus is out of phase adjustment. **B,** Phase annulus moved so that it is nearly aligned. **C,** Alignment: phase annulus is superimposed on phase absorption ring.

shade of light passing through them. The end result is that one can observe unstained wet preparations with good resolution and detail, as shown in Fig. 5-11. In the clinical laboratory, phase contrast is especially useful for counting platelets and for observing cellular structures and casts in wet preparations of urinary sediment and vaginal smears. Owing to its superior visualization and ease of operation, the phase-contrast microscope has become a common tool in routine urinalysis. However, the microscopist must be proficient in changing from brightfield to phase contrast, as in a given specimen some structures are better visualized with phase contrast and others with brightfield.

Interference-Contrast Microscope

Another illumination technique gaining in clinical use is interference-contrast illumination. This technique gives the viewer a three-dimensional image of the object under study. Like phase contrast, it is especially useful for wet preparations such as urinary sediment, showing finer details without the need for special staining techniques. The brightfield microscope is modified by the addition of a special beam-splitting (Wollaston) prism to the condenser. The two split beams are then polarized; one passes through the specimen, which alters the amplitude (or height) of the light wave, and the other (which serves as a reference) does not pass through the specimen. The two

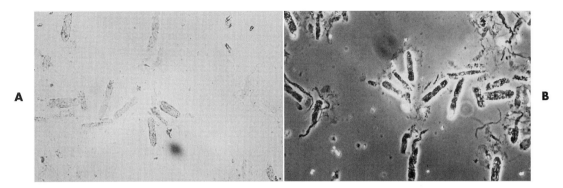

FIG 5-11. Brightfield versus phase-contrast illumination. **A,** Several casts with brightfield illumination. **B,** Same field with phase-contrast illumination. Casts are now clearly visible.

dissimilar light beams then pass separately through the objective and are recombined by a second Wollaston (beam-combining) prism. This recombination of light waves gives the three-dimensional image to the additive or subtractive effects of the light waves as they are combined.

Polarizing Microscope

Another useful adaptation of the brightfield microscope is the polarizing microscope. A **polarizer** (or polarizing filter) may be thought of as a sieve that takes ordinary light waves, which vibrate in all orientations (or directions), and allows only light waves of one orientation (say north-south or east-west) to pass through the filter (Fig. 5-12, *A*). In a polarizing microscope, a polarizing filter is placed between the light source (bulb) and the specimen. A second polarizing filter (called an **analyzer**) is placed above the specimen, between the objective and the eyepiece (either at some point in the microscope tube or in the eyepiece). One of the polarizers is then rotated until the two are at right angles to each other (Fig. 5-12, *B*). When one is looking through the eyepieces, this will be seen as the extinction of light (one sees a dark or black field), since all light is blocked out of the light path when the polarizing filters are at right angles to each other. However, certain objects have a property termed **birefringence,** which means that

they rotate (or polarize) light. An object that polarizes bends light, so that it can be visualized when viewed through crossed polarizers. Objects that do not bend light will not be observed in the microscope. An object that polarizes light (or is birefringent) will appear light against a dark background (Fig. 5-13).

A further modification of the polarizing microscope involves the use of **compensated polarized light.** A compensator, also referred to as a first-order red plate (filter) or full-wave retardation plate, is placed between the two crossed polarizing filters and positioned at 45 degrees to the crossed polarizer and analyzer (Fig. 5-12, *C* and *D*). With this addition the field background appears red or magenta, while objects that are birefringent (polarize light) appear yellow or blue in relation to their orientation to the compensator and their optical properties.

The compensated polarized microscope is especially useful clinically for differentiating between monosodium urate (MSU) and calcium pyrophosphate dihydrate (CPPD) crystals in synovial fluid. It is also becoming useful in the routine study of urinary sediment and in some histologic work. Polarizing microscopy is commonly used in geology for particle analysis, and clinically in forensic medicine. With the polarizing microscope the optical properties of an object can be determined.

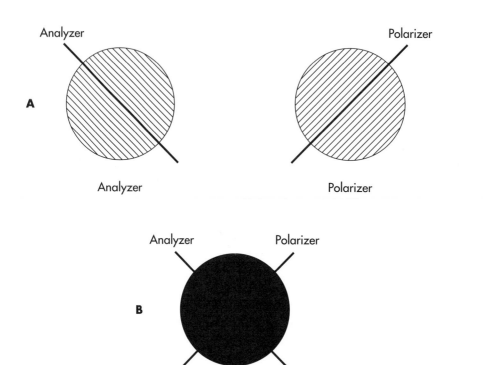

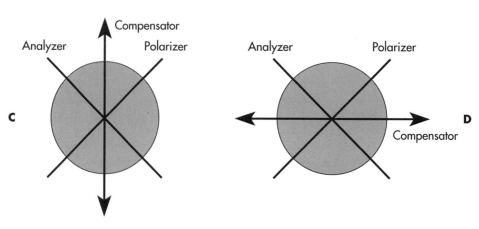

FIG 5-12. Principle of polarized light and compensated polarized light. **A,** Polarizing lenses or filters. Polarizer is placed between light source and specimen; analyzer is placed between specimen and eye of the observer. **B,** Polarized light. This is obtained by placing analyzer and polarizer at right angles to each other. The position of the analyzer is fixed, and the polarizer is rotated until light is extinguished (seen as a black or dark background). **C,** Compensated polarized light. The compensator is placed at 45 degrees to the crossed polarizers, resulting in a red or magenta background color. In this case, the direction of the slow wave of compensation is in a north-south (N-S) orientation. **D,** Compensated polarized light. In this case, the direction of the slow wave of compensation is in an east-west (E-W) orientation.

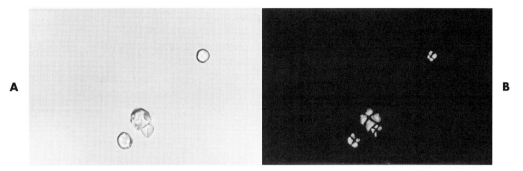

FIG 5-13. Brightfield versus polarized light. **A,** Starch granules viewed with brightfield illumination. **B,** Starch granules viewed with polarized light (crossed polarizing filters). Starch is birefringent; therefore it is visible with polarized light.

Darkfield Microscope

With darkfield microscopy, a special substage condenser is used that causes light waves to cross on the specimen rather than pass in parallel waves through the specimen. Thus, when one looks through the microscope, the field in view will be black, or dark, as no light passes from the condenser to the objective. However, when an object is present on the stage, light will be deflected as it hits the object and will pass through the objective and be seen by the viewer. As a result, the object under study appears light against a dark background. Any brightfield microscope may be converted to a darkfield microscope by use of a special darkfield condenser in place of the usual condenser.

The darkfield microscope has long been used in the routine clinical laboratory to observe spirochetes in the exudates from leptospiral or syphilitic infections. A more recent use, facilitated by newer microscope design technology, is as a low-power scanner for urinary sediment. A darkfield effect may be achieved by using a mismatched phase annulus and phase objective, such as a low-power phase objective with a high-power phase annulus.

Fluorescence Microscope

The transmitted light fluorescence microscope is a further refinement of the darkfield microscope. It is basically a darkfield microscope with wavelength selection. Certain objects have the ability to fluoresce. This means that they absorb light of certain very short (ultraviolet) wavelengths and emit light of longer (visible) wavelengths. In fluorescence microscopy with transmitted light and a compound microscope, the darkfield condenser is preceded by a special exciter filter, which allows only shorter-wavelength blue light to pass and cross on the specimen plane. If the specimen contains an object that fluoresces (either naturally or because of staining or labeling with certain fluorescent dyes), it will absorb the blue light and emit light of a longer yellow or green wavelength. A special barrier filter is placed in the microscope tube or eyepiece. This barrier filter will pass only the desired wavelength of emitted light for the particular fluorescent system. Thus, the fluorescence technique shows only the presence or absence of the fluorescing object. The barrier filter used must be carefully chosen so that only light of the desired wavelength will be passed through the microscope to the observer. Objects in the specimen that do not fluoresce will not emit light of that wavelength and will not be seen.

Fluorescence techniques, in particular fluorescent antibody (FA) techniques, are especially useful in the clinical laboratory. They are used particularly in the clinical microbiology laboratory and for various immunologic studies. Different fluorescent antibody techniques may be used in the primary identification of microorganisms, or in the final identification of bacteria (such as group A streptococci), replacing older serologic methods. Such techniques have the advantage of saving time, which results in earlier diagnosis for the patient, and they are often more sensitive than other techniques. They may also be useful in the identification of organisms that cannot be cultured, such as *Treponema pallidum.*

Electron Microscope

The limit of magnification with any of the variations of the light microscope is about $1,500\times$ to $2,000\times$. Above this, there is decreased resolving power. However, for magnification up to about $50,000\times$ the electron microscope may be used with good resolution.

In general, the principle of the electron microscope is the same as for the light microscope. Rather than a beam of light, the specimen is illuminated with a beam of electrons, produced by an electron gun. The electrons are accelerated by a high-voltage potential and pass through a condenser lens system, usually composed of two magnetic lenses. The electron beam is concentrated onto the specimen, and the objective lens provides the primary magnification. The final image is not visible and cannot be viewed directly; rather it is projected onto a fluorescent screen or a photographic plate. This is the principle of the **transmission electron microscope (TEM).**

Another variation is the **scanning electron microscope (SEM).** It looks at the surface of the specimen and produces a three-dimensional image by striking the sample with a focused beam of electrons. Electrons emitted from the surface of the sample, in addition to deflected electrons from the focused beam of electrons, are focused onto a cathode ray tube or photographic plate and are visualized as a three-dimensional image.

In both cases, specimens need special preparation that is not done in routine clinical laboratories. Specimens must be extremely thin; with TEM the electron beam must pass through the specimen, and electrons have a very poor penetrating power. With SEM the specimen is thicker, since the beam of electrons does not pass through the specimen. In either case, it is impossible to study living cells with electron microscopy because of the high vacuum to which the specimen is subjected and because the electron beam itself is highly damaging to living tissue. However, much of the knowledge of cell structure and function has come from electron microscopy.

BIBLIOGRAPHY

Brown BA: *Hematology: Principles and Procedures*, ed 6. Philadelphia, Lea & Febiger, 1993.

Freeman JA, Beeler MF: *Laboratory Medicine/Urinalysis and Medical Microscopy*, ed 2. Philadelphia, Lea & Febiger, 1983.

Physician's Office Laboratory Procedure Manual: Tentative Guidelines, Villanova, Pa, National Committee for Clinical Laboratory Standards, 1995, POL 1/2-T3 and POL 3-R.

STUDY QUESTIONS

1. **Which is the preferred method of obtaining maximum resolution with sufficient contrast when one is observing a wet preparation using the high-power objective?**

   a. Focus the condenser, utilizing the field diaphragm; then reduce the amount of light presented to the objective to 70% to 80% by closing the aperture iris diaphragm.

   b. Adjust the condenser position to be as far from the specimen slide as possible, and close the field diaphragm.

   c. Keep the condenser height as close to the slide as possible, and open the aperture iris diaphragm as far as possible; then reduce the amount of light to the objective with the intensity-control device.

2. **What is the total magnification of an item under study with a 10× ocular and a 40× objective?**

3. **Where is the aperture iris diaphragm located, and what is its function?**

4. **Where is the field diaphragm located, and what is its function?**

5. **Match the following common working distances (1 to 3) with their objectives (A to C).**

   1. 4 mm
   2. 1.8 mm
   3. 16 mm

   _____ A. Oil-immersion objective
   _____ B. High-power objective
   _____ C. Low-power objective

6. **Match the following objectives (1 to 3) with their common numerical apertures (A to C), and tell how the condenser should be positioned (D to F), assuming the NA of the condenser is 0.85.**

   1. Oil-immersion objective
   2. High-power objective
   3. Low-power objective

   _____ A. 0.25 NA
   _____ B. 0.85 NA
   _____ C. 1.2 NA
   _____ D. Highest possible position or very slightly decreased
   _____ E. Highest possible position
   _____ F. Decreased to 1 or 2 mm below the slide

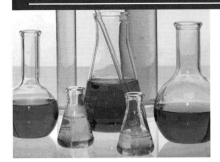

Photometry

Learning Objectives

From study of this chapter, the reader will be able to:

➤ Compare and contrast components of the filter photometer, the absorbance spectrophotometer, and the reflectance spectrophotometer.

➤ Describe light and explain how the observed color of a solution is related to the wavelengths of light absorbed.

➤ Explain how the intensity of color in a substance can be used to measure its concentration.

➤ Define Beer's Law.

➤ Discuss the differences between plotting concentration against percent transmittance and plotting concentration against absorbance and between the use of linear graph paper and the use of semilogarithmic paper.

➤ Use a standard curve to obtain the concentration of an unknown.

➤ Describe the components of a flame photometer.

INTRODUCTION TO PHOTOMETRY

In the clinical laboratory there is a continual need for the use of quantitative techniques. By use of a quantitative method, the exact amount of an unknown substance can be determined accurately, and this is the basis for many laboratory determinations, especially in the chemistry department. Various methods for measuring substances quantitatively are discussed in Chapter 4. One of the techniques used most frequently in the clinical laboratory is photometry, or, specifically, absorbance or reflectance spectrophotometry. **Photometry**, or **colorimetry**, employs color and color variation to determine the concentrations of substances. A photometric component is employed in many of the automated analyzers currently in use in the clinical laboratory, and any person doing clinical laboratory techniques should know and understand thoroughly the principles of photometry in general.

ABSORBANCE SPECTROPHOTOMETRY

Principle of Absorbance Spectrophotometry

The use of **spectrophotometry**, or colorimetry, as a means of quantitative measurement depends primarily on two factors, the color itself and the intensity of the color. Any substance to be measured by spectrophotometry must be colored to begin with or must be capable of being colored. An example of a substance that is colored to begin with is hemoglobin (determined by use of spectrophotometry in the hematology laboratory). Sugar, specifically glucose, is an example of a substance that is not colored to begin with but is capable of being colored by the use of certain reagents and reactions. Sugar content can therefore be measured by spectrophotometry.

When spectrophotometry is used as a method for quantitative measurement, the unknown colored substance is compared with a similar substance of known strength (a standard solution), according to the principle that the intensity of the color is directly proportional to the concentration of the substance present.

In **absorbance spectrophotometry**, the absorbance units or values for several different concentrations of a standard solution are determined by spectrophotometry and are plotted on graph paper. The resulting graph is known as a **standard calibration curve** or a Beer's law plot. Unknown specimens can then be read in the spectrophotometer and, by use of their absorbance values, their concentrations determined from the calibration curve. Standard solutions are also discussed in Chapter 8.

The Nature of Light

To understand the use of absorbance spectrophotometry (and photometry in general), one must first understand the fundamentals of color. To understand color, one must also understand the nature of light and its effect on color as we see it. Light is a type of radiant energy, and it travels in the form of waves. The distance between waves is the **wavelength of light**. The term light is used to describe radiant energy with wavelengths visible to the human eye or with wavelengths bordering on those visible to the human eye. The human eye responds to radiant energy, or light, with wavelengths between about 380 and 750 nm. A nanometer is 1×10^{-9} m. With modern photometric apparatus, shorter (ultraviolet) or longer (infrared) wavelengths can be measured.

The wavelength of light determines the color of the light seen by the human eye. Every color that is seen is light of a particular wavelength. A combination, or mixture, of light energy of different wavelengths is known as daylight, or white light. When light is passed through a filter, a prism, or a diffraction grating, it can be broken into a spectrum of visible colors ranging from violet to red. The **visible spectrum** consists of the following range of colors: violet, blue, green, yellow, orange, and red. If white light is diffracted or partially absorbed by a filter or a prism, it becomes visible as certain colors. The different portions of the spectrum may be identified by wavelengths ranging from 380 to 750 nm for the visible colors. Wavelengths below approximately 380 nm are ultraviolet, and those above 750 nm are infrared; these light waves are not visible to the human eye. To compare and contrast the colors of the visible spectrum in terms of their respective wavelengths, see Table 6-1.

The color of light seen in the visible spectrum depends on the wavelength that is not absorbed. When light is not absorbed, it is transmitted. A colored solution has color because of its physical properties, which result in its absorbing certain wavelengths and transmitting others. When white light is passed through a solution, part of the light is absorbed and that remaining is transmitted light. A rainbow is seen when there are droplets of moisture in the air that refract or filter certain rays of the sun and allow others to pass through. The colors of the rainbow range from red to violet—the visible spectrum.

Absorbance and Transmittance of Light: Beer's Law

Many solutions contain particles that absorb certain wavelengths and transmit others. Solutions appear to the human eye to have characteristic colors. The wavelength of light transmitted by the solution is recognized as color by the eye. See Table 6-1 for the visible colors of the spectrum and their respective approximate wavelength ranges.[1] A blue solution appears blue because particles in the solution absorb all the wavelengths except blue; the blue is the color transmitted and seen. A red solution appears red because all other wavelengths except red have been absorbed by the solution, while the red wavelength passes through.

Measurement by spectrophotometry is based on the reaction between the substance to be measured and a reagent, or chemical, used to produce color. The amount of color produced in a reaction between the substance to be measured and the reagent depends on the concentration of the substance. Therefore, the intensity of the color is proportional to the concentration of the

TABLE 6-1

Observed Colors of the Visible Spectrum and Their Corresponding Wavelengths[1]

Approximate Wavelength (in nm)	Color Observed
<380	Not visible (ultraviolet light)
380-440	Violet
440-500	Blue
500-580	Green
580-600	Yellow
600-620	Orange
620-750	Red
>750	Not visible (infrared light)

substance. **Beer's law** states this relationship: color intensity at a constant depth is directly proportional to concentration. Beer's law is the basis for the use of photometry in quantitative measurement. If one saw a solution with a very intense red color, one would be correct in assuming that the solution had a high concentration of the substance that made it red. Another way of stating Beer's law is that any increase in the concentration of a color-producing substance will increase the amount of color seen.

As the law states, the depth at which the color is determined must be constant. The depth of the solution is regulated by the **cuvette** or container used to hold it. Increasing the depth of the solution through which the light must pass (by using a cuvette with a larger diameter) is the same as placing more particles between the light and the eye, thereby creating an apparent increase in the concentration, or intensity, of color. To avoid this alteration of the actual concentration, only cuvettes with a constant diameter can be used—or a flow-through apparatus, which eliminates the use of cuvettes.

Expressions of Light Transmitted or Absorbed

There are two common methods of expressing the amount of **light transmitted** or **light**

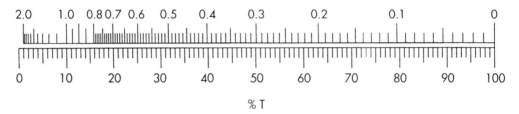

FIG 6-1. Viewing scales showing divisions for reading percent transmittance versus absorbance. Absorbance is the measure of light stopped or absorbed. Percent transmittance is the measure of light transmitted through the solution. (From Campbell JB, Campbell JM: *Laboratory Mathematics: Medical and Biological Applications*, ed 5. St Louis, Mosby, 1997, p 211.)

absorbed by a solution. The units used to express the readings obtained by the electronic measuring device (see under Parts Essential to All Spectrophotometers) are either **absorbance (A) units** or **percent transmittance (%T) units**. Another term for absorbed light is **optical density (OD)**; this term is generally not used. Most spectrophotometers give the readings in both units. Absorbance units are sometimes more difficult to read directly from the reading scale because it is divided logarithmically rather than in equal divisions (Fig. 6-1). **Absorbance** is an expression of the amount of light absorbed by a solution. Absorbance values are directly proportional to the concentration of the solution, and therefore they may be plotted on **linear graph paper** to give a straight line (Fig. 6-2, *A*). Most spectrophotometers also give the percent transmittance readings on the viewing scale. **Percent transmittance** is the amount of light that passes through a colored solution compared with the amount of light that passes through a blank or standard solution. The blank solution contains all the reagents used in the procedure, but it does not contain the unknown substance being measured (see also under Ensuring Reliable Results: The Quality Control Program, in Chapter 8). Standard solutions will be discussed later in this chapter. Percent transmittance varies from 0 to 100 (it is usually abbreviated %T), with equal divisions on the viewing scale (see Fig. 6-1). As the concentration of the colored solution increases,

the amount of light absorbed increases and the percentage of the light transmitted decreases. The transmitted light does not decrease in direct proportion to the concentration or color intensity of the solution being measured. Percent transmittance readings plotted against concentration will not give a straight line on linear graph paper (see Fig. 6-2, *B*). There is a logarithmic relationship between percent transmittance and concentration, so when percent transmittance is plotted against concentration, **semilogarithmic graph paper** is used to obtain a straight line (Fig. 6-3). Absorbance and percent transmittance are related in the following way:

$$\text{Absorbance} = 2 \text{ minus the logarithm of the percent transmittance}$$

or

$$A = 2 - \log \%T$$

Therefore, 2 is the logarithm of 100%T. It is possible to obtain a convenient conversion table for transmittance and absorbance from a standard chemistry reference textbook.

Preparation of a Standard Curve (Standardizing a Procedure)

The use of standard curves in today's clinical laboratory has declined with the advent of computerized instrumentation, which includes the

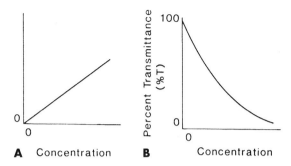

FIG 6-2. Relationships of absorbance **(A)** and percent transmittance **(B)** to concentration when plotted using linear graph paper. (From Kaplan LA, Pesce AJ: *Clinical Chemistry: Theory, Analysis, and Correlation*, ed 3. St Louis, Mosby, 1996, p 88.)

steps formerly done with graph paper to calculate the relationship between any spectrophotometer eadings for the standards and those for the unknowns. It is nevertheless important to understand how standard curves are constructed and used.

For each analytic method utilizing photometry, specific standard solutions must be prepared and used in the procedure. **Standard solutions** of varying concentrations are prepared using high levels of accuracy in their preparation (high-grade chemicals, analytical weighing, and volumetric dilution). Once a series of standard tubes have been read in the spectrophotometer, the galvanometer readings and standard concentrations are plotted on graph paper. The readings for the unknown solutions are then compared with those of the standard solution by use of the **standard curve**. The preparation of a standard curve is also an important component of examining laboratory data for validity. It can indicate abnormalities or variations in the analytic systems being used by the laboratory (see also Ensuring Reliable Results: The Quality Control Program, in Chapter 8).

Types of Graph Paper

Linear graph paper can be used to plot absorbance readings, since absorbance of wave-

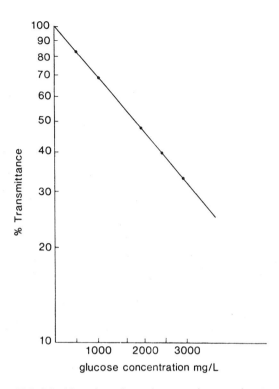

FIG 6-3. Use of semilogarithmic graph paper showing percent transmittance plotted against concentration. (From Kaplan LA, Pesce AJ: *Clinical Chemistry: Theory, Analysis, and Correlation*, ed 3. St Louis, Mosby, 1996, p 42.)

lengths of light is directly proportional to the concentration of the colored solution being read. **Semilogarithmic graph paper** is used to plot percent transmittance readings from the photometer, since there is a logarithmic relationship between percent and concentration, as described. The horizontal axis of semilogarithmic graph paper is a linear scale, and the vertical axis is a logarithmic scale (Fig. 6-3). The concentrations of the standard solutions being used are plotted on the horizontal axis. The transmittance or absorbance readings from the photometer are plotted along the vertical axis. When percent transmittance readings are used, these can be plotted directly on the logarithmic scale of the semilogarithmic graph paper (the horizontal axis), as the concentration is proportional to the logarithm of the galvanometer reading. In this way, percent transmittance readings are converted to the appropriate numbers on the logarithmic scale. Using semilogarithmic graph paper is simple and convenient for most laboratory purposes. When percentages are plotted against concentrations on semilogarithmic graph paper, the proportional relationship is direct, and the necessary straight-line graph is obtained when the individual standard points are connected.

The criteria for a good standard curve are that the line is straight, that the line connects all points, and that the line goes through the origin, or intersect, of the two axes. The origin of the graph paper is the point on the vertical and horizontal axes where there is 100%T and zero concentration (see Fig. 6-3).

Another type of graph paper, called linear graph paper, is available for plotting standard curves. This graph paper has linear scales on both the horizontal and vertical axes. If linear graph paper is used to construct a standard curve and only percent transmittance readings are available, these readings must first be converted to logarithmic values and the logarithmic values plotted on the vertical axis. Absorbance units can be plotted directly against the concentration on the linear graph paper to obtain a straight-line graph (Beer's law is followed). To eliminate the conversion of percent transmittance to absorbance in order to obtain the necessary straight-line graph, the use of semilogarithmic graph paper is suggested.

Plotting a Standard Curve

When points are plotted on graph paper, whether they represent concentrations or galvanometer readings, care must be taken to note the intervals on the graph paper. Many errors result from carelessness in the initial plotting of points on the graph paper. When a standard curve is prepared, the axes must also be properly labeled, as well as other information labeling or defining the graph specifics (see Fig. 6-4).

Using a Standard Curve

Once the standard curve has been plotted, it is used to calculate the concentrations of any unknowns that were included in the same batch as the standards used to make the graph. To find the concentration of a solution, there must be some way of comparing it with a solution of known concentration.

A simplified example of the construction and use of a standard curve is given in Figure 6-4. In the example shown, three standard solutions are prepared with the following concentrations: standard 1 (S1), 0.02 mg; standard 2 (S2), 0.04 mg; and standard 3 (S3), 0.06 mg. These concentrations are plotted on the linear, horizontal, scale of the semilogarithmic graph paper. The three standard tubes are read in a photometer, giving the following readings in percent transmittance: S1, 76^2; S2, 58^3, and S3, 45^1%T. The percent transmittance readings are plotted under their respective concentrations on the logarithmic, vertical, scale of the paper. The points are connected, using a ruler. An undetermined substance gives a reading of 63^2%T. Using the graph in Fig. 6-4, the 63^2%T point on the vertical scale is found, followed horizontally to the graph line just drawn, and then followed vertically to the concentration scale. The degree of accuracy with which an unknown concentration can be read depends on the concentrations of the standards used. The accuracy of the unknown can be no greater than the accuracy of the standard solutions used. Standard solutions are usually weighed to the fourth decimal place. In this example, if the graph lines were present, the unknown concentration would be read as 0.0343 mg (the figure in the fourth decimal place is approximate).

Using standard solutions to standardize the analyses of each batch, rather than relying on a permanently established calibration curve, allows the clinical laboratory to produce more reliable results. It compensates for variables such as time, temperature, the age of the reagents, and the condition of the instruments. It is always best to use several different concentrations of the standard solution, not just one. To obtain reliable

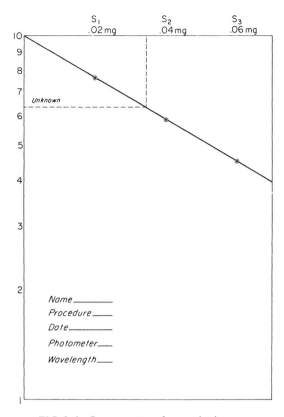

FIG 6-4. Construction of a standard curve.

photometric information about the concentration of a substance, standard solutions must be used as the basis for comparison.

Instruments Used in Spectrophotometry

The instrument used to show the quantitative relationship between the colors of the undetermined solution and the standard solution is called a **spectrophotometer**, or **colorimeter**.

Most of the instruments used in photometry have some means of isolating a narrow wavelength, or range, of the color spectrum for measurements. Instruments using filters for this purpose are referred to as filter photometers, while those using prisms or gratings are called spectrophotometers or photoelectric colorimeters. Both types are used frequently in the clinical laboratory. In older colorimetric procedures, visual

comparison of the color of an unknown with that of a standard was used. In general, visual colorimetry has been replaced by the more specific and accurate photoelectric methods.

One current application of visual colorimetry is employed in the various dry reagent strip tests, which are so prevalent in many clinical chemistry tests—dry reagent strip tests used in urinalysis, for example. These strips can be read visually, although instruments are also available to electronically read the color developed.

There are many types of spectrophotometers in common use in the clinical laboratory. The principle of most of these instruments is the same, in that the amount of light transmitted by the standard solution is compared with the amount of light transmitted by the solution of unknown concentration.

Precise, accurate methods are needed to accomplish the numerous determinations required in today's clinical laboratory. The spectrophotometer is one piece of equipment that is essential and can be considered to be of prime importance in quantitative analysis. Spectrophotometers are also known as photoelectric colorimeters or photometers. The many available spectrophotometers have their own technical variations, but all operate according to the same general principles. For teaching purposes, the Coleman Junior Spectrophotometer has proved to be very satisfactory (Fig. 6-5). In general, photometers employing filters are called filter photometers, and those with diffraction gratings are called spectrophotometers. Photometers utilize an electronic device to compare the actual color intensities of the solutions measured. As the name implies, a spectrophotometer is really two instruments in a single case: a spectrometer, a device for producing light of a specific wavelength, the monochromator; and a photometer, a device for measuring light intensity. Because of its common use, the operation of the Coleman Junior Spectrophotometer is described in Procedure 6-1. Any spectrophotometric instrument should be used only by following the manufacturer's instructions.

In the automated analyzing instruments used in many laboratories, a photometer is still a

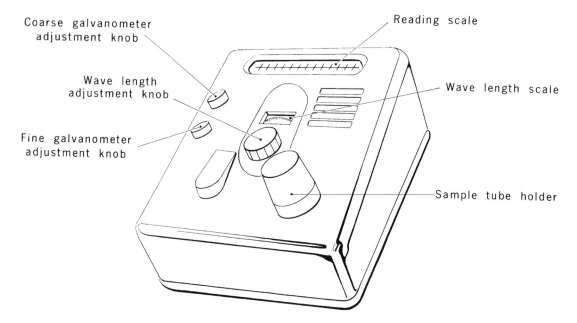

Coarse galvanometer adjustment knob

Wave length adjustment knob

Fine galvanometer adjustment knob

Reading scale

Wave length scale

Sample tube holder

FIG 6-5. Coleman Junior Spectrophotometer.

necessary component, so that absorbance values for unknown and standard solutions can be determined. Some instruments contain a filter wheel, which allows for the measurement of absorbance at any wavelength for which there is a filter on the wheel. Microprocessors control the location of the correct filter for the particular analyte being measured. From the absorbance information, the computer microprocessor calculates the unknown concentration.

Parts Essential to All Spectrophotometers

There are parts necessary to all spectrophotometers (Fig. 6-6). These are as follows:

1. *Light source.* Each spectrophotometer must have a light source. This can be a light bulb constructed to give the optimum amount of light. The light source must be steady and constant; therefore, use of a voltage regulator or an electronic power supply is recommended. The light source may be movable or stationary.

2. *Wavelength isolator.* Before the light from the light source reaches the sample of solution to be measured, the interfering wavelengths must be removed. A system of isolating a desired wavelength and excluding others is called a monochromator; the light is actually being reduced to a particular wavelength. Filters can be used to accomplish this. Some are very simple, composed of one or two pieces of colored glass. Some are more complicated. The more complicated filters are found in the better spectrophotometers. The filter must transmit a color that the solution can absorb. A red filter transmits red, and a green filter transmits green. Filters are available to cover almost any point in the visible spectrum, and each filter has inscribed on it a number that indicates the wavelength of light that it transmits. For example, a filter inscribed with 540 nm absorbs all light except that of wavelengths around 540 nm. Since the filter must transmit a color that the solution can absorb, for a red solution the filter chosen should not be red (all colors except red are absorbed). The wavelength of light transmitted is, then, the important thing to consider in choosing the correct filter for a procedure.

PROCEDURE 6-1

Operation of the Coleman Junior Spectrophotometer

1. Mount the selected scale panel in the galvanometer viewing window. A general purpose scale panel is usually used. There are several types of scale panels available, depending on the use to which the spectrophotometer is to be put. The scale panel is calibrated both in percent transmittance and in absorbance (optical density).

2. Insert into the cuvette well the cuvette adapter of the proper size to accommodate the type of cuvette specified in the analytic procedure.

3. Turn on the switch located on the back of the instrument. Allow the instrument to warm up for 5 minutes.

4. Verify the galvanometer zero setting, and readjust if necessary. The indicator line on the galvanometer spot should register at zero on the percent transmittance scale. The zero adjustment level for this instrument is located under the raised housing just to the left of the cuvette well. If the spectrophotometer is not disturbed and its position is not altered, this galvanometer adjustment remains very stable.

   a. To check the zero position, darken the photoelectric cell by inserting into the cuvette well a cuvette adapter turned 90 degrees from the calibration marker. In this position, the body of the adapter completely blocks the pathway of light. A piece of opaque paper may also be slipped into the adapter well; in this way the light pathway is also completely stopped.

   b. Cover the well with the light shield or other suitable cover.

   c. With a pencil point move the galvanometer adjusting lever so that the indicator line on the galvanometer spot reads zero on the left zero index of the selected scale panel.

   d. Complete the adjustment by sliding the scale panel until the index is exactly at zero on the scale.

5. Adjust the wavelength control so that the specific wavelength is set. Different procedures will call for different wavelengths. The wavelength to be used will be specified in the procedure.

6. Cuvettes used for reading in the spectrophotometer must be free from scratches. Before the cuvette is placed in the adapter for reading, it must be free of finger marks and bubbles; the spectrophotometer does not recognize the cause of light impediment and will respond similarly to a scratched tube, lint, bubbles, finger marks, and the absorbance of the solution being examined. Therefore, wipe the cuvettes with a clean, dry, soft cloth or gauze before reading. All cuvettes must contain a certain volume of solution, called the minimum volume. Different sizes of cuvettes need different minimum volumes to ensure that the light passes through the solution rather than through the empty space in the tube.

7. Place the cuvette containing the reagent blank in the adapter first. For more information on the use of blank solutions, see Chapter 8. The calibration mark (or trademark, if precalibrated Coleman cuvettes are used) must face the light source to ensure constancy of the light path. Adjust the galvanometer control knobs (labeled *GALV Coarse* and *GALV Fine*) until the galvanometer index on the viewing scale reads 100%T for the "blank" tube.

8. Remove the blank tube.

Continued

PROCEDURE 6-1

Operation of the Coleman Junior Spectrophotometer—cont'd

9. Place the next polished cuvette containing the solution to be read in the adapter well, again taking note of the calibration mark. Place this mark in a position facing the light source.

10. Record the galvanometer reading to the nearest ¼%T reading.

11. Remove the cuvette, and reinsert the blank tube.

12. Observe the reading for the blank tube on the galvanometer scale. It should still read 100%T. If it does, remove the blank tube and proceed with the next tube to be read. If the blank tube does not read exactly 100%T, adjust it to read 100%T with the GALV Coarse and GALV Fine knobs. Then read the next tube. The blank tube should be reinserted between all readings, and it should always read 100%T.

13. Read all tubes, and record results to the nearest ¼%T reading. Fractional parts (in fourths) of percent transmittance readings are recorded with the numerator figure only. For example, if a reading is 75½ (= 75 ²⁄₄), the result is recorded as 75²%T. For a reading of 75¾ the result is recorded as 75³, and for a reading of 75¼ the result is recorded as 75¹.

14. When finished, return the galvanometer index to the original position by turning both the *GALV Coarse* and *GALV Fine* knobs completely counterclockwise, and turn off the machine switch.

15. Clean up the area around the instrument, wipe up anything spilled on the machine, and cover the spectrophotometer with the protective cover provided. For cleaning cuvettes, see under Cleaning Laboratory Glassware and Plastic Ware, discussed previously in Chapter 4.

From Operating Directions for the Coleman Model 6A and 6C Junior Spectrophotometer. Maywood, Ill, Coleman Instruments Corp, September 1966.

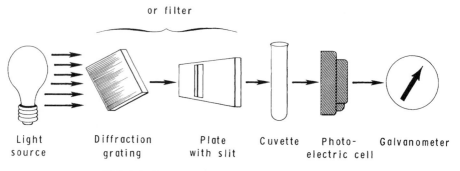

FIG 6-6. Parts essential to all spectrophotometers.

Light of a desired wavelength can also be provided by other means. One of the more commonly used instruments employs a diffraction grating with a special plate and slit to reduce the spectrum to the desired wavelength. The grating consists of a highly polished surface with numerous lines on it that break up white light into the spectrum. By moving the spectrum behind a slit (the light source must be movable), only one particular portion of the spectrum is allowed to pass through the narrow slit. The particular band of light, or wavelength, that is transmitted through the slit is indicated on a viewing scale on the machine. Certain wavelengths are more desirable than others for a particular color and procedure. The wavelength chosen is determined by running an absorption curve and selecting the correct wavelength after inspecting the curve obtained. Only when new methods are being developed is it necessary to run an absorption curve.

3. *Cuvettes, absorption cells, or photometer tubes.* Any light (of the wavelength selected) coming from the filter or diffraction grating will next pass on to the solution in the cuvette. Glass cuvettes are relatively inexpensive and are satisfactory, provided they are matched or calibrated. **Calibrated cuvettes** are tubes that have been optically matched so that the same solution in each will give the same reading on the photometer. In using calibrated cuvettes, the depth factor of Beer's law is kept constant. Depending on the concentration and thus the color of the solution, a certain amount of light will be absorbed by the solution and the remainder will be transmitted. The light not absorbed by the solution is transmitted. This light next passes on to an electronic measuring device of some type. Alternatively, to eliminate the cuvette entirely, a flow-through apparatus can be used.

4. *Electronic measuring device.* In the more common spectrophotometers, the electronic measuring device consists of a photoelectric cell and a galvanometer. The amount of light transmitted by the solution in the cuvette is measured by a **photoelectric cell**. This cell is a most sensitive instrument, producing electrons in proportion to the amount of light hitting it. The electrons are passed on to a **galvanometer**, where they are measured. The galvanometer records the amount of current (in the form of electrons) that it receives from the photoelectric cell on a special viewing scale on the spectrophotometer (see Fig. 6-1). The results are reported in terms of percent transmittance. In some cases, the readings are made in terms of absorbance. The percent transmittance is dependent on the concentration of the solution and its depth. If the solution is very concentrated (the color appearing intense), less light will be transmitted than if it is dilute (pale). Therefore, the reading on the galvanometer viewing scale will be lower for a more concentrated solution than for a dilute solution. This is the basis for the comparison of color intensity with the spectrophotometer.

Flow-Through Adaptation

A special adaptation available for Coleman Junior Spectrophotometers is called a Coleman Vacuvette Cell Assembly. This is designed to increase the speed with which samples can be introduced into and discharged from the photometer. Another name for an assembly of this kind is a flow-through apparatus. Instead of separate cuvettes being used for each sample read in the photometer, the sample is poured directly into a specially designed cuvette incorporating a funnel for easy pouring. The sample is read in the same way as in the regular cuvette method and is then evacuated from the photometer by means of a capillary tubing attached to a discard bottle. When a suitable vacuum system is attached to the cuvette-capillary tubing assembly, rapid and automatic discarding of the sample is possible. This assembly apparatus must be periodically cleaned to maintain its proper operation. A flow-through apparatus can be used for reading samples when the sample can be discarded. It cannot be used to read multiple values on the same sample because the sample is lost once it is poured into the special cuvette. The Coleman Instruments Corporation manufactures this specially designed cuvette in various sizes so that varying amounts of sample may be read in the photometer. This device is another example of how many laboratory functions have been made more efficient so that time can be saved and results can be obtained and reported more quickly.

Care and Handling of Spectrophotometers

In the use of a spectrophotometer, error caused by color in the reagents used must be eliminated. Since color is so important and since the color produced by the undetermined substance is the desired one, any color resulting from the reagents themselves or from interactions between the reagents could cause confusion and error. By use of a blank solution, a correction can be made for any color resulting from the reagents used. The blank solution contains the same reagents as the unknown and standard tubes, with the exception of the substance being measured. The use of blank solutions is discussed further in Chapter 8.

A spectrophotometer, as is the case with any expensive, delicate instrument, must be handled with care. The manufacturer supplies a manual of complete instructions on the care and use of a particular machine. Care should be taken not to spill reagents on the spectrophotometer. Spillage could damage the delicate instrument, especially the photoelectric cell. Any reagents spilled must be wiped up immediately. Spectrophotometers with filters should not be operated without the filter in place, since the unfiltered light from the light source may damage the photoelectric cell and the galvanometer. A spectrophotometer should be placed on a table with good support, where it will not be bumped or jarred.

Tests of Quality Control for Spectrophotometers

The spectrophotometer must be tested periodically to ensure that it is functioning properly. Wavelength calibration can be checked by use of a rare-earth glass filter such as didymium. The wavelength calibration can also be checked by use of a stable chromogen solution. Calibration

at two wavelengths is necessary for instruments with diffraction gratings and at three wavelengths for instruments with prisms.

Photoelectric accuracy can be checked by reading standard solutions of potassium dichromate or potassium nitrate. As an alternative, the National Bureau of Standards (NBS) has sets of three neutral-density glass filters that have known absorbance at four wavelengths for each filter. These filters are not completely stable, however, and require periodic recalibration.

Calibration of Cuvettes for the Spectrophotometer

If cuvettes are used, it is essential that their diameters be uniform; that is, it is necessary that the depth of the cuvettes or tubes used in the spectrophotometer be constant for Beer's law to apply. Cuvettes for the spectrophotometer can be purchased precalibrated. Precalibrated cuvettes must be checked before being put into actual use in the laboratory. Calibrated cuvettes are optically matched so that the same solution in each will give the same percent transmittance reading on the galvanometer viewing scale.

In checking cuvettes for use in spectrophotometry, the cuvette is carefully observed to see that the solution in it gives the same reading in that cuvette as it did in other calibrated cuvettes. To check cuvettes for uniformity, the same solution, such as a stable solution of copper sulfate or cyanmethemoglobin, is read in many cuvettes. Readings are taken, and cuvettes that match within an established tolerance are used.

If new plain glass tubes are being calibrated to be used as cuvettes, since all tubes may not be perfectly round, the tubes are rotated in the cuvette well to observe any changes in reading with the position in the well. The cuvette is etched at the point where the reading corresponds with the established tolerance for the absorption reading. Cuvettes that do not agree or do not correspond are not used for spectrophotometry.

Different sizes of cuvettes can be used, depending on the spectrophotometer. The Coleman Junior Spectrophotometer can be adapted to use several different sizes cuvettes in the same machine. For each size, a special cuvette adapter is used, enabling the cuvette to fit securely in the cuvette holder. Only when the cuvette fits securely will the readings obtained be precise and accurate.

REFLECTANCE SPECTROPHOTOMETRY

Reflectance spectrophotometry is another quantitative spectrophotometric technique; the light reflected from the surface of a colorimetric reaction is used to measure the amount of unknown colored product generated in the reaction. A beam of light is directed at a flat surface, and the amount of light reflected is measured. A photodetector measures the amount of reflected light directed to it. This technology has been employed in many of the handheld instruments for bedside testing and smaller instruments used in physicians' offices and clinics.

Principle of Technology Employed in Reflectance Spectrophotometry

Different surfaces have different optical properties. The optical properties of plastic strips or test paper are different from those of dry film. To use a reflectance spectrophotometer, the system must use a standard with the same specific surface optical properties as the specific surface used in the test system. The use of reflectance spectrophotometry provides the quantitative measurement of reactions on surfaces such as strips, cartridges, and dry film.

The amount of light reflected and then measured depends on the specific instrumentation employed. Variables are: angles at which the reflected light is measured and the area of the surface being used for the measurement. Since employment of this technology depends on the use of products manufactured for use in the specific instrumentation, manufacturing processes (quality-control considerations) or shipping and handling or storage problems can affect the resulting measurements.

Quality control for single test instruments—using instrument-based systems—has been integrated into the instruments by the manufacturers. As long as the reagent packs or tabs have been properly stored and are used within the stated outdate, the manufacturer assures the user that calibration of the instrument will function automatically, crucial quality-control information has been encoded via the bar code on the unit packs, and real-time processing is monitored. Use of the usual quality-control measures in place for the laboratory can be problematic for this technology, because when the single-test, instrument-based systems are used, each time a new cartridge, pack, or strip is inserted into the instrument, a new test system is created.

Parts of a Reflectance Spectrophotometer

The instrumentation necessary for a reflectance spectrophotometer is similar to that of a filter photometer, in which the filter serves to direct the selected wavelength for the methodology. A lamp generates light, which passes through the filter and a series of slits and is focused on the test surface (Fig. 6-7). As in the case of a filter photometer, some light is absorbed by the filter; in the reflectance spectrophotometer, the remaining light is reflected. The light that is reflected is analogous to the light transmitted by the filter spectrophotometer. The reflected light passes next through a series of slits and lenses and on to the photodetector device, where the amount of light is measured and recorded as a signal. The signal is then converted to an appropriate readout.

Instruments Used in Reflectance Spectrophotometry

A major use for reflectance spectrophotometry is for the many instruments now available for point-of-care testing (POCT), including analyzers used in physicians' offices and clinics. Common bedside testing and self-testing instruments used for quantitation of blood glucose (employing a single-test methodology) for maintaining

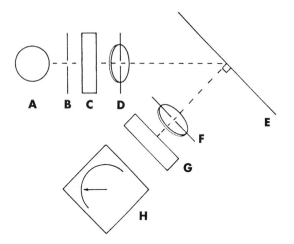

FIG. 6-7. Diagram of reflectance spectrophotometer. **A,** Light source; **B,** slit; **C,** filter or wavelength selector; **D,** lens or slit; **E,** test surface; **F,** lens or slit; **G,** detector/photodetector device; **H,** readout device. (From Kaplan LA, Pesce AJ: *Clinical Chemistry: Theory, Analysis, and Correlation,* ed 3. St Louis, Mosby, 1996, p 94.)

good diabetic control are one example. Chemistry and therapeutic drug monitoring analyzer systems also employ this technology, an example being the Reflotron,* for which reagents have been integrated into disposable unit-dose devices. The Reflotron system uses dry reagent tabs containing a magnetic code to identify the tests, reaction parameters, and calibration curve for each assay done. These reagent tabs have a long shelf-life—up to two years in some cases. In this system, blood is placed on a glass-fiber pad, the plasma is separated from the red cells and the plasma transported away from the red cells by capillary action, the required plasma sample volume is added to the reagent at a temperature of 37° C, excess plasma is removed, and the concentration of the desired analyte is determined by reflectance spectrophotometry. The Reflotron system is a single-test system, and blood used for it can be obtained by capillary puncture of the finger or heel. The ability to perform quantitative analyses on only a few microliters of whole

blood is a significant benefit of the use of this technology.

In urinalysis testing, the Clinitek Atlas* uses dry reagent reflectance spectrophotometry technology.

FLAME EMISSION PHOTOMETRY

Use and Principle of Flame Emission Photometry

Flame emission photometry is used most commonly for the quantitative measurement of lithium, sodium, and potassium in body fluids. In flame emission analysis by emission photometry, a solution containing metal ions is sprayed into a flame. The metal ions are energized to emit light of a characteristic color. Atoms of many metallic elements, when given sufficient energy (such as that supplied by a hot flame), will emit this energy at wavelengths characteristic of the elements. Lithium produces a red, sodium a yellow, potassium a violet, and magnesium a blue color in a flame. Sodium and potassium are the metal ions most commonly measured in biological specimens, but lithium, which is not normally present in serum, may also be measured in connection with the use of lithium salts in the treatment of some psychiatric disorders. The intensity of the color is proportional to the amount of the element burned in the flame. **Flame photometers** are laboratory instruments that make use of this principle. Details of the operation of a specific flame photometer should be obtained from the manufacturer, but a few general principles and components are common to most instruments.

Essential Parts of Flame Photometer

An atomizer is needed to spray the sample as fine droplets into the flame. Another name for atomizer is nebulizer (Fig. 6-8). The atomizer creates a fine spray of the sample and feeds this spray into a burner. The fine spray is produced

---

*Boehringer Mannheim Diagnostics, Indianapolis, Ind.

*Bayer Corp, Diagnostic Division, Tarrytown, NY.

FILTER AND PLATES WITH SLITS

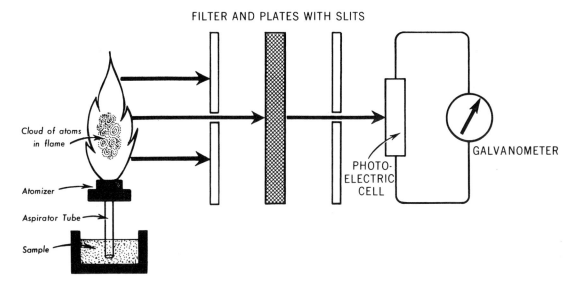

FIG 6-8. Essential parts of a flame emission photometer.

by combining a stream of sample with a stream of air. A total-consumption burner feeds the entire sample directly into the flame. A premix atomizer mixes the fuel gases and the sample in a mixing chamber before sending this mixture to the flame. Both types of atomizers are available.

In most flame photometers the fuel usually consists of various combinations of acetylene, propane, oxygen, natural gas, and compressed air. The combinations and types of fuel used determine the temperature of the flame. For sodium and potassium determinations, a propane–compressed air flame appears entirely adequate. The atomizer and the flame are critical components of a flame photometer. The most important variable in the flame itself is the temperature, since the energy emitted by the metal ions is measured and the number of energized metal ions is dependent on the temperature of the flame. Frequent standardization of flame photometers is essential, because thermal changes occur and affect the operation of the instrument and subsequent measurements with it.

Flame photometers must also have a filter, prism, grating, or other device for selecting light of the appropriate wavelength for the element to

be measured. These devices spread or disperse the light into its spectral components. The desired wavelength is selected by means of a narrow slit. In this respect the flame photometer is similar to the spectrophotometer. However, the light source described for the spectrophotometer has been replaced with an atomizer-flame combination in the flame photometer. The flame photometer must also have an electronic measuring device to detect the intensity of the emitted light. Photocells or photo tubes are used to detect the light intensity by converting the light into an electrical current. The amount of current generated is proportional to the quantity of light that reaches the detector. The amount of current is measured by a galvanometer or other recording device (see under Absorbance Spectrophotometry).

Types of Flame Photometers

An example of a flame photometer that operates according to an absolute or direct principle is one in which the intensity of color is proportional to the amount of the element burned in the flame. When an unknown sample is being measured, its intensity of color is compared with that of a standard solution of the element being measured. For example, a standard solution of potassium is used for measuring potassium.

In another commonly used method of flame photometry, the principle of the **internal standard** is applied. Most currently used flame photometers employ an internal standard. In this method, another element, usually lithium, is added to all solutions analyzed—blanks, standards, and unknowns. Lithium is usually absent from biological fluids, and it has a high emission intensity. It also emits at a wavelength sufficiently distant from that of potassium or sodium to permit spectral isolation. In flame photometry using the internal standard principle, the emission of the unknown element (sodium or potassium) is compared with that of the reference element lithium. By measuring the ratios of the emissions, any change in gas or air pressure, line voltage, flame temperature, rate of atomization, or other small variable will be minimized because both the unknown element and the reference element are affected simultaneously. A specially designed adaptation of the machine is used for this purpose, and the ratio of the reference lithium and unknown metal emissions is measured by two detectors. Two filter systems are set up, one for the unknown and one for the lithium reference. Lithium does not function as a "true" standard in its use as a reference solution. Therefore, various known concentrations of potassium or sodium are prepared and used to establish calibration curves. The use of lithium as the reference solution can cause problems, however, because lithium salts are given to patients being treated for manic-depressive states. In these patients, the lithium level must be measured.

REFERENCES

1. Burtis CA, Ashwood ER (eds): *Tietz Fundamentals of Clinical Chemistry*, ed 4. Philadelphia, WB Saunders Co, 1996, p 55.

BIBLIOGRAPHY

Campbell JB, Campbell JM: *Laboratory Mathematics: Medical and Biological Applications*, ed 5, St Louis, Mosby, 1997.

Henry JB (ed): *Clinical Diagnosis and Management by Laboratory Methods*, ed 19. Philadelphia, WB Saunders Co, 1996.

Kaplan LA, Pesce AJ: *Clinical Chemistry: Theory, Analysis, and Correlation*, ed 3. St Louis, Mosby, 1996.

STUDY QUESTIONS

1. A. Complete the following: In a colored solution, the intensity of the color at a constant depth is directly proportional to the _____ of the substance present.
   B. What is this principle called?

2. What is the approximate range of wavelengths of light that is visible to the human eye?

3. For a substance to be measured by photometry, what physical capability must be present in the substance?

4. What determines the color of light seen by the human eye?

5. If a solution appears green in absorbance spectrophotometry, which colors are being absorbed and which are being transmitted?

6. Match each of the following photometry instruments (1 to 3) with its most general use (A to C):

   1. Absorbance spectrophotometer
   2. Flame photometer
   3. Reflectance spectrophotometer

_____ A. To measure the concentration of sodium or potassium in a body fluid or serum

_____ B. To measure the concentration of glucose in blood by using dry film technology

_____ C. To measure the concentration of hemoglobin in a solution

7. **Match each of the following ways of plotting the concentration of a substance (1 and 2) with the type of graph paper used to obtain a straight line on the graph (A and B):**

1. Concentration plotted against percent transmittance
2. Concentration plotted against absorbance

   _____ A. Linear graph paper; plot is a linear relationship

   _____ B. Semilogarithmic graph paper; plot is not a linear relationship

8. **List two or three uses for reflectance spectrophotometric technology.**

CHAPTER 7

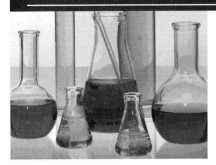

Laboratory Mathematics

Learning Objectives

From study of this chapter, the reader will be able to:

➤ Use proportions and ratios.
➤ Know the rules for rounding off numbers and for the use of significant figures.
➤ Use exponents.
➤ Describe the procedures for making a single dilution and a serial dilution.
➤ Calculate the amount of one solution needed to make a solution of a lesser concentration from it.
➤ Differentiate the expressions of solution concentration weight per unit weight, weight per unit volume, and volume per unit volume.
➤ Know how to prepare a percent solution.
➤ Describe the differences between molar and normal solutions and be able to calculate how to prepare solutions of a given volume and normality or molarity.

IMPORTANCE OF LABORATORY CALCULATIONS

With the advent of computerized instrumentation in many laboratories, the formerly repetitious calculations that were necessary are now done via the computer interfaced with the analytic instrument. It remains important for the persons using these instruments, however, to know the way mathematics is applied to obtain the results achieved. It is important for any person involved in doing clinical laboratory analyses to understand not only how the necessary calculations are done but also why the mathematical concepts work as they do. The principles on which a particular formula is based must be understood and not only the formula itself. If principles are understood thoroughly, modifications can be made, when necessary.

A sound background in basic mathematics (including algebra), an understanding of the units in which quantities are expressed, and a knowledge of the methods of analysis are all necessary in performing laboratory calculations. There are no simple formulas for solving all such problems, but certain fundamentals are a part of many of the problems encountered in a clinical laboratory.

PROPORTIONS AND RATIOS

The use of proportions involves a commonsense approach to problem solving. **Proportions** are used to determine a quantity from a given ratio. A **ratio** is an amount of something compared to an amount of something else.

Ratios always describe a relative amount, and at least two values are always involved. For example, 5 g of something dissolved in 100 mL of something else can be expressed by the ratio 5/100, 5:100, or 5 ÷ 100, or by the decimal 0.05. Proportion is a means of saying that two ratios are equal. Thus, the ratio 5:100 is equal, or proportional to, the ratio 1/20. This proportion can be expressed as 5:100 = 1:20. In the laboratory, proportions and ratios are useful when it is necessary to make more (or less) of the same thing.

However, ratios and proportions can be used only when the concentration (or any other kind of relationship) does not change.

The following is an example of a proportion or ratio problem: A formula calls for 5 g of sodium chloride (NaCl) in 1000 mL of solution. If only 500 mL of solution is needed, how much NaCl is required?

$$\frac{5\ g}{1,000\ mL} = \frac{x\ g}{500\ mL}$$

$$x = \frac{5\ g \times 500\ mL}{1,000\ mL}$$

$$x = 2.5\ g\ NaCl$$

In setting up ratio and proportion problems, the two ratios being compared must be written in the same order and they must be in the same units.

When specimens are diluted in the various laboratory analyses, the ratio principle is applied. This use of dilutions is described later in this section.

Relating Concentrations of Solutions

To relate different concentrations of solutions that contain the same amount of substance (or solute), a basic relationship, or ratio, is used. The volume of one solution (V_1) times the concentration of that solution (C_1) equals the volume of the second solution (V_2) times the concentration of the second solution (C_2), or:

$$V_1 \times C_1 = V_2 \times C_2$$

If any three of the values are known, the fourth may be determined. This relationship shows that when a solution is diluted, the volume is increased as the concentration is decreased. However, the total amount of substance (or solute) remains unchanged. Several applications of this relationship are used in the clinical laboratory, some of them being in titrations (see under Titration in Chapter 4), in dilution of specimens, and in the preparation of weaker solutions from stronger solutions.

An example of making a less concentrated solution from one more concentrated is as follows: A sodium hydroxide (NaOH) solution is available that has a concentration of 10 g of NaOH per deciliter (dL) of solution (1 dL = 100 mL). To calculate the volume of the 10 g/dL NaOH solution required to prepare 1,000 mL of 2 g/dL NaOH:

$$V_1 \times C_1 = V_2 \times C_2$$
$$x \text{ mL} \times 10 \text{ g/dL} = 1,000 \text{ mL} \times 2 \text{ g/dL}$$
$$x = \frac{2 \text{ g/dL} \times 1,000 \text{ mL}}{10 \text{ g/dL}} = 200 \text{ mL}$$

Note that this relationship is not a direct proportion; instead, it is an inverse proportion. As this is a proportion problem, it is important to remember that the concentrations and volumes on both sides of the equation must be expressed in the same units.

DILUTIONS

It is often necessary **to make dilutions** of specimens being analyzed or to make weaker solutions from stronger solutions in various laboratory procedures. It is therefore necessary to be capable of working with various dilution problems and **dilution factors.** In these problems one must often be able to determine the concentration of material in each solution, the actual amount of material in each solution, and the total volume of each solution. All dilutions are a kind of ratio. Dilution is an indication of relative concentration.

Diluting Specimens

In most laboratory determinations, a small sample is taken for analysis, and the final result is expressed as concentration per some convenient standard volume. In a certain procedure, 0.5 mL of blood is diluted to a total of 10 mL with various reagents, and 1 mL of this dilution is then analyzed for a particular chemical constituent. The final result is to be expressed in terms of the concentration of that substance per 100 mL of blood.

Dilution Factor

A dilution factor is used to correct for having used a diluted sample in a determination rather than the undiluted sample. The result (answer) using the dilution must be multiplied by the reciprocal of the dilution made.

For example, a dilution factor by which all determination answers are multiplied to give the concentration per 100 mL of sample (blood) may be calculated as follows:

First determine the volume of blood that is actually analyzed in the procedure. By use of a simple proportion, it is evident that 0.5 mL of blood diluted to 10 mL is equivalent to 1 mL of blood diluted to 20 mL.

$$\frac{0.5 \text{ mL blood}}{10 \text{ mL solution}} = \frac{1 \text{ mL blood}}{x \text{ mL solution}}$$
$$x = \frac{1 \text{ mL} \times 10 \text{ mL}}{0.5 \text{ mL}} = 20 \text{ mL}$$

In other words, there is a 1:20 dilution of blood in this procedure—that is, 1 mL of blood diluted to a total volume of 20 mL with the desired diluent (usually saline or deionized water) or reagents. This is the same as 1 mL of blood plus 19 mL of diluent.

The concentration of specimen (blood) in each milliliter of solution may be determined, by the use of another simple proportion, to be 0.05 mL of blood per milliliter of solution:

$$\frac{1 \text{ mL blood}}{20 \text{ mL solution}} = \frac{x \text{ mL blood}}{1 \text{ mL solution}}$$
$$x = \frac{1 \text{ mL} \times 1 \text{ mL}}{20 \text{ mL}} = 0.05 \text{ mL}$$

Since 1 mL of the 1:20 dilution of blood is analyzed in the remaining steps of the procedure, 0.05 mL of blood is actually analyzed (1 mL of the dilution used × 0.05 mL/mL = 0.05 mL of blood analyzed).

To relate the concentration of the substance measured in the procedure to the concentration in 100 mL of blood (the units in which the result is to be expressed), another proportion may be used:

$$\frac{100 \text{ mL (volume of blood desired)}}{0.05 \text{ mL (volume of blood used)}} =$$

$$\frac{\text{Concentration desired}}{\text{Concentration used or determined}}$$

Concentration desired =

$$\frac{100 \text{ mL} \times \text{Concentration determined}}{0.05 \text{ mL}}$$

Concentration desired = 2,000 × Value determined

In other words, the concentration of the substance being measured in the volume of blood actually tested (0.05 mL) must be multiplied by 2,000 in order to report the concentration per 100 mL of blood.

The preceding material may be summarized by the following statement and equations. In reporting results obtained from laboratory determinations, one must first determine the amount of specimen actually analyzed in the procedure and then calculate the factor that will express the concentration in the desired terms of measurement. Thus, in the previous example the following equations may be used:

$$\frac{0.5 \text{ mL (volume of blood used)}}{10 \text{ mL (volume of total dilution)}} =$$

$$\frac{x \text{ mL (volume of blood analyzed)}}{1 \text{ mL (volume of dilution used)}}$$

x = 0.05 mL (volume of blood actually analyzed)

$$\frac{100 \text{ mL (volume of blood required for expression of result)}}{0.05 \text{ mL (volume of blood actually analyzed)}}$$

= 2,000 (dilution factor)

Single Dilutions

When the concentration of a particular substance in a specimen is too great to be accurately determined, or when there is less specimen available for analysis than the procedure requires, it may be necessary to dilute the original specimen, or to further dilute the initial dilution (or filtrate). Such **single dilutions** are usually expressed as a ratio, such as 1:2, 1:5, or 1:10, or as a fraction, ½,

⅕, or ¹⁄₁₀. These ratios or fractions refer to 1 unit of the original specimen diluted to a final volume of 2, 5, or 10 units, respectively. A **dilution** therefore refers to the volume or number of parts of the substance to be diluted in the total volume, or parts, of the final solution. A dilution is an expression of concentration; it indicates the relative amount of substance in solution—not an expression of volume. Dilutions can be made singly or in series.

To calculate the concentration of a single dilution, multiply the original concentration by the dilution expressed as a fraction.

Calculation of the Concentration of a Single Dilution

A specimen contains 500 mg of substance per deciliter of blood. A 1:5 dilution of this specimen is prepared by volumetrically measuring 1 mL of the specimen and adding 4 mL of diluent (usually distilled water or saline). The concentration of substance in the dilution is:

$$500 \text{ mg/dL} \times \tfrac{1}{5} = 100 \text{ mg/dL}$$

Note that the concentration of the final solution (or dilution) is expressed in the same units as that of the original solution.

To obtain a dilution factor that can be applied to the determination answer in order to express it as a concentration per standard volume, proceed as follows. Rather than multiply by the dilution expressed as a fraction, multiply the determination value by the reciprocal of the dilution fraction. In the case of a 1:5 dilution, the dilution factor that would be applied to values obtained in the procedure would be 5, since the original specimen was five times more concentrated than the diluted specimen tested in the procedure.

Use of Dilution Factors

A 1:5 dilution of a specimen is prepared, and an **aliquot** (one of a number of equal parts) of the dilution is analyzed for a particular substance. The concentration of the substance in the aliquot is multiplied by 5 to determine its concentration in the original specimen. If the concentration of the dilution is 100 mg/dL, the concentration of the original specimen is:

100 mg/dL × 5 (the dilution factor) = 500 mg/dL in blood

Serial Dilutions

As mentioned previously, dilutions can be made singly or in series, in which case the original solution is further diluted. A general rule for calculating the concentrations of solutions obtained by dilution in series is to multiply the original concentration by the first dilution (expressed as a fraction), this by the second dilution, and so on until the desired concentration is known.

Several laboratory procedures, especially serologic ones, make use of a dilution series in which all dilutions, including or following the first one, are the same. Such dilutions are referred to as **serial dilutions.** A complete dilution series

usually contains five or ten tubes, although any single dilution may be made directly from an undiluted specimen or substance. In calculating the dilution or concentration of substance or serum in each tube of the dilution series, the rules previously discussed apply.

A five-tube twofold dilution may be prepared as follows (see Fig. 7-1): A serum specimen is diluted 1:2 with buffer. A series of five tubes are prepared, in which each succeeding tube is rediluted 1:2. This is accomplished by placing 1 mL of diluent into each of four tubes (tubes 2 to 5). Tube 1 contains 1 mL of undiluted serum. Tube 2 contains 1 mL of undiluted serum plus 1 mL of diluent, resulting in a 1:2 dilution of serum. A 1-mL portion of the 1:2 dilution of serum is placed in tube 3, resulting in a 1:4 dilution of serum ($\frac{1}{2} \times \frac{1}{2} = \frac{1}{4}$). A 1-mL portion of the 1:4 dilution from tube 3 is placed in tube 4, resulting in a 1:8 dilution ($\frac{1}{4} \times \frac{1}{2} = \frac{1}{8}$). Finally, 1 mL of the 1:8 dilution from tube 4 is added to tube 5, re-

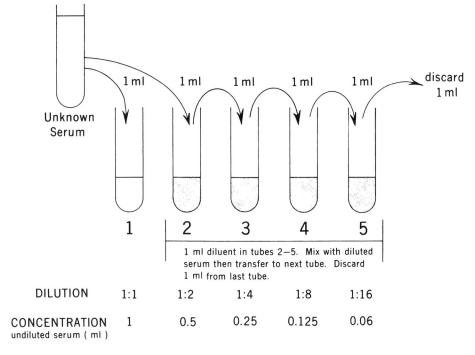

DILUTION	1:1	1:2	1:4	1:8	1:16
CONCENTRATION undiluted serum (ml)	1	0.5	0.25	0.125	0.06

FIG 7-1. Five-tube twofold dilution.

sulting in a 1:16 dilution ($\frac{1}{8} \times \frac{1}{2} = \frac{1}{16}$). One milliliter of the final dilution is discarded so that the volumes in all the tubes are equal. Note that each tube is diluted twice as much as the previous tube and that the final volume in each tube is the same. The undiluted serum may also be given a dilution value, namely 1:1.

The concentration of serum in terms of milliliters in each tube is calculated by multiplying the previous concentration (mL) by the succeeding dilution. In this example tube 1 contains 1 mL of serum, tube 2 contains 1 mL $\times \frac{1}{2} = 0.5$ mL of serum, and tubes 3 to 5 contain 0.25, 0.125, and 0.06 mL of serum, respectively.

Other serial dilutions might be fivefold or tenfold; that is, each succeeding tube is diluted five or ten times. A fivefold series would begin with 1 mL of serum in 4 mL of diluent and a total volume of 5 mL in each tube, while a tenfold series would begin with 1 mL of serum in 9 mL of diluent and a total volume of 10 mL in each tube. Other systems might begin with a 1:2 dilution and then dilute five succeeding tubes 1:10. The dilutions in such a series would be 1:2, 1:20 ($\frac{1}{2} \times \frac{1}{10} = \frac{1}{20}$), 1:200 ($\frac{1}{20} \times \frac{1}{10} = \frac{1}{200}$), 1:2,000, 1:20,000, and 1:200,000.

Calculation of the Concentration After a Series of Dilutions

A working solution is prepared from a stock solution. In so doing, a stock solution with a concentration of 100 mg/dL is diluted 1:10 by volumetrically adding 1 mL of it to 9 mL of diluent. The diluted solution (intermediate solution) is further diluted 1:100 by volumetrically measuring 1 mL of intermediate solution and diluting to the mark in a 100-mL volumetric flask. The concentration of the final or working solution is:

$$100 \text{ mg/dL} \times \frac{1}{10} \times \frac{1}{100} = 0.1 \text{ mg/dL}$$

SIGNIFICANT FIGURES

Using more digits than are necessary to calculate and report the results of a laboratory determination has several disadvantages. It is important that the number used contain only the digits necessary for the precision of the determination. Using more digits than necessary is misleading in that it ascribes more accuracy to the determination than is actually the case. There is also the danger of overlooking a decimal point and making an error in judging the magnitude of the answer. Digits in a number that are needed to express the precision of the measurement from which the number is derived are known as **significant figures.** A significant figure is one that is known to be reasonably reliable. Judgment must be exercised in determining how many figures should be used. Some rules to assist in making such decisions are as follows:

1. Use the known accuracy of the method to determine the number of digits that are significant in the answer, and, as a general rule, retain one more figure than this. An example is: A urea nitrogen result was reported as 11.2 mg/dL. This would indicate that the result is accurate to the nearest tenth and that the exact value lies between 11.15 and 11.25. In reality, the accuracy of most urea nitrogen methods is ±10%, so that the result reported as 11.2 mg/dL could actually vary from 10 to 12 mg/dL and should be reported as 11 mg/dL. In addition, if the decimal point were omitted or overlooked, the result could be taken as 112 mg/dL.

2. Take the accuracy of the least accurate measurement, or the measurement with the least number of significant figures, as the accuracy of the final result. In doing so, certain things must be done in the addition and subtraction or multiplication and division of numerals. An example of addition or subtraction is as follows: In order to add

$$
\begin{array}{r}
206.1 \\
7.56 \\
\underline{0.8764}
\end{array}
$$

rewrite it as

$$
\begin{array}{r}
206.1 \\
7.6 \\
\underline{0.9}
\end{array}
$$

In this example, the least accurate figure is accurate to one decimal place; this is therefore the determining factor. In determining the least accurate figure, the following rule is utilized: in a column of addition or subtraction, in which the decimal points are placed one above the other, the number of significant figures in the final answer is determined by the first digit encountered going from left to right that terminates any one numeral.

An example of multiplication or division is as follows: In the division of

$$32.973 \div 4.3 =$$

the result should be reported as 7.7. This is determined by utilizing the following general rule: the number of significant figures in the final product or quotient should not exceed the smallest number of significant figures in any one factor.

Rounding Off Numbers

Test results sometimes produce insignificant digits. It is then necessary to **round off the numbers** to a chosen number of significant value in order not to imply an accuracy of precision greater than the test is capable of delivering.

The following general rule may be used in rounding off decimal values to the proper place: When the digit next to the last one to be retained is less than 5, the last digit should be left unchanged. When the digit next to the last one to be retained is greater than 5, the last digit is increased by 1. If the additional digit is 5, the last digit reported is changed to the nearest even number. Examples are as follows:

2.31463 g is rounded off to 2.3146 g.
5.34659 g is rounded off to 5.3466 g.
23.5 mg is rounded off to 24 mg.
24.5 mg is rounded off to 24 mg.

EXPONENTS

Exponents are used to indicate that a number must be multiplied by itself as many times as is indicated by the exponent. The number that is to be multiplied by itself is called the base. Usually the exponent is written as a small superscript figure to the immediate right of the base figure and is sometimes referred to as the power of the base. The exponent figure can have either a plus sign or a minus sign before it. The plus sign is usually implied and does not actually appear.

A **positive exponent** indicates the number of times the base is to be multiplied by itself.

Examples of exponents with no sign or a plus sign (positive exponents) are as follows:

$$10^2 = 10 \times 10 = 100$$
$$10^5 = 10 \times 10 \times 10 \times 10 \times 10 = 100,000$$
$$5^3 = 5 \times 5 \times 5 = 125$$

A **negative exponent** indicates the number of times the reciprocal of the base is to be multiplied by itself—in other words, a negative exponent indicates a fraction.

Examples of exponents with a minus sign (negative exponents) are as follows:

$$10^{-1} = \frac{1}{10} = 0.1$$

$$10^{-4} = \frac{1}{10} \times \frac{1}{10} \times \frac{1}{10} \times \frac{1}{10} \times \frac{1}{10,000} = 0.0001$$

EXPRESSIONS OF SOLUTION CONCENTRATION

Solutions are made up of a mixture of substances. In making up a solution, there usually are two main parts, the substance that is being dissolved (the **solute**) and the substance into which the solute is being dissolved (the **solvent**). In working with solutions, it is necessary to know, or to be able to measure, the relative amounts of the substance in solution—known as the **concentration of the solution.** Concentration is the amount of one substance relative to the amounts of the other substances in the solution.

Solution concentration is expressed in several different ways. The most common methods used in clinical laboratories involve either weight per unit weight (w/w), also known as mass per unit mass (m/m); weight per unit volume (w/v), also known as mass per unit volume (m/v); or volume per unit volume (v/v). Weight is the term commonly used, although mass is really what is being measured. Mass is the amount of matter in something, and weight is the force of gravity on something. The most accurate measurement is weight per unit weight, since weight (or mass) does not vary with temperature as does volume. Probably the most common measurement is weight per unit volume. The least accurate measurement is volume per unit volume, because of the changes in volume resulting from temperature changes. Volume per unit volume is used in the preparation of a liquid solution from another liquid substance. A few concentrations are expressed as a proper name, such as Wright's stain (used in hematology) or the Sudan III stain (used to demonstrate fat).

Proper Name

There are very few instances in which a solution is described by a proper name as far as its concentration is concerned. This solution is prepared with specific amounts of ingredients according to a series of instructions or directions. When Wright's stain is needed, one knows exactly what is meant and what chemicals in which amounts are used in its preparation.

Weight (Mass) per Unit Volume (w/v)

The most common way of expressing concentration is by **weight (mass) per unit volume (w/v).** When weight (mass) per unit volume is used, the amount of solute (the substance that goes into solution) per volume of solution is expressed. Weight per unit volume is used most often when a solid chemical is diluted in a liquid. The usual way to express weight per unit volume is as grams per liter (g/L) or milligrams per milliliter (mg/mL). If a concentration of a certain solution is given as 10 g/L, it means that there are 10 g of solute for every liter of solution. If a solution with a concentration of 10 mg/mL is desired and 100 mL of this solution is to be prepared, the use

of a proportion formula can be applied. An example follows:

$$\frac{10 \text{ mg}}{1 \text{ mL}} = \frac{x \text{ mg}}{100 \text{ mL}} = 1{,}000 \text{ mg, or } 1 \text{ g}$$

One gram of the desired solute is weighed and diluted to 100 mL (see under Reagents Used in Laboratory Assays, in Chapter 4).

In working with standard solutions, it will be seen that their concentrations, almost without exception, are expressed as milligrams per milliliter (mg/mL).

Volume per Unit Volume (v/v)

Another way of expressing concentration is by **volume per unit volume (v/v).** Volume per unit volume is used to express concentration when a liquid chemical is diluted with another liquid; the concentration is expressed as the number of milliliters of liquid chemical per unit volume of solution. The usual way to express volume per unit volume is as milliliters per milliliter (mL/mL) or milliliters per liter (mL/L). The number of milliliters of liquid chemical in 1 mL or 1 L of solution utilizes the volume per unit volume expression of concentration. If 10 mL of alcohol is diluted to 100 mL with water, the concentration is expressed as 10 mL/100 mL, or 10 mL/dl, or 0.1 mL/mL, or 100 mL/L. If a solution with a concentration of 0.5 mL/mL is desired and 1 L is to be prepared, a proportion can again be used to solve the problem. An example follows:

$$\frac{0.5 \text{ mL}}{1 \text{ mL}} = \frac{x \text{ mL}}{1{,}000 \text{ mL}}$$
$$x = 500 \text{ mL}$$

Thus 500 mL of the liquid chemical is measured accurately and diluted to 1,000 mL (1 L).

To express concentration in milliliters per liter, one needs to know how many milliliters of liquid chemical there are in 1 L of the solution.

Any chemical (liquid or solid) can be made into a solution by diluting it with a solvent. The usual solvent is deionized or distilled water (see under Laboratory Reagent Water, in Chapter 4). If the desired chemical is a liquid, the amount needed is measured in milliliters or liters (on occasion liquids are weighed, but the usual method is to measure their volume); if the desired chemical is a solid, the amount needed is weighed in grams or milligrams.

Weight per Unit Weight (w/w)

Another way of expressing concentration is by **weight per unit weight** or **mass per unit mass (m/m)**. This expression is not commonly used. Not many reagents are prepared by using only solid chemicals and no liquid solvent. When the desired chemical is a solid and it is mixed with, or diluted with, another solid, the expression of concentration is mass per unit mass. The usual way to express mass per unit mass is as milligrams per milligram (mg/mg), grams per gram (g/g), or grams per kilogram (g/kg). The number of milligrams or grams of one solid in the total number of milligrams or grams of the dry mixture is the mass per unit mass.

Percent

Another expression of concentration is the percent solution (%), although in the SI system the preferred units are kilograms (or fractions thereof) per liter (w/v) or milliliters per liter (v/v). A description of the percent solution follows, as this expression of concentration is still used in some instances. **Percent** is defined as parts per hundred parts (the part can be any particular unit). Unless otherwise stated, a percent solution usually means grams or milliliters of solute per 100 mL of solution (g/100 mL or mL/100 mL). Recall that 100 mL is equal to 1 deciliter (dL). Percent solutions can be prepared by using either liquid or solid chemicals. Percent solutions can be expressed either as weight per unit volume percent (w/v%) or as volume per unit volume percent (v/v%), depending on the state of the solute (chemical) used—that is, whether it is a solid

or a liquid. When a solid chemical is dissolved in a liquid, percent means grams of solid in 100 mL of solution. If 10 g of NaCl is diluted to 100 mL with deionized water, the concentration is expressed as 10% (10 g/dL). If 2.5 g is diluted to 100 mL, the concentration is 2.5% (2.5 g/dL).

The following is an example of concentration expressed in percent: Ten grams of NaOH is diluted to 200 mL with water. What is the concentration in percent? A proportion can be set up to solve this problem:

$$\frac{10 \text{ g}}{200 \text{ mL}} = \frac{x \text{ g}}{100 \text{ mL}}$$

x = 5% solution (preferably expressed as 5 g/dL)

Remember that the percent expression is based on how much solute is present in 100 mL (or 1 dL) of the solution.

Some concentrations of solutions are expressed as milligrams of solute in 100 mL of solution (mg%). When this method of expression is used, mg% is always specifically stated. If 25 mg of a chemical is diluted to 100 mL, the concentration in milligrams percent would be 25 mg% (preferably expressed as 25 mg/dL).

If a liquid chemical is used to prepare a percent solution, the concentration is expressed as volume per unit volume percent, or milliliters of solute per 100 mL of solution. If 10 mL of hydrochloric acid (HCl) is diluted to 100 mL with water, the concentration is 10% (preferably expressed as 10 ml/dL). If 10 mL of the same acid is diluted to 1 L (1,000 mL), the concentration is 1% (preferably expressed as 1 mL/dL).

Molarity

The **molarity of a solution** is defined as the gram-molecular mass (or weight) of a compound per liter of solution. This is a weight per unit volume method of expressing concentration. A basic formula follows:

Molecular weight $\times$ Molarity = Grams/liter

Another way to define molarity is as the number of moles per liter (mol/L) of solution. A mole is the molecular weight of a compound in grams (1 mole equals 1 gram-molecular weight). The number of moles of a compound equals the number of grams divided by the gram-molecular weight of that compound. One **gram-molecular weight** equals the sum of all atomic weights in a molecule of the compound, expressed in grams.

To determine the gram-molecular weight of a compound, the correct chemical formula must be known. When this formula is known, the sum of all the atomic weights in the compound can be found by consulting a periodic table of the elements or a chart with the atomic masses of the elements.

Examples of Molarity Calculations

1. Sodium chloride has one sodium ion and one chloride ion; the correct formula is written as NaCl. The gram-molecular weight is derived by finding the sum of the atomic weights:

$$Na = 23$$
$$Cl = 35.5$$
$$\text{Gram-molecular weight} = 58.5$$

If the gram-molecular weight of NaCl is 58.5 g, a 1 molar (1M) solution of NaCl would contain 58.5 g of NaCl per liter of solution, because molarity equals moles per liter, and 1 mol of NaCl equals 58.5 g.

2. For barium sulfate ($BaSO_4$), the gram-molecular weight equals 233 (the formula indicates that there are one barium, one sulfur, and four oxygen ions).

$$1\ Ba = 137 \times 1 = 137$$
$$1\ S = 32 \times 1 = 32$$
$$4\ O = 16 \times 4 = \frac{64}{233}$$

Since the gram-molecular weight is 233, a 1M solution of $BaSO_4$ would contain 233 g of $BaSO_4$ per liter of solution.

The quantities of solutions needed will not always be in units of whole liters, and often fractions or multiples of a 1M concentration will be desired. Parts of a molar solution are expressed as decimals. If a 1M solution of NaCl contains 58.5 g of NaCl per liter of solution, a 0.5M solution would contain one half of 58.5 g, or 29 g/L, and a 3M solution would contain 3 times 58.5 g, or 175.5 g/L.

What is the molarity of a solution containing 30 g of NaCl per liter? Molarity equals the number of moles per liter, and the number of moles equals the grams divided by the gram-molecular weight.

Step 1: Find the gram-molecular weight of NaCl. It is 58.5 g (Na = 23 and Cl = 35.5).

Step 2: Find the moles per liter.

$$\frac{30\ \text{g/L}}{x} = \frac{58.5\ \text{g/L}}{1\ \text{mol}}$$

$$x = \frac{30\ \text{g/L} \times 1\ \text{mol}}{58.5\ \text{g/L}} = 0.513\ \text{mol NaCl}$$

Step 3: The number of moles per liter of solution equals the molarity; the solution in the example is therefore 0.513M, rounded off to 0.5M.

Equations might prove useful to some in working with molarity solutions. However, all of these equations can be derived by applying a common sense proportion approach to molarity problems, as described above under Proportions and Ratios. Some of these equations are listed below.

$$\text{Molarity} = \frac{\text{Moles of solute}}{\text{Liters of solution}}$$

$$\text{Molarity} = \frac{\text{Grams of solute}}{\text{Gram-molecular weight}} \times \frac{1}{\text{Liters of solution}}$$

$$\text{Moles of solute} = \text{Molarity} \times \text{Liters of solution}$$

Grams of solute =
$$\text{Molarity} \times \text{Gram-molecular weight} \times \text{Liters of solution}$$

Note: These equations are all on the basis of 1 L of solution; if something other than 1 L is used, refer back to the 1-L basis (500 mL = 0.5 L, or 2,000 mL = 2 L, for example).

Molarity does not provide a basis for direct comparison of strength for all solutions. For example, 1 L of 1M NaOH will exactly neutralize 1 L of 1M HCl, but it will neutralize only 0.5 L of 1M sulfuric acid (H_2SO_4). It is therefore more convenient to choose a unit of concentration that will provide a basis for direct comparison of strengths of solutions. Such a unit is referred to as an equivalent (or equivalent weight or mass), and this term is used in describing normality.

Millimolarity

A **milligram molecular weight** (the molecular weight expressed in milligrams) is a **millimole (mmole)**. This is in contrast to the molarity described above, which is the number of moles per liter. The following formulas compare the two:

$$\text{Molarity (moles/liter)} = \frac{\text{g/L}}{\text{Molecular weight}}$$

$$\text{Millimoles/liter} = \frac{\text{mg/L}}{\text{Molecular weight}}$$

Normality

Normality is defined as the number of equivalent weights per liter of solution. The **equivalent (equiv) weight** is the mass in grams that will liberate, combine with, or replace one gram-atom (g atom) of hydrogen ion (H^+). By using equivalents, the numbers of units of all substances involved in a reaction are made numerically equal. Normality is expressed as a weight per unit volume concentration.

Examples of Normality Calculations

Reaction 1:

I equiv NaOH + I equiv HCl →
I equiv H_2O + I equiv NaCl

Reaction 2:

I equiv NaOH + I equiv H_2SO_4 →
I equiv H_2O + I equiv Na_2SO_4

The balanced equation for this reaction is:

$$2NaOH + IH_2SO_4 \rightarrow 2H_2O + INa_2SO_4$$

This same reaction expressed using moles is:

I mol NaOH + 0.5 mol H_2SO_4 →
I mol H_2O + 0.5 mol $NaSO_4$

One equivalent of any acid will neutralize one equivalent of any base.

In discussing molarity, the term moles per liter (mol/L) is used; in units of normality, the terms equivalents per liter (equiv/L), milliequivalents per milliliter (mEq/mL), and milliequivalents per liter (mEq/L) are used. The normality of a solution is defined as the number of gram-equivalents (or equivalent weights) per liter of solution, or the number of milliequivalents per milliliter of solution.

Equivalent Weight

The **equivalent weight** (or **mass**) is the weight in grams that will liberate, combine with, or replace one gram-atom of hydrogen. The equivalent weight may be found by dividing the gram-molecular weight (GMW) by the total combining power, or **valence**, of the positive ion (ions) of the substance. As a general rule, the equivalent weight of a compound or substance (element) is equal to the molecular weight divided by the valence. The SI system prefers the use of molarity (mol/L) to express the amount of substance in chemical units. A disadvantage of the concept of normality is that a particular solution may have more than one normality, depending on the reaction in which it is used, while it will always have the same molarity, since there is only one molecular weight for any substance.

Examples of Equivalent Weights. Hydrochloric acid has one atom of H^+ and one atom of Cl^-; therefore, the gram-equivalent weight equals the molecular weight.

Hydrogen sulfide (H_2S) has two atoms of H^+ and only one atom of S^{2-}, or one atom of H^+ and one-half atom of S^{2-}; therefore, the equivalent weight equals one-half the molecular weight, or:

$$\frac{\text{Molecular weight}}{\text{Total positive valence}} = \frac{34}{2} = 17$$

NaCl has one atom of Cl^- and one atom of Na^+ (Na^+ replaces H^+); therefore, the gram-equivalent weight equals the gram-molecular weight.

A liter of a 1N solution of H_2SO_4 contains the same number of equivalents as 1 L of 1N HCl, or 1N NaOH, or 1N barium hydroxide ($Ba[OH]_2$). Again, equations might prove useful in working with normality solutions. Some of these are:

$$\text{Normality} = \frac{\text{Equivalents of solute}}{\text{Liters of solution}}$$

$$\text{Normality} = \frac{\text{Grams of solute}}{\text{GMW/combining power (valence)}} \times$$

$$\frac{1}{\text{Liters of solution}}$$

where GMW is gram-molecular weight.

$$\text{Normality} = \frac{\text{Moles}}{\text{Combining power}} \times \frac{1}{\text{Liters of solution}}$$

$$\text{Normality} = \frac{\text{Grams of solute}}{\text{Equivalent weight}} \times \frac{1}{\text{Liters of solution}}$$

$$\text{Normality} = \frac{\text{Equivalents}}{\text{Liters}}$$

$$\text{Normality} = \frac{\text{Milliequivalents}}{\text{Milliliters}}$$

Milliequivalent Weight. Just as a millimole relates to a mole, the milliequivalent (mEq) relates to the equivalent. A **milliequivalent weight** (the equivalent weight in milligrams) = 1 mEq. The following formulas apply:

$$\frac{\text{mg}}{\text{eq. wt.}} = \text{mEq}$$

$$1 \text{ eq} = 1,000 \text{ mEq}$$

$$1 \text{ mEq} = \frac{1}{1000} \text{ eq}$$

Interconversion of Molarity and Normality

On occasion, it is necessary to convert an expression of concentration in molarity to one in normality and vice versa. Two simple formulas are available for this purpose:

$$\text{Molarity} = \frac{\text{Normality}}{\text{Total positive combining power (valence)}}$$

$$\text{or } \frac{N}{\text{Valence}}$$

$$\text{Normality} = \text{Molarity} \times \text{Total positive}$$
$$\text{combining power (valence) or M} \times \text{Valence}$$

To prepare 1 L of a 2N NaCl solution, first calculate the gram-molecular weight, using the known formula for the compound: Na = 23; Cl = 35.5; the gram-molecular weight thus is 58.5 g. In working with normality problems, the gram-equivalent weight is used; therefore, the next step is to calculate this. The gram-equivalent weight equals the gram-molecular weight divided by the valence, or 58.5 g divided by 1; the gram-equivalent weight is therefore 58.5 g. For 1 L of a 1N solution of this compound, 58.5 g would be weighed; for 1 L of a 2N solution, 58.5 g × 2, or 117 g, of NaCl is needed per liter. An example of another such problem follows.

Prepare 200 mL of a 0.5N calcium chloride ($CaCl_2$) solution.

Step 1: Calculate the gram-molecular weight.

$$Ca = 40 \times 1 = 40$$

$$Cl = 35.5 \times 2 = \frac{71}{111 \text{ g}} = \text{Total gram-molecular weight}$$

Step 2: Calculate the gram-equivalent weight.

$$\text{Equivalent weight} = \frac{\text{GMW}}{\text{Valence}} = \frac{111}{2} = 55.5 \text{ g}$$

Step 3: Solve for normality. A 1N solution would contain 55.5 g/L. A 0.5N solution would contain only half as much chemical per liter of solution, or

27.8 g. A proportion could be set up to solve this:

$$\frac{55.g}{1N\ solution} = \frac{x\ g}{0.5N\ solution} = 27.8\ g$$

However, only 200 mL of this solution is needed. Therefore another proportion could be set up for this:

$$\frac{27.8\ g}{1,000\ mL} = \frac{x\ g}{200\ mL} = 5.6\ g$$

Step 4: In the actual preparation of solution, 5.6 g of $CaCl_2$ is weighed and diluted to 200 mL volumetrically (see under Reagents Used in Laboratory Assays, in Chapter 4).

Osmolarity

Osmolarity is defined as the number of osmoles of solute per liter of solution. An osmole (osm) is the amount of a substance that will produce 1 mol of particles having osmotic activity. An osmole of any substance is equal to 1 gram-molecular weight (1 mol) of the substance divided by the number of particles formed by the dissociation of the molecules of the substance. For materials that do not ionize, 1 osm is equal to 1 mol. This gives an estimate of the osmotic activity of the solution—the relative number of particles dissolved in the solution. Osmolarity is an expression of weight per unit volume concentration.

For a solution of glucose, a substance that does not ionize or dissociate in aqueous solution, 1 osm of glucose is equal to 1 mol of glucose For a solution of sodium chloride, which does ionize, 1 osm of sodium chloride is equal to 1 gram-molecular weight divided by the number of particles formed upon ionization. Sodium chloride completely ionizes in water to form one sodium ion and one chloride ion, or a total of two particles. The molecular weight of NaCl is 58.5. To calculate the osmolarity of NaCl, the following formula is used:

$$1\ osm\ NaCl = \frac{58.5}{2} = 29.25\ g$$

Density

Density is defined as the amount of matter per unit volume of a substance. All substances have this property, not only solutions. An example of the expression of density is the specific gravity of a substance. Specific gravity is defined as the ratio between the mass of a substance and the mass of an equal volume of water, or:

$$Specific\ gravity = \frac{Mass\ of\ substance}{Mass\ of\ equal\ volume\ of\ water}$$

BIBLIOGRAPHY

Campbell JB, Campbell JM: *Laboratory Mathematics: Medical and Biological Applications*, ed 5. St Louis, Mosby, 1997.

STUDY QUESTIONS

1. **Match the following terms (1 to 5) with their definitions (A to E):**

   1. Ratio
   2. Concentration
   3. Normality
   4. Molarity
   5. Dilution

   _____ A. The amount of one substance relative to the amounts of other substances in the solution

   _____ B. An indication of relative concentration

   _____ C. The gram-molecular mass (or weight) of a compound per liter of solution

   _____ D. An amount of something compared with an amount of something else

   _____ E. The number of equivalent weights per liter of solution

2. How would each of the following numbers be rounded off to 1 fewer decimal place?

   A. 63.24
   B. 15.568
   C. 10.021
   D. 25.5
   E. 24.5

3. How much of a 5 g/dL (dL = 100mL) solution of NaCl is needed to prepare 1,000 mL (1 L) of a 2 g/dL solution?

4. Express each of the following as the corresponding whole number, decimal, or fraction.

   A. 4^5
   B. 3^{-3}
   C. 10^3

5. How would you dilute a serum specimen 1:10?

6. How would you prepare 100 mL of a 5% (w/v) solution of NaCl?

7. If there are 20 g of NaCl per liter of solution, what is the molarity of the solution?

8. How would you prepare 1000 mL of a 0.5M solution of NaCl?

9. How much of a 2M solution can be made from 50 mL of a 5M solution?

10. How would you prepare 500 mL of a 0.5N solution of $CaCl_2$?

CHAPTER 8

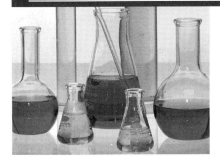

Quality Assurance in the Clinical Laboratory

Learning Objectives

From study of this chapter, the reader will be able to:

➤ Understand how federal, state, and local regulations require the implementation of quality assurance programs in the clinical laboratory, to ensure that the results reported are of medical use to the physician.

➤ Identify the components necessary to a laboratory's quality assurance program, including its quality control program and the use of control specimens.

➤ Assess the diagnostic usefulness of results reported, which requires an understanding of accuracy and precision, and specificity and sensitivity, for laboratory tests and methodologies.

➤ Understand the sources of variance or error in a laboratory procedure.

➤ Appreciate the use of reference values, including the use of the mean and the standard deviation in determination of the reference range.

➤ Appreciate the importance of a quality control program, including the use of control samples, the determination of the control range, and the use of quality control charts.

INTRODUCTION

Quality can be defined as satisfaction of the needs and expectations of the users of a service. In a clinical laboratory, the assurance of quality results for the various analyses is critical and is an important component of the operation of every good laboratory. Analytic results obtained through laboratory determinations are used by the physician both to discover the existence of disease in a patient and to follow the progress of treatment. It is the responsibility of the clinical laboratory, to both patient and physician, to ensure that the results reported are reliable and to give the physician an estimate of what constitutes "normal." The dimension of quality assurance (QA) and the improvement of quality— quality improvement, total quality improvement (TQI)—are driven by both public and private pressures and by the need to contain the cost of the service.

STANDARDS SET BY THE JOINT COMMISSION ON ACCREDITATION OF HEALTHCARE ORGANIZATIONS

The public's focus on health care delivery is relevant to most areas of work done in clinical laboratories. Agencies from public and medical communities, as well as from the government, are continually reexamining health care facilities. Standards have been set by the **Joint Commission on Accreditation of Healthcare Organizations (JCAHO),** reflecting the commission's focus on **quality assurance programs.** These standards require the monitoring and evaluation of quality and appropriateness of services to patients and the resolution of any identified problems. The JCAHO has published a ten-step monitoring process for quality assurance programs.[1] These steps are:

1. Assign responsibility for a quality assurance plan.
2. Define the scope of patient care.
3. Identify the important aspects of care.
4. Construct indicators.
5. Define the thresholds for evaluation.
6. Collect and organize the data.
7. Evaluate the data.
8. Develop a corrective action plan.
9. Assess actions; document improvement.
10. Communicate relevant information.

No concern is of greater importance than quality assurance. As defined by the JCAHO ten-step plan, **quality assurance** is an overall and continuing process by which the hospital or health care facility monitors all areas that contribute to providing the highest quality and most appropriate care for the patient. Quality assurance requires a planned, systematic process of monitoring all aspects of patient care. As part of the health care team, the clinical laboratory must also have an ongoing quality assurance process for monitoring its analytic results. The analytic results of the test or tests done on a clinical specimen must be as accurate as possible so that the physician can rely on the data and use the information in the diagnostic and treatment plan for the patient. This is the service provided by the clinical laboratory to the total health care plan for the patient. An ongoing, active, comprehensive quality assurance program is an essential component for hospital accreditation. Because quality assurance has become so important, other regulatory groups, such as the College of American Pathologists (CAP), have included quality assurance activities as necessary components of accreditation standards.[6]

COMPONENTS OF QUALITY ASSURANCE PROGRAMS

The documentation of an ongoing quality assurance program in clinical laboratories is mandated by the CLIA '88 regulations.[3]

Commitment

It is essential that all persons working in the clinical laboratory be totally committed to the concepts of the quality assurance process as it is defined by the specific health care facility. The dedication of sufficient planning time to quality assurance and the implementation of the program in the total laboratory operation are critical. All persons working in the clinical laboratory must be willing to work together to make the quality of service to the patient their top priority. Because the total laboratory staff must be involved in carrying out any quality assurance process, it is important to develop a comprehensive program to include all levels of laboratorians.

Facilities and Resources

The physical location and layout of the laboratory are an important aspect of quality assurance. Since the product of the laboratory is the analytic result for the patient's specimen, it is vital that the physical laboratory site be conducive to good performance by the laboratorians working there. A safe working site with adequate, properly maintained equipment and supplies is essential to ensure that high-quality analytic results are a reasonable expectation.

Technical Competence

The competence of personnel is an important determinant of the quality of the laboratory result. Crucial to any quality assurance process is the maintenance of a high level of performance by the laboratorians doing the analyses. Only well-trained, competent personnel should be carrying out the testing processes. CLIA '88 requirements for laboratory personnel in regard to levels of education and experience or training must be followed for laboratories doing moderately complex or highly complex testing (see under Regulation of the Clinical Laboratory, in Chapter 1). In addition to the actual performance of analytic procedures, competent laboratory personnel must be able to perform quality control activities, maintain instruments, and keep accurate and systematic records of reagents and control specimens, equipment maintenance, and patient and analytic data. For new laboratory personnel, a thorough orientation to the laboratory procedures and policies is vital.

Periodic opportunities for personal upgrading of technical skills and for obtaining new relevant information should be made available to all persons working in the laboratory. This can be accomplished through in-service training classes, opportunities to attend continuing education courses, and by encouraging independent study habits by means of scientific journals and audiovisual materials.

Personnel performance should be monitored with periodic evaluations and reports. Quality assurance demands that the results of daily work be monitored by a supervisor and that all analytic reports produced during a particular shift be evaluated for errors and omissions. Quality control measures are used to monitor possible human error in performing laboratory analyses. Quality control is one aspect of the quality assurance process and is discussed in more detail below.

Quality Assurance Procedures

Quality assurance programs monitor test requesting procedures; patient identification, specimen procurement, and labeling; specimen transportation and processing procedures; laboratory personnel performance; laboratory instrumentation, reagents, and analytic test procedures; turnaround times; and the accuracy of the final result. Complete documentation of all procedures involved in obtaining the final analytic result for the patient sample must be maintained and monitored in a systematic manner. Some of these procedures are described in the following sections.

Test Requesting

The request form for each patient's laboratory work must be completed by the physician directing the patient's care. The form must include the patient identification data, the time and date of specimen collection, the source of the specimen, and the analyses requested to be done. The complete request form must accompany the specimen. It is of interest to the laboratory to note the time of receipt of the specimen. This information is necessary for the monitoring of turnaround times—the interval between receipt of the specimen in the laboratory and release of the analytic result when the test has been completed and the result verified. The request form must be clean and legible. The information on the accompanying specimen container must match exactly the patient identification on the request slip. The information needed by the physician to assist in ordering tests is included in a database or handbook described in the following section.

Patient Identification, Specimen Procurement, and Labeling

A process of educating physicians, nurses, laboratorians, and other health care personnel who are involved in collecting clinical specimens is extremely important. A computerized (electronic) database or handbook of specimen requirement information, in an easily accessible format and location, is one of the first steps in establishing a quality assurance program for the clinical laboratory. This information must be made available on the patient care units or any other place where patient specimens are collected, and it must be kept current. Information about obtaining appropriate specimens, special collection requirements for special kinds of tests, ordering tests correctly, and transporting and processing specimens appropriately is included in this information. Any changes in content must be communicated to those persons needing the information.

Patients must be carefully identified. For hospitalized patients, the most convenient way to do so is to have the patient wear a wristband with the necessary information printed on it.

Using established specimen requirement information, the clinical specimens must be properly labeled or identified once they have been obtained from the patient. The practice of using standard precautions in collecting specimens cannot be overemphasized. All specimens should be handled as though they contained a hazardous agent or pathogen (see also Standard Precautions, in Chapter 2).

The laboratory can accept only properly labeled specimens. Computer-generated labels assist in making certain that proper patient identification is noted on each specimen container sent to the laboratory. Improperly labeled or unlabeled specimens cannot be accepted by the laboratory. All containers must be labeled by the person doing the collection, to make certain that each specimen has been collected from the patient whose identification is noted on the label. An important rule to remember is that the analytic result can only be as good as the specimen received (see also Specimen Collection, in Chapter 3).

Specimen Transportation and Processing

Specimens must be transported to the laboratory in a safe, timely, and efficient manner. It is important that a central receiving and processing area be set aside in the laboratory to monitor and record all incoming specimens and the request forms accompanying them. The documentation of specimen arrival times in the laboratory as well as other specific test request data is an important aspect of laboratory organization and an essential part of the quality assurance process. It is important that the specimen status can be determined at any time—that is, where in the laboratory processing system a given specimen can be found. Turnaround time is an important factor; specimen processing, analyses, and reporting of results within an acceptable time frame constitute a part of the quality assurance process as a whole (see also Specimen Collection, in Chapter 3).

Quality Control

Quality control activities include monitoring the performance of laboratory instruments, reagents, other testing products, and equipment. In the process of quality assurance, it is important to document the effectiveness of quality control measures. The written record of quality control activities for each procedure or function should also include details of deviation from the usual results, problems, or failures in functioning or in the analytic procedure, as well as any corrective action taken in response to these problems.

Instruments for quality control can include preventive maintenance records, temperature charts, and other records of performance such as quality control charts for specific analytic procedures. All products and reagents used in the analytic procedures must be carefully checked before actual use in testing patient samples. Use of quality control specimens, proficiency testing, and standards depends upon the specific requirements of the accrediting agency of the health care facility. General use of control specimens, proficiency testing programs, and reference values is described later in this chapter.

Sometimes laboratories are asked to assist other departments in the health care facility in their quality control measures. This could include checking the effectiveness of autoclaves in surgery or in the laundry, or providing aseptic checks for the pharmacy, blood bank, or dialysis service.

External quality control activities include periodic inspections by the various accrediting agencies involved in the regulation of clinical laboratories. It is for these inspections that well-monitored, well-documented quality assurance records are maintained.

Laboratory Procedure Manuals

A complete **laboratory procedure manual** for all analytic procedures performed within the laboratory must be provided. The National Committee for Clinical Laboratory Standards (NCCLS) recommends that these procedure manuals follow a specific pattern in how the procedures in the manual are organized. Each assay done in the laboratory must be included in the manual, beginning with the title of the test, or the test name, along with the principle of the procedure. The manual should also contain the following: specimen requirements such as patient preparation (if needed) and special collection or processing details; test request information; other criteria for performing the test; procedural information (how to perform the test), including the reagents and control specimens used and the cal-

ibration of instruments and maintenance checks performed; quality control data; limitations of the procedure; details about reference values; and information about reporting of results. These manuals must be reviewed regularly by the supervisory staff and updated, as needed. In the process of quality assurance, the documentation of laboratory procedural information is as important as documentation of quality control activities, specimen receiving data, or reporting of the laboratory result itself. The NCCLS has set guidelines for writing laboratory procedure manuals.[2]

Problem-Solving Mechanisms

Since an important aspect of quality assurance is **documentation,** CLIA '88 regulations mandate that any problem or situation that might affect the outcome of a test result must be recorded and reported. All such incidents must be documented in writing, including the changes proposed and their implementation, and follow-up monitored. These incidents can involve specimens that are improperly collected, labeled, or transported to the laboratory, or problems concerning prolonged turnaround times for test results. There must be a reasonable attempt to correct the problems or situation, and all steps in this process must be documented.

Continuous Quality Improvement

The ongoing process of making certain that the correct laboratory result is reported for the right patient in a timely manner and cost is known as **continuous quality improvement,** or **CQI.** This is a process of assuring the clinician ordering the test that the testing process has been done in the best possible way to provide the most useful information in diagnosing or managing the particular patient in question. **Quality assurance indicators** are evaluated as part of the CQI process. These indicators monitor the performance of the laboratory. Each laboratory will set its own indicators, depending on the specific goals of the laboratory. Any quality assurance indicators should be appreciated as a tool to ensure that reported results are of the highest quality.

Test Result and Information Processing Systems

With the use of laboratory computer systems and information processing, record keeping can be done in a fast, efficient manner. Quality assurance programs require documentation, and computer record-keeping capability assists in doing this. Patient test results, by dates performed, as well as quality control data for the same dates, must be recorded. When control results are within the acceptable limits established by the laboratory, these data provide the necessary link between the control and patient data, thus giving reassurance that the patient results are reliable, valid, and reportable. This information is necessary in order to document that uniform protocols have been established and that they are being followed. The data can also support the proper functioning capabilities of the test systems being used at the time patient results are produced.

CAP Quality Assurance Programs

The College of American Pathologists (CAP) provides assistance to the clinical laboratory in organizing and managing its **CAP quality assurance program.** As described in the CAP's *Physician Office Laboratory Policy and Procedure Manual,* "All laboratories must have a quality assurance program with the proper documentation defining the goals of the program, the procedures necessary to achieve the goals, and specific records showing that procedures have been carried out. A comprehensive quality assurance program must be designed to monitor and evaluate the ongoing and overall quality of the total testing process (preanalytic, analytic, and postanalytic). The laboratory's quality assurance program must evaluate the effectiveness of its policies and procedures; identify and correct problems; assure the accurate, reliable and prompt reporting of test results; and assure the adequacy and competency of the staff."[5] Quality

assurance programs are not without cost, but they are an essential part of health care.

Components of a CAP Quality Assurance Program

According to the College of American Pathologists, a comprehensive quality assurance program should include the following components:

Patient test management
Procedure manuals
Quality control assessment
Proficiency testing
Comparison of test results
Relationship of patient information to test results
Personnel assessment
Communications

DIAGNOSTIC VALUE OF RESULTS REPORTED: DESCRIPTORS USED

The ability of the laboratory results reported to substantiate a diagnosis, lead to a change in diagnosis, or follow the management for a diagnosis already made is what makes the laboratory test useful to the clinician. The diagnostic usefulness of a test and its procedure is assessed by using statistical evaluations such as description of the accuracy and reliability of the test and its methodology. To describe the reliability of a particular procedure, two terms are commonly used: **accuracy** and **precision. The reliability of a procedure** depends on a combination of these two factors, although they are different and are not dependent on each other. **Variance** is another general term that describes the factors or fluctuations that affect the measurement of the substance in question. Statistical methods available also can assess the usefulness of a test result in terms of its **sensitivity,** its **specificity,** and its **predictive value.**

Accuracy versus Precision

The **accuracy** of a procedure refers to the closeness of the result obtained to the true or actual value, while **precision** refers to repeatability or reproducibility—that is, the ability to get the same value in subsequent tests on the same sample. It is possible to have great precision, with all laboratory personnel who perform the same procedure arriving at the same answer, but without accuracy if the answer does not represent the actual value being tested for. The precision of a test, its **reproducibility,** may be expressed as **standard deviations (SD)** or the **derived coefficient of variation (CV).** A procedure may be extremely accurate, yet so difficult to perform that individual laboratory personnel are unable to arrive at values that are close enough to be clinically meaningful.

In very general terms, accuracy can be aided by the use of properly standardized procedures, statistically valid comparisons of new methods with established reference methods, the use of samples of known values (controls), and participation in proficiency testing programs.

Precision can be ensured by the proper inclusion of standards, reference samples, or control solutions; statistically valid replicate determinations of a single sample; or duplicate determinations of sufficient numbers of unknown samples. Day-to-day and between-run precision is measured by inclusion of blind samples and control specimens.

Coefficient of Variation

The coefficient of variation can be used to compare the standard deviations of two samples. Standard deviations cannot be compared directly without considering the mean. The CV can be used to compare one day's work with that of a similar day or to compare test results from one laboratory with the same type of test results from another laboratory. The coefficient of variation in percent is equal to the standard deviation divided by the mean:

$$CV\% = \frac{SD}{Mean} \times 100$$

Sources of Variance or Error

In general, it is impossible to obtain exactly the same result each time a determination is per-

formed on a particular specimen. This may be described as the **variance (or error) of a procedure.** These factors include limitations of the procedure itself and limitations related to the sampling mechanism used.

Sampling Factors

One of the major difficulties in guaranteeing reliable results involves the **sampling procedure.** Only a very small amount of sample is taken— for example, 5 to 10 mL of a total blood volume of 5 to 6 L, approximately one thousandth of the total blood volume. Other sources of variance that involve the sample include the time of day when the sample is obtained, the patient's position (lying down or seated), the patient's state of physical activity (in bed, ambulatory, or physically active), the interval since last eating (fasting or not), and the time interval and storage conditions between the obtaining of the specimen and its processing by the laboratory. The aging of the sample is another source of error.

Procedural Factors

Still other sources of variance involve aging of chemicals or reagents; personal bias or limited experience of the person performing the determination; and laboratory bias because of variations in standards, reagents, environment, methods, or apparatus. There may also be experimental error resulting from changes in the method used for a particular determination, changes in instruments, or changes in personnel.

Sensitivity and Specificity of a Test

Laboratory results that give medically useful information, including the specificity and sensitivity of the tests being ordered and reported, are important. Both specificity and sensitivity are desirable characteristics for a test, but in different clinical situations, one is generally preferred over the other. For assessing the sensitivity and specificity of a test, four entities are needed: tests positive, tests negative, disease present (positive), or disease absent (negative). **True positives** are those subjects who have a positive test result and who also have the disease in question. **True negatives** represent those subjects who have a negative test result and who do not have the disease. **False positives** are those subjects who have a positive test result yet do not have the disease. **False negatives** are those subjects who have a negative test result yet do have the disease.

Sensitivity

The **sensitivity** of a test is defined as the proportion of cases with a specific disease or condition that give a positive test result (that is, the assay correctly predicts with a positive result):

$$\text{Sensitivity \%} = \frac{\text{True positives}}{\text{True positives} + \text{False negatives}} \times 100$$

Practically, sensitivity represents how much of a given substance is measured; the more sensitive the test, the smaller the amount of assayed substance that is measured.

Specificity

The **specificity** of a test is defined as the proportion of cases with absence of the specific disease or condition that gives a negative test result (that is, the assay correctly excludes with a negative result):

$$\text{Specificity \%} = \frac{\text{True negatives}}{\text{False positives} + \text{True negatives}} \times 100$$

Practically, specificity represents what is being measured. A highly specific test measures only the assay substance in question; it does not measure interfering or similar substances.

Predictive Values

To assess the predictive value (PV) for a test, the sensitivity, specificity, and prevalence of the disease in the population being studied must be known. The **prevalence** of a disease is the proportion of a population that has the disease. This is in contrast to the **incidence** of a disease, which is the number of subjects found to have the dis-

ease within a defined time period, such as a year, in a population of 100,000.

A **positive predictive value** for a test indicates the number of patients with an abnormal test result who have the disease, compared with all patients with an abnormal result:

Positive PV =

$$\frac{\text{Number of patients with disease and with abnormal test results}}{\text{Total number of patients with abnormal test results}}$$

$$\text{Positive PV} = \frac{\text{True positives}}{\text{True positives} + \text{False positives}}$$

A **negative predictive value** for a test indicates the number of patients with a normal test result who do not have the disease, compared with all patients with a normal (negative) result:

$$\text{Negative PV} = \frac{\text{True negatives}}{\text{True negatives} + \text{False negatives}}$$

Reference Values
Definition of "Normal"

Before physicians can determine whether a patient is diseased, they must have an idea of what is normal. This is not an easy task, yet it is the responsibility of the clinical laboratory to supply the physician with this information. Much attention is being paid to the description of what constitutes normal, yet our knowledge remains quite limited. Many factors enter into this determination. There are variations because of such factors as age, sex, race, geographic location, and ethnic, cultural, and economic characteristics, plus internal factors related to the actual analytic methods and practices used by a particular laboratory. To complicate matters, an individual may show daily physiologic variations within his or her normal range, to say nothing of normal changes with age. **Biometrics** (the science of statistics applied to biological observations) is a rapidly expanding field that attempts to describe these variations. The selection of a group on which to base "normals" is another problem confronting the individual laboratory. Traditionally, normals have been defined by testing such groups as blood donors, persons who are working and "feeling healthy," medical students, student nurses, and medical technologists. Many of the old established normals reported in the medical literature have questionable validity because of such factors as poor sampling techniques, questionable selection of the normal group, and questionable use of clinical methods. In developing normal values or reference values, the proper statistical tools of sampling, selection of the normal comparison group, and analysis of data must be used. Such statistical tools are relatively well defined, but a discussion of them here is beyond the scope of this book.

Reference Range Statistics

Statistically, the **reference range** for a particular measurement is in most cases related to a normal bell-shaped curve (Fig. 8-1). This **gaussian curve** or **distribution** has been shown to be correct for virtually all types of biological, chemical, and physical measurements. A statistically valid series of individuals who are thought to represent a normal healthy group are measured, and the average value is calculated. This mathematical average is defined as the **mean ($\overline{X}$, called the X-bar).** The distribution of all values around the average for the particular group measured is described statistically by the **standard deviation (SD).**

Mean. The mean is a term used often in laboratory measurements—it is a mathematical average calculated by dividing the sum of all individual values by the number of values.

Median. The median is the middle value of a body of data. In a body of data, if all the variables are arranged in order of increasing magnitude, the median is that variable which falls halfway between the highest and the lowest.

Mode. The mode is the value that occurs most commonly in a mass of data.

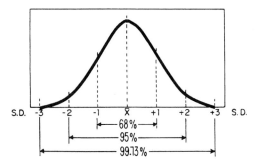

FIG 8-1. Normal bell-shaped gaussian curve.

How the mean, the median, and the mode are used is explained in the following example: A series of results reported for a laboratory test done on 7 different specimens is: 7, 2, 3, 6, 5, 4, and 2.

The mean is the mathematical average and is calculated by taking the sum of the values (29) and dividing by the number of values (7) in the list. The mean is 4.1 (rounded off to 4).

The median equals the middle value. To find the median, the list of numbers must first be ranked according to magnitude: 2, 2, 3, 4, 5, 6, 7, There are seven values in the list, and the median is the middle value in the list. In this example, the median is 4.

The mode is the value most frequently occurring, or 2 in this example.

Standard Deviation. The **standard deviation (SD)** is the square root of the variance of the values in any one observation or in a series of test results. In any normal population, 68% of the values will be clustered above and below the average and defined statistically as falling within the first standard deviation (±1 SD) (see Fig. 8-1). The second standard deviation represents 95% of the values falling equally above and below the average, while 99.7% will be included within the third standard deviation (±3 SD). (Again, variations occur equally above and below the average value [or mean] for any measurement.) Thus, in determining reference values for a particular measurement, a statistically valid series of people are chosen and assumed to represent a healthy population. These people are then tested, and the results are averaged. The term **reference range** therefore means the range of values that includes 95% of the test results for a healthy reference population. The term replaces "normal values" or "normal range." The limits (or range) of normal are defined in terms of the standard deviation from the average value.

In evaluating an individual's state of health, values outside the third standard deviation value are considered clearly abnormal. When the distribution is gaussian, the reference range closely approximates the mean ±2 SD. Values within the first (68%) and second (95%) standard deviation limits are considered normal, while those between the second (95%) and third (99.7%) standard deviation limits are questionable. Thus, **normal** or **reference values** are stated as a range of values. This stated range is in terms of standard deviation units.

Confidence Intervals. When the reference range is expressed using 2 SD on either side of the mean, with 95% of the values falling above and below the mean (see Fig. 8-1), the term **confidence interval** or **confidence limits** is used. This interval should be kept in mind when there are day-to-day shifts in values for a particular analytic procedure. The **95% confidence interval** is used, in part, to account for certain unavoidable error due to sampling variability and imprecision of the methods themselves.

As an example, for a population study, the 95% confidence interval can be interpreted in the following way: if the procedure or experiment is repeated many times and a 95% confidence interval is constructed each time for the parameter being studied, then 95% of these intervals will actually include the true population parameter and 5% will not.

Reference Values for a Specific Laboratory

It is important to realize that reference values will vary with innumerable factors, but especially between laboratories and between geo-

graphic locations. Thus, it is necessary for each laboratory to give the physician information concerning the range of reference values for that particular laboratory. The values will be related to an overall normal, yet they may be more refined or narrow and they may be skewed in the particular situation in question. Although several textbooks are available that describe reference values for virtually all laboratory measurements, and generally accepted reference values are given in such books, the most important indicator of disease is the situation in the clinician's particular institution and locale.

It is hoped that increasing standards and improving the quality of all clinical laboratories will bring all of these reference values closer to an overall value, while parameters describing what constitutes a physiologically normal situation will become established as biometry is further advanced.

ENSURING RELIABLE RESULTS: THE QUALITY CONTROL PROGRAM

Some type of control system to ensure reliable results in the clinical laboratory is essential, a fact that has been proved by numerous laboratory accuracy surveys. A means of ensuring that a particular procedure is performed in such a way that the day-to-day results are within the established precision for the procedure and that the values reported to the physician represent the true clinical condition of the patient is essential for quality assurance. According to CLIA '88, "The laboratory must establish and follow written quality control procedures for monitoring and evaluating the quality of the analytical testing process of each method to assure the accuracy and reliability of patient test results and reports."[3]

Control of laboratory error is influenced and maintained by several factors. The physician depends on the laboratory values and might be misled if these values are not those expected from the clinical diagnosis. Thus, the laboratory must be sure that the results it gives for any analysis are clinically correct. This is done primarily through the use of a **quality control program,** which makes use of standards and control samples. Other factors influencing the control of laboratory variance are expanding state and federal regulations and participation in various proficiency testing programs, either voluntarily or because of legal mandate.

The control system that is used in most laboratories is the quality control program. The quality control program for the laboratory makes use of a **control specimen,** which is similar in composition to the unknown specimen and is included in every batch or run. It must be carried through the entire test procedure and be treated in exactly the same way as any unknown specimen; it is affected by any or all of the variables that affect the unknown specimen. Control specimens have long been routinely included in the clinical chemistry laboratory as well as in routine hemoglobin determinations. All clinical laboratory departments, such as the chemistry or urinalysis laboratories, recognize the need for quality control programs and the use of control specimens as a part of the quality assurance process as mandated by CLIA '88.[3,4]

The quality control program established by a laboratory involves more than only the use of control samples. The use of standards, blanks, duplicates, and recoveries is a part of the quality control program, and they are discussed separately. The use of automated procedures in place of manual methods often requires the inclusion of additional standards and controls, both between specimens and at the end of the run.

In controlling the reliability of laboratory determinations, the objective is to reject results when there is evidence that more than the permitted amount of error has occurred. The clinical laboratory has several ways of controlling the reliability of the results it turns out. When chemical determinations are performed, the term batch or run is often used. A **batch** or **run** is a collection of any number of specimens to be analyzed plus any or all of the following aids for ensuring reliable results (that is, controlling the variance of the procedure): standard solutions,

blanks (these are used only for photometric procedures), control specimens, duplicates, and recoveries (these are used only occasionally).

Proficiency testing programs are still another means for verification of laboratory accuracy. Periodically a specimen is tested which has been provided by a government agency, a professional society, or a commercial company. Identical samples are sent to a group of laboratories participating in the proficiency testing program; each laboratory analyzes the specimen, reports the results to the agency, and is evaluated and graded on those results in comparison to results from other laboratories. In this way, quality control between laboratories is monitored (see also Quality Assurance Under CLIA Regulations, in Chapter 1).

Standard Solutions

To determine the concentration of a substance in a specimen, there must be a basis of comparison. For analyses that result in a colored solution, a spectrophotometer is used to make this comparison (see also under Chapter 6). The buret is also used in the clinical laboratory in titration for volumetric analysis (see Measurement of Volume: Pipetting and Titration, in Chapter 4).

A **standard solution** is one that contains a known, exact amount of the substance being measured. It is prepared from high-quality reference material with measured, known amounts of a fixed and known chemical composition that can be obtained in a pure form. The standard solution is measured accurately and then treated in the testing procedure as if it were a specimen whose concentration is to be determined. Standard solutions are purchased "ready-made," already prepared from high-quality chemicals, or they can be prepared in the laboratory from high-quality chemicals that have been dried and stored in a desiccator. The standard chemical is weighed on the analytical balance and diluted volumetrically. This standard solution is usually most stable in a concentrated form, in which case it is usually referred to as a stock standard. Working standards are prepared from the stock, and sometimes an intermediate form is prepared. The working standard (a more dilute form of the stock standard) is the one employed in the actual determination. Stock and working standards are usually stored in the refrigerator. The accuracy of a procedure is absolutely dependent on the standard solution used; therefore extreme care must be taken whenever these solutions are prepared or used in a clinical laboratory.

Standards Used in Spectrophotometry

To use the standard solution as a basis of comparison in quantitative analysis with the spectrophotometer, a series of calibrated cuvettes (or tubes) are prepared. Each cuvette contains a known different amount of the standard solution. In this way, a series of cuvettes is available containing various known amounts of the standard. Standard cuvettes are carried through the same developmental steps as cuvettes containing specimens to be measured. This set of standard cuvettes is read in the spectrophotometer, and the galvanometer readings are recorded. These readings can be recorded in percent transmittance or in absorbance units (see Chapter 6). Standard solutions are also included in automated analytic methods.

Blanks

For every procedure using the spectrophotometer, a blank solution must be included in the batch. The **blank solution** contains reagents used in the procedure, but it does not contain the substance to be measured. It is treated with the same reagents and processed along with the unknown specimens and the standards. The blank solution is set to read 100% T on the galvanometer viewing scale. In other words, the blank tube is set to transmit 100% of the light. The other cuvettes in the same batch (unknown specimens and standards, for example) transmit only a fraction of this light, because they contain particles that absorb light (particles of the unknown substance), and thus only part of the 100% is transmitted (see also Chapter 6). Using a blank solution corrects for any color that may be present because of the reagents used or an interaction between those reagents.

Control Specimens

The use of control specimens is based on the fact that repeated determinations on the same or different portions (or aliquots) of the same sample will not, as a rule, give identical values for any particular constituent. Many factors can produce variations in laboratory analyses. However, with a properly designed control system, it is possible to be aware of the variables and to keep them under control.

A **control specimen** is a material or solution with a known concentration of the analyte being measured in the testing procedure. For the control specimen to have meaning in terms of the reliability of all results reported by the laboratory, it must be treated exactly like any unknown specimen. It is of no value to the patient and the physician to have the control specimen within the allowable range if the value reported for the unknown is not accurate and precise. The use of quality control specimens is an indication of the overall reliability (both accuracy and precision) of the results reported by the laboratory, a part of the quality assurance process. According to CLIA '88 regulations, a minimum of two control specimens (negative or normal and positive or increased) must be run in every 24-hour period when patient specimens are being run; or, when automated analyzers are in use, the bi-level controls are run once every eight hours of operation (or once per shift).[3]

If the value of the **quality control specimen** for a particular method is not within the predetermined acceptable range, it must be assumed that the values obtained for the unknown specimens are also incorrect, and the results are not reported. After the procedure has been reviewed for any indication of error, and the error has been found and corrected, the batch must be repeated until the control value falls within the acceptable range.

If the control value in a determination is out of the acceptable range (out of control), one or more of the following factors may be responsible: (1) deterioration of reagents or standards, (2) faulty instrument or equipment, (3) dirty glassware, (4) lack of attention to timing or incubation temperature, (5) use of a method not suited to the needs and facilities of the laboratory, (6) use of poor technique by the person doing the test, owing to carelessness or lack of proper training, and (7) statistics: a certain percentage of all determinations will be statistically out of control.

The control sample may be obtained commercially or may be prepared by the individual laboratory. The most important consideration is that control samples be routinely included with each group of laboratory determinations as previously described and mandated by CLIA '88.

Commercial Control Specimens

Commercially prepared controls can be purchased from a manufacturer. These control solutions are obtained in small samples, called aliquots, prepared originally from a large pooled supply of serum or plasma. Commercial controls are usually obtained in a lyophilized (or dried) form. Care must be taken in reconstituting the material to add exactly the correct amount of diluent (usually deionized or distilled water) and to make certain that the material is completely dissolved and well mixed. Commercial control solutions generally have an expiration date, the date by which they must be used in order to give reliable results. Controls should not be used after the expiration date. Reconstituted control solutions must be used within a relatively short period of time, which is generally specified by the manufacturer.

Commercial control material may be purchased either assayed or unassayed. Assayed control preparations have been tested by the manufacturer, and stated values are given for each of the constituents. The manufacturer should provide information concerning the analytic method and statistical procedures used in arriving at the stated values, so that the laboratory can determine the appropriateness of the material for its particular methods and practices.

If unassayed control preparations are used, the laboratory will have to establish its own range of acceptable results for each constituent being measured. The method of arriving at this acceptable range is the same as that used in establishing limits for "laboratory-made" control solutions, to be described next. Tentative standards for manufacturers of control preparations were established in 1972 by the NCCLS.

Control Solutions Prepared by the Laboratory

In rare circumstances, control solutions can also be prepared by the individual laboratory. In the case of control specimens for certain chemistry determinations, serum or plasma is pooled using blood obtained from known donors. The blood is tested for hepatitis B and human immunodeficiency virus (HIV) pathogens. Only disease-free blood is used. Blood is processed and serum frozen. In most laboratories, the commercially prepared product is preferable. After a sufficient pool of the serum or plasma has accumulated, the control specimens for daily use can be made. Only normal serum or plasma is used (i.e., not lipemic or hemolyzed). When enough serum has been saved, it is thawed and mixed thoroughly. After thorough mixing, the pool is divided into aliquots of a convenient size. Aliquots of 2 to 3 mL in a small tube or vial are satisfactory. These samples are then stored in a freezer. Every effort must be made to exclude from the pool serum from patients with blood-borne diseases.

Determination of Control Range

Once a control solution has been prepared or if purchased unassayed, it is necessary for the laboratory to determine the **acceptable control range** for a particular analysis. There are various ways of establishing such a range, and one commonly employed method will be described; however, any method must adhere to statistically acceptable methods. In establishing the control range, an aliquot of the control serum being tested is processed along with the regular batch of tests for 15 to 25 days. It is imperative to thoroughly mix the thawed aliquot, since the sample layers as it freezes. In testing the control sample, it is important that it be treated exactly like an unknown specimen; it must not be treated any more or less carefully than the unknown specimen.

As described previously, repeated determinations on different aliquots of the same sample will often not give identical values for any particular constituent. However, it has been shown that if a sufficient number of repeated determinations are made, the values obtained will fall into a normal bell-shaped curve, as described above (see Fig. 8-1). When a statistically sufficient number of determinations have been run (the number is different for averaged duplicate determinations and single tests), the mathematical mean ($\overline{X}$) or average value can be calculated. The acceptable limits or variation from the mean for the control solution are then calculated on the basis of the standard deviation from the mean, using statistical formulas. Most laboratories use 2 SD above and below the mean as the allowable range of the control specimen, while others use this range as a warning limit. According to the normal bell-shaped curve (see Fig. 8-1), setting 2 SD as the allowable range for the control sample means that 95% of all determinations on that sample will fall within the allowable range, while 5% will be out of control. It may not be desirable to disallow this many batches, so the third standard deviation may be chosen as the limit of control, or the action limit. Once the range of acceptable results has been established, one of the control specimens is included in each batch of determinations. If the control value is not within the limits established, the procedure must be repeated, and no patient results may be reported to the physician until the control value is within the allowable range.

Quality Control Chart

It is conventional in most laboratories to plot the daily control specimen values on a **quality control chart,** such as the Levy-Jennings control chart (Fig. 8-2). The control chart is made on a rectangular sheet of linear graph paper. Monthly control charts are prepared, with the days of the month marked on the horizontal axis and units of concentration for the determination in question marked on the vertical axis. The mean value for the determination in question is then indicated on the chart, in addition to the limits of acceptable error. Control limits are generally set at ±2 SD or ±3 SD on either side of the mean. The 2- and 3-SD values might be indicated, with the 2-SD value as a warning limit and the 3-SD value as an action limit. Each day the control value is plotted on the chart, and any value falling out of control can easily be seen. The control chart serves as visual documentation of the information derived from using control specimens. A different control chart is plotted for each substance being determined. It is possible to observe trends leading toward trouble by plotting the control values daily. When procedural changes, such as the addition of new reagents, standards, or instruments, are made, they are also noted on the control chart. Such a chart can assist in preventing difficulties and can aid in troubleshooting. If all is going well, the plotted control values should be distributed equally above and below the established mean value. A regular weekly visual inspection of the control chart is particularly useful for observing trends before control specimen values are actually out of the established acceptable limits. Generally, an excess of more than five control value results on one side of the mean indicates a trend, although not all such trends need action. The use of quality control programs, including the control chart, is a part of the process of laboratory quality assurance.

Duplicate Determinations

In each batch of determinations, one of the specimens is measured in duplicate. This specimen is chosen at random from those to be tested. Often control specimens are measured in duplicate. If this is done, the allowable range for duplicates is less than that for single determinations. The use of **duplicate determinations** checks the technique used—that is, the precision, or repeatability, of the method. Duplicates do not measure

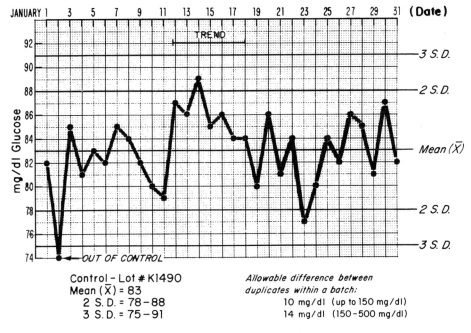

FIG 8-2. Quality control chart for glucose (Levy-Jennings type).

accuracy. It is possible to have grossly inaccurate duplicate results that agree perfectly. The allowable difference between duplicate determinations varies and must be established for each determination performed by the laboratory. This is done by using statistical formulas; the standard deviation is calculated from the differences between a number of duplicate determinations. Duplicate determinations are also part of a quality control and assurance program.

Recovery Solutions

Recovery solutions are used as an indicator of the accuracy of a particular determination. To a specimen in the batch (or to a control solution), in addition to the regular specimens, a measured amount of the pure substance being analyzed is added. Theoretically, the amount of substance added should be recovered at the end of the determination if the method is an accurate one. Recoveries are not used routinely with most proce-

dures, but are often used to evaluate new procedures. Recovery solutions are another part of quality control programs.

Other Components of Quality Control
Specimen Appearance

First, consider the specimen itself—how it is collected, transported to the laboratory, received, identified, processed, and stored. The specimen should be visually inspected for hemolysis or lipemia, as these might affect or invalidate certain determinations. The presence of an abnormal appearance in the specimen should be recorded with the final result. In photometric procedures, the laboratorian should observe the final solution in the cuvette for turbidity or inappropriate color development.

Validating New Procedures

Another part of the quality control program concerns the way new procedures are validated before they are included among the methods routinely used by the laboratory. Each laboratory must determine the reproducibility (or confidence limits) for each procedure used and establish acceptable limits of variation for control specimens. The quality control program includes calculation of the mean (or average value) and standard deviation and the preparation of control charts for each procedure.

Control of Human Error

The quality control program should include a means of independent monitoring to minimize bias on the part of the person doing the tests. This may be done by using blind controls, such as commercial control solutions labeled as patient unknowns, or by dividing patient specimens into different aliquots to be processed blindly and independently on the same day, or carried over to another day if the constituent is stable.

Correlation of Test Results

Another valuable quality control technique is to look at the data generated for each patient and inspect them for relationships between them. There are many relationships, such as the mathematical relationship between anions and cations in the electrolyte report, the correlation between protein and casts in urine, and the relationship between hemoglobin and hematocrit and the appearance of the blood smear in hematologic studies.

Evaluation of Procedures

Each laboratory must have an assessment routine for all procedures, to be done on a daily, weekly, and monthly basis to detect problems such as trends and shifts in the established mean values. When such problems are indicated, it is most important that they be corrected as soon as possible. Many of the components of the quality control program are the responsibility of the laboratory supervisor or director. However, every person working in the laboratory has an important role in ensuring reliable laboratory results, by carefully doing the analysis itself, including control samples, and by calling potential problems to the attention of the supervisor.

Proficiency Testing

In addition to the use of internal quality control programs, each laboratory should participate in at least one external control program. These are known as proficiency testing programs and are a required provision of the CLIA '88 regulations.[3,4]

Proficiency surveys are a means of establishing quality control between laboratories. Both state and national agencies have established programs to help laboratories maintain their quality control programs. Proficiency testing programs are available through the CAP, the Centers for Disease Control and Prevention (CDC), and various state health departments. These programs periodically send specimens to laboratories that participate in them. Each laboratory analyzes its sample, using its routine procedures, and sends the results to the program administrator. Each participating laboratory is furnished with an evaluation of its results that compares them with those of all other laboratories participating in the survey. Participation in at least one proficiency survey is an important part of a laboratory's quality control program.

REFERENCES

1. *Accreditation Manual for Pathology and Clinical Laboratory Services: Standards and Scoring Guidelines.* Chicago, Joint Commission on Accreditation of Healthcare Organizations, 1993.
2. *Clinical Laboratory Technical Procedure Manual: Approved Guideline*, ed 3. Villanova, Pa, National Committee for Clinical Laboratory Standards, 1996, NCCLS Document GP2-A3.
3. Department of Health and Human Services, Health Care Financing Administration: Clinical Laboratory Improvement Amendments of 1988. *Federal Register*, February 28, 1992. CLIA '88, Final Rule. 42 CFR. Subpart K, 493.1201.
4. Department of Health and Human Services, Health Care Financing Administration: Clinical Laboratory Improvement Amendments of 1988. *Federal Register*, vol 60, no 78, April 24, 1995. Final rules with comment period.

5. *Physician Office Laboratory Policy and Procedure Manual.* Northfield, Ill, 1993, College of American Pathologists, Section 4, p 1.
6. *Standards for Laboratory Accreditation, Laboratory Accreditation Program,* Northfield, Ill, College of American Pathologists, 1996.

BIBLIOGRAPHY

Burtis CA, Ashwood ER (eds.): *Tietz Textbook of Clinical Chemistry,* ed 4. Philadelphia, WB Saunders Co, 1996.

Campbell JB, Campbell JM: *Laboratory Mathematics: Medical and Biological Applications,* ed 5. St Louis, Mosby, 1997.

Henry JB (ed): *Clinical Diagnosis and Management by Laboratory Methods,* ed 19. Philadelphia, WB Saunders Co., 1996.

Meisenheimer CG: *Quality Assurance: A Complete Guide to Effective Programs.* Rockville, Md, Aspen Publications, 1985.

NCCLS: *Continuous Quality Improvement: Essential Management Approaches and Their Use in Proficiency Testing, Proposed Guideline.* Villanova, Pa, National Committee for Clinical Laboratory Standards, 1997, Document GP22-P.

Revision of the laboratory regulations for Medicare, Medicaid and Clinical Laboratories Improvement Act of 1967 programs, final rule. *Federal Register* 1990; 55(March 14):50.

STUDY QUESTIONS

1. **Define quality assurance.**

2. **Which regulations mandate the inclusion of a quality assurance program in the clinical laboratory?**

3. **Which activities of the laboratory are to be included in a quality assurance program?**

4. **Match each of the following terms (1 to 6) with the best definition (A to F):**

   1. Accuracy
   2. Precision
   3. Sensitivity
   4. Specificity
   5. Prevalence
   6. Proficiency testing program
      _____ A. Repeatability or reproducibility of a procedure
      _____ B. Allows monitoring of quality control between laboratories
      _____ C. The proportion of cases with a specific disease that gives a positive test result
      _____ D. Closeness of a result to the true or actual value
      _____ E. The proportion of a population that has the disease being studied
      _____ F. The proportion of cases without disease that gives a negative test result

5. **A new pregnancy screening test (test A) is being compared with the test now in use (test B). Ten known pregnant women and ten known nonpregnant women participate in the testing. The following are the test results for these women:**

	Test A	Test B
Pregnant women	7 of 10 positive	9 of 10 positive
Nonpregnant women	1 of 10 positive	3 of 10 positive

   A. What would be the sensitivity of tests A and B?
   B. What would be the specificity of tests A and B?

6. **For the following numbers: 10, 12, 15, 18, 20, 18, 14**

   A. Calculate the mean.
   B. Calculate the median.
   C. Calculate the mode.

7. **According to a gaussian curve, if the reference range for a test result is expressed as 2 SD on either side of the mean, what percentage of values would fall within that range?**

8. Define "standard solution."

9. Match each of the following terms (1 to 3) with the best definition (A to C):

1. Standard solution
2. Blank solution
3. Control specimen

_____ A. Material or solution with a known concentration of the analyte being measured

_____ B. Reference material that is prepared with measured, known amounts of a fixed and known chemical composition that can be obtained in a pure form

_____ C. Contains reagents used in the procedure, but does not contain the substance to be measured

10. What is the use for a quality control chart?

CHAPTER 9

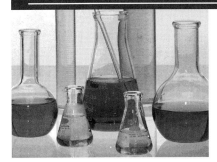

Automation in the Clinical Laboratory

Learning Objectives

From study of this chapter, the reader will be able to:

➤ Compare and contrast the various types of automated instruments available for chemistry, hematology, and urinalysis.

➤ Outline the steps involved in the process of general automation of laboratory testing.

➤ Define terms used in describing the various automated analytical systems and their methodologies.

➤ Appreciate both the benefits and the potential problems resulting from the use of automated instruments.

INTRODUCTION TO AUTOMATION

More and more laboratory tests per patient are ordered every year; the variety of tests available has also increased, and test results are generated more quickly, providing the physician with medically useful information. The fast turnaround time required in today's medical practices has affected the instrumentation required, including the devices used for point-of-care testing (POCT). One of the major technologic changes in the clinical laboratory has been the introduction of automated analysis. An automated analytic instrument provides a means of transfer of a specimen within its complex assembly to a series of self-acting components, each of which carries out a specific process or stage of the process, ending in the analytic result being produced.

USE OF AUTOMATION

In general, laboratory automation has centered on handling the sample after it has been received in the laboratory. Laboratory automation actually begins with the physician ordering the test and ends when the results are reported back to the physician. The sequence of the process includes test ordering, sample collection and transport to the laboratory, sample processing and analysis by the laboratory, quantitating the result, and test reporting (Fig. 9-1). The discussion in this chapter will center primarily on the steps in the sequence from the receipt of the specimen in the laboratory to the results being reported back to the physician. Automation of specimen transfer from patient care units to the laboratory is accomplished in many health care facilities by means of a vacuum tube transport system.

The demand for medically useful laboratory data has grown to such an extent that automation has become essential to process the increasing number of requests for laboratory determinations. Automation provides a means by which an increased workload can be processed rapidly and reproducibly. It does not necessarily improve the accuracy of the results. Ideally, automated testing would use whole blood for analysis, as it would eliminate the need for centrifugation and the problems associated with it. Whether whole blood, serum, or plasma is used, the specimen should be pipetted directly from the primary collection tube. This would prevent specimen mix-ups when samples are transferred from the tube to the sample cups for analysis. Closed-tube sampling is also best—it eliminates possible splashing of the biologic material being tested. Centrifugation and the aliquoting of specimens are manual, time-consuming tasks, which are best automated if possible.

The first practical automated system was introduced into the clinical laboratory in 1957. Numerous other instruments for automation have been devised since that first system, employing the continuous-flow principle, was conceived by L.T. Skeggs.[3] This system was introduced commercially as the AutoAnalyzer* and has since been used extensively by many laboratories. It has undergone several refinements and modifications, so that the latest units have much more versatility than the original instrument. In the **continuous-flow analyzer,** samples flow in sequence through a channel; each sample in the batch or run is subjected to the same analytic reaction. Another group of instruments employs the principle of discrete-sample processing. The **discrete-sample analyzer** processes each specimen separately, generally in steps, somewhat as in a conventional manual method. In the discrete analyzer, each sample undergoes analysis on a discretionary basis; only selected tests are run on each sample. A third group makes use of centrifugal force to transfer and mix samples and reagents.

Originally, automation was used for the tests done most frequently in the clinical laboratory. Automation is now used in many areas of the laboratory, and in many larger laboratories very few procedures are done manually. Perhaps the chemistry department is the area in which the advent of automation has made the greatest difference. In hematology, automation has also

---

*Technicon Instruments Corp, Tarrytown, NY.

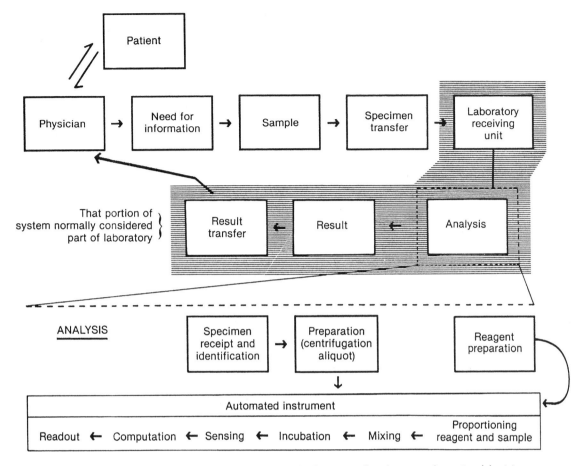

FIG 9-1. Example of a sequence for specimen and information flow between the patient/physician and the clinical laboratory. Lower portion shows the steps in sample processing and analysis in the laboratory. (From Kaplan LA, Pesce AJ: *Clinical Chemistry: Theory, Analysis, and Correlation*, ed 3. St Louis, Mosby, 1996, p 294.)

made a great change in the way work is done. Electronic cell counters have replaced manual counting of blood cells even in clinics and physicians' office laboratories. There is an automated system for Wright's staining of blood smears. For coagulation studies several automated and semiautomated systems are available. Prothrombin time and activated partial thromboplastin time determinations can be done automatically on various instruments. Semiautomatic instruments are also used, especially for dilution steps. Several instruments are available for precise and convenient diluting, which both aspirate the sample and wash it out with the diluent. Some automatic diluters dispense and dilute in separate processes. There also are automated instruments for performing routine urinalysis determinations, for identification of bacterial organisms, and for setting up and reading blood cultures in the microbiology laboratory.

If an automated system is basically sound and in good working order, there are many advantages to its use: large numbers of samples may be processed with minimal personnel time, two or more methods may be performed simultaneously, precision is superior to that of a manual method, and calculations may not be required. Sometimes the automatic systems are so impressive in their appearance that laboratory personnel put too much faith in them and are misled about their shortcomings. These machines must be appreciated, and yet their potential problems must be noted.

The fact that automation has found its way into the clinical laboratory does not mean that the laboratorian responsible for the work is no longer important. There still are many laboratories in which manual procedures are used, especially in smaller hospitals, where the number of laboratory determinations does not always justify the purchase of an automated system. Many smaller hospital laboratories do lease these units, however, and so the size of the hospital does not always limit the use of automated equipment. Back-up manual procedures are always necessary in case of equipment failure, and these procedures must be set up and ready to use when needed. The emphasis in the laboratory has turned to faster turnaround times for results, with accuracy and precision being maintained. Automation has enabled the laboratory to accommodate the increased demand for increased numbers of tests.

Disadvantages of Automation

Some problems that may arise with many automated units are as follows: (1) there may be limitations in the methodology that can be used (sometimes a compromise must be made that results in less accurate, although often more precise, values than are obtained with manual methods); (2) with automation, laboratorians are often discouraged from making observations and using their own judgment about potential problems; (3) many systems are impractical for small numbers of samples, and therefore manual methods are still necessary as back-up procedures for emergency individual analyses; (4) back-up procedures must be available in case of instrument failures; (5) automated systems are expensive to purchase and maintain—regular maintenance requires personnel time as well as the time of trained service personnel; and (6) there is often an accumulation of irrelevant data because it is so easy to produce the results—tests are run that are not always necessary.

COMPONENTS OF AN AUTOMATED LABORATORY ANALYZER

Automation can be applied to any or all of the steps used to perform any manual assay. Automated systems include some kind of device for sampling the patient's specimen or other samples to be tested (such as blanks, controls, and standard solutions), a mechanism to add the necessary amounts of reagents in the proper sequence, incubation modules when needed for the specific reaction, monitoring or measuring devices such as photometric technology to quantitate the extent of the reaction, and a recording mechanism to provide the final reading or permanent record of the analytic result. Most analyzers are capable of processing serum, plasma, urine, and cerebrospinal fluid, but not whole blood. A few instruments are designed to process whole blood.

The steps included in the analytic process can be performed manually or with automated instruments. Generally the automated analyzers employ the same steps as the manual methods, using the same reagents and principles. The precision is greater in automated systems, however, because the operation of the instrument is under better control and manual intervention has been replaced by mechanical intervention. Automated systems perform essentially the same types of analyses as the manual methods do. Almost any manual method can be adapted to one that is automated. As with any piece of laboratory apparatus, the manufacturer's directions must always be followed carefully. Automation of analyses generates test results rapidly and accurately and provides data that can be sent to the requesting physician in a timely manner to affect the medical decisions concerning the patient.

GENERAL FUNCTIONS PERFORMED BY AUTOMATED ANALYZERS

Whether a laboratory determination is done manually or automatically, certain individual steps are necessary. It is generally advisable to perform as many steps as possible without manual intervention, to increase efficiency. Several of these steps can be automated for faster and more accurate results. Some methods and procedures have been partially automated, or semiautomated, by use of mechanical pipetting and diluting devices. Full automation reduces the possibility of human errors that arise from repetitive and boring manipulations done by laboratorians, such as pipetting errors in routine procedures.

Collection, Identification, and Preparation of the Sample

The specimen must be collected properly, labeled, and transported to the laboratory for analysis. Specimen handling and processing are a vital step in the total analytic process (see Chapter 3). Automation of specimen preparation steps can include the use of bar-coded labels on samples, which allow electronic identification of the samples and the tests requested. **Bar coding** is a sample or product recognition system that, when coupled with a bar-code reader, can identify a sample and the reagents or analyses needed and relay this information to the automated analyzer. This can prevent clerical errors that could result in improperly entering patient data for analysis.

Sample and Reagent Measurements and Mixing: Proportioning

Automated instruments measure, aspirate, and introduce samples into the analyzer reagents. Automation combines reagents and sample in a prescribed manner to yield a specific final concentration. This combination of predetermined amounts of reagent and sample is termed **proportioning.** It is important that the proper amounts of reagents be introduced to the sample and in specific sequences for the analysis to be carried through correctly. In most systems, the sample is introduced into the analyzer with a thin probe made from stainless steel. The probe passes into the sample either by directly penetrating the primary collection tube cap/stopper or after the stopper is removed from the tube. Mixing of reagents and sample can be done by stirring, agitation, or some other device.

Incubation

In automated analyzers, incubation is simply a waiting period in which the test mixture is allowed time to react. This is done at a specified, constant temperature controlled by the analyzer.

Monitoring or Sensing the Reaction Result

This can be done by optical, thermal, or electrical means. Chemical reactions can be monitored either at one time point or at many. Some measurements can be done in the vessel, cell, or cuvette where the reaction has taken place; this is known as **in situ monitoring.** If the sample has been transferred from the reaction vessel to the sensing device, the monitoring is external. Different instruments employ different monitoring mechanisms.

Quantitating the Reaction Result: Computation

Quantitating by automated computation can be done by either the digital or the analog format.

Analog Computation

In analog computation, the microprocessor uses an electrical signal from the sensor, as from the photoelectric cell, and compares it with a reference signal, as for the blank solution. It then compares the two signals and takes the logarithm of the result as the final result for the unknown sample. **Analog computation** is derived directly from a signal from the instrument, usually in a graphic form.

Digital Computation

Digital computation is usually restricted to certain mathematical functions (such as addition or subtraction). A digital computer needs an analog-to-digital converter in order to process the signals received from the many types of sensing or monitoring devices used in the automated instruments. This converter changes the voltage or current signal into a digital form, which can then be processed by the computer so that the data are available in discrete units or from calculations made from these data.

Visualizing the Result: Results Reporting

A common and easy way to visualize an instrument readout is with the use of a television monitor (cathode-ray tube) or light-emitting diodes. Data can be visualized before results are accepted. This visualized readout can be converted to hard copy by means of a paper or tape printout. This data printout information must then be transferred or transcribed to laboratory report slips or other permanent records. If the **data** (results) are **interfaced** with, or connected to, a laboratory computer, this transcription process is done quickly and without errors, which may occur when transcription is done manually. If this interfacing is available, when the laboratorian has verified the results, they are immediately available electronically to the ordering physician.

Standardization of Methods and Use of Controls

To ensure the accuracy of results obtained with automated systems, there must be frequent standardization of methods. Once the standardization has been done, a well-designed automated system maintains or reproduces the prescribed conditions with great precision. Frequent standardization and running of control specimens are essential to ensure this accuracy and precision. CLIA '88 regulations have mandated the use of control specimens for certain tests. For laboratories doing moderately complex or highly complex testing using automated analyzers, a minimum of two control specimens (negative or normal and positive or increased) must be run once every eight hours of operation or once per shift when patient specimens are being run[1] (see also Chapter 8).

KINDS OF AUTOMATED ANALYZERS

Many analyzers are being manufactured for use in the clinical laboratory. The choice of which type of instrument to use is dependent on several factors: the volume of determinations done in the laboratory, the type of data profile to be generated, the level of staffing, the initial cost of the instrument, the cost of its upkeep and operation, and the amount of time it takes for each analysis. Automated instruments have been designed to perform the most frequently ordered tests because it is known that six tests make up 50% of the workload of the average chemistry laboratory and that another 14 tests make up an additional 40%.[2] Versatility and flexibility are often just as important as high volume and speed of testing, however, as automation is also desirable for the more rarely ordered tests. Automated chemistry analyzer systems can be based on chemistry reactions and methodologies along with their appropriate quantitating systems, or on immunoassay systems. Some of the most common automated instruments or categories of automated instruments are described in the following paragraphs.

Automated Chemistry
Automated Batch Analyzers

Batch analyzers can test a batch of samples simultaneously for one particular analyte at a time. Batch analyzers can also be designed to analyze a number of different analytes. They are controlled by a microprocessor that can change the program for each different analyte to be measured. It is possible to have a batch analyzer capable of measuring 30 or more analytes, one analyte at a time. For these systems, generally there is a reagent delivery apparatus for each reagent needed. This type of analyzer does not require that every sample be tested for every analyte.

Random Access or Selective Analyzers

The **random access analyzer** does all the selected determinations on a patient sample before it goes on to the next sample. These analyzers can process different assay combinations for individual specimens. The microprocessor enables the analyzer to perform up to 30 determinations. The selected tests are ordered from the menu, and the testing is begun, with the unordered tests being left undone. A sampling device begins the process by measuring the exact amount of sample into the required cells. The microprocessor controls the addition of the necessary diluents and reagents to each cell. After the proper reacting period, the microprocessor begins the spectrophotometric measurements of the various cells, the reaction results are calculated, control values are checked, and the results are reported. Some analyzers of this type have a circular configuration utilizing an analytic turntable device for the various cells. Other random access analyzers have a parallel configuration.

Discrete Analyzers

Instruments that compartmentalize each sample reaction are **discrete analyzers.** In these analyzers, the sample aliquot and the reagent are contained in a single cuvette that is physically separated from all other cuvettes. Most of the commonly used laboratory chemistry analyzers are of the discrete type.

Du Pont Automated Clinical Analyzers

The automated clinical analyzers (ACA) introduced by Du Pont* are designed to perform analyses in prepackaged plastic bags. They are discrete, selective analyzers. The sample is automatically discharged into the pack, the reagents that are compartmentalized in the pack are released and mixed with the sample, and the functions that are necessary to carry out a particular analysis are carried out. Samples can be serum, plasma, urine, or cerebrospinal fluid. For some methods, measurement is made photoelectrically; for end-point methods, the measurement is done bichromatically. A Du Pont ACA requires a separate reagent pack for each test, which also serves as the reaction cuvette. The reagent packs allow introduction of the sample into various reagent compartments, where different stages of reagent mixing and reactions occur, depending on the analysis to be done. The pack moves to the photometer, where the amount of absorbance for the particular constituent being measured is noted electronically. The instrument's computer calculates the concentration for the unknown along with the concentrations for the necessary controls and standards.

A Du Pont ACA can serve as a general chemistry analyzer in small hospital laboratories. It can also be used in medium-sized laboratories as a specialty analyzer. Any combination of tests can be run on any sample at any time.

Vitros Clinical Chemistry Analyzer

There are various models of the Vitros Clinical Chemistry Analyzer*; they are generally discrete, selective analyzers that use a random access design. This instrument was formerly known as Ektachem, an Eastman Kodak product. The Vitros Clinical Chemistry Analyzer utilizes dry film technology, in which the dry reagents are impregnated into Vitros Clinical Chemistry Slides. A thin layer of gelatin is mounted on plastic slides to which the dry reagent is added. The addition of the sample provides the necessary solvent (water) to rehydrate the dry reagents. The slides are composed of multiple layers of film, some of which serve as ultrafilters for the sample. Others provide reactive reagents for the particular analysis being performed.

Samples are pipetted from bar-coded primary collection tubes or from sample cups on a turntable. The sample cups are covered with a top that can be penetrated by the automatic robotic device attached to a disposable pipette. This robotic device applies the measured sample to the

---

selected dry reagent slide. Slides are automatically dispensed from method-specific cartridges. Slides are incubated while color development takes place. For methods utilizing reflectance photometry, after the reaction has taken place on the slide and incubation has occurred, reflected radiant energy is read, with the measured energy being relayed to a microprocessor. The reflected energy is converted into concentration units. Used slides are automatically dropped into containers for disposal. Printouts are available with results for unknown samples and controls.

Abbott IMx

The IMx* is a bench top immunoassay system capable of producing 40 results per hour. It combines two assay technologies in one system: **latex-microparticle enzyme immunoassay (MEIA) technology** and fluorescence polarization immunoassay. A robotic probe assembly dispenses the sample into either a predilution well for some assays or a reaction well for others. Diluent and reagent with a latex particle suspension are also dispensed into the reaction well by the probe. A bar-code reader scans the reagent pack to select the assay chosen to be done. During the incubation step that follows, an immunocomplex forms. The incubation time is assay specific. After incubation, the reaction mixture (the immunocomplex) is transferred to a capture surface, where the microparticles, together with the bound analyte, adhere to the inert glass-fiber matrix, where they are bound irreversibly to the matrix. After a washing step, an alkaline phosphatase conjugate and substrate are added and the reaction is allowed to continue. The fluorescence of the product formed is measured and related to quantitation of the analyte being assayed.

Automated Analyzers for the Physician's Office

Since physicians' office laboratories are performing many tests, and since the number of these laboratories is expected to increase over the next few years, many automated or semiautomated analyzers have been introduced for use outside the traditional hospital laboratory setting. The criteria used by the physician to select the appropriate instrument(s) for a particular laboratory include the type of practice or specialty, the volume of tests to be done, whether single tests or chemistry profiles are needed, the turnaround time available, and the cost of the analyzer and its reagents.

In a physician's office laboratory, ideally the specimen to be tested would be whole blood and the automatic pipetting of the specimen and necessary reagents would be done by the analyzer, eliminating as much interaction by laboratory personnel as possible. The use of instruments with stable calibration curves is important, and a quality control program should be available from the manufacturer. Data computation from the analyzing instruments should be interfaced with a computer, if possible, to provide the necessary documentation of laboratory results. Quality control information can also be stored in the computer. The instrument should be easy to use, and, because in many physicians' office laboratories there will be persons working who have little or no laboratory training, the instrument should require only a limited user training period. The reagents, whether wet or dry, should be bar coded, prepackaged, and stable for at least 6 months.

Dry Reagent Systems. In dry-film technology systems, the reagents are already proportioned in the required amounts and only the sample must be added. The sample may be added volumetrically or by saturation addition, in which an excess of the sample is exposed to the dry-film reagent and the pores of the film allow only a fixed amount of sample to be absorbed—this is its proportioning mechanism. Several systems are available for physicians' offices that use this technology. They include the Seralyzer*; the DT System,† which is similar to

---

*Abbott Laboratories, Diagnostics Division, Irving, Tex.

*Bayer Corp, Diagnostics Division, Tarrytown, NY.
†Johnson & Johnson Clinical Diagnostics, Rochester, NY.

the larger Vitros technology; the i-STAT*; the Analyst system†; and the Reflotron system.‡ Each has slightly different testing reagents, but the principle of use is similar. The Reflotron system is described here.

Reflotron System. The solid-phase reagent test tabs used in this system are bar coded to identify the tests, the reaction parameters, and the calibration curves for each assay. The manufacturer establishes the calibration curve for each lot of reagent strips, eliminating the need for calibration by the laboratory. The reagent strips have a shelf life of from 1 to 2 years. In this system, whole blood from a finger or heel stick can be used for analysis. The blood is placed on the reagent strip, made up of a glass fiber pad that separates the plasma from the red cells. The separation of cells from plasma is accomplished by capillary action, leaving the required plasma to react with the reagent in the strip at a temperature of 37° C. Excess plasma is removed from the reaction site. The analyte concentration is determined by reflectance photometry and recorded visually or interfaced with a laboratory computer.

Wet Chemistry Reagent Systems. One system utilizing wet reagent chemistry is the Vision system,§ which is described in this section.

Vision System. This automated system uses specially designed reagent packs, which are disposable. The reagent pack is a self-contained unit with a cuvette, liquid reagents, and bar codes to identify the assay to be done. Blood can be obtained by finger or heel stick and placed in a special tube provided by the manufacturer. This special tube can then be inserted directly into the reagent pack, eliminating the step of pipetting the sample from the capillary tube into the analyzer. Two drops of blood, serum, or plasma are placed in the multichambered reagent pack, and the packs are placed in the ten-position rotor in the analyzer. The red cells, if whole blood is used, are separated from plasma by centrifugal force. Next the packs are rotated to a 90-degree angle, allowing the premeasured amount of sample and the reagents to be transferred into the cuvette. The reaction occurs at 37° C; it is monitored, and the absorbances are measured bichromatically. The reagents for this system are stable for several months, and one to ten analytes can be measured. The Vision system is suitable for doing batches of tests, profiles, or stat procedures.

Automated Hematology

The best source of information about the various instruments available is the manufacturers' product information literature. The continual advances in commercial instruments for hematologic use and their variety preclude an adequate description of them in this chapter. Some basic, general information follows, however.

Automated Cell Counters

Automated cell counters are used extensively in hematology to identify and enumerate the blood cells in a given patient sample. Even the simplest instruments can identify and count red blood cells, white blood cells, and platelets. In more sophisticated instruments, the types of white blood cells can be identified and counted. These instruments are known as **flow cytometers.**

Most automated cell counters can be classified as one of two types, those using electrical resistance and those using optical methods with focused laser beams, in which cells cause a change in the deflection of a beam of light. In the cell counters using **optical methods,** the deflections are converted to measurable pulses by a photo multiplier tube. Both types of instruments count thousands of cells in a few seconds, and both decrease the coefficient of variation and increase the precision of cell counts as compared with manual methods.

In the **electrical resistance cell counters,** blood cells passing through an aperture through which a current is flowing cause a change in elec-

---

*i-STAT Corp, Princeton, NJ.
†Du Pont Medical Products, Wilmington, Del.
‡Boehringer Mannheim Diagnostics, Indianapolis, Ind.
§Abbott Laboratories, Diagnostics Division, Irving, Tex.

trical resistance that is counted as voltage pulses. The voltage pulses are amplified and can be displayed on an oscilloscope screen. Each spike indicates a cell. Several manufacturers employ this principle in instruments for cell counting; these include Coulter,* Abbott,[†] and Nova.[‡]

Alternative systems using **capillary tube density gradient** methodology are available; these systems measure red blood cells, white blood cells, and platelets in a manner similar to the way in which microhematocrits are measured after centrifugation, in which cell layers are noted. One system employing this methodology is the QBC II Plus.[§] In this methodology, the different types of blood cells have different densities, so after centrifugation, they will settle in separate layers. By use of further mechanical expansion and optical magnification, augmented by supravital fluorochrome staining, other measurements are derived.

Automated Differential Counters

Automated differential counters utilize the impedance method to construct a size-distributed histogram of white blood cells. In most of these instruments, three subpopulations of white cells are counted: lymphocytes, other mononuclear cells, and granulocytes. A computer calculates the number of particles in each area as a percentage of the total white blood cell count histogram. Any abnormal histograms are flagged for review.

Automated Urinalysis

Instruments are available to automate the routine urinalysis (UA), or parts of it, and most can be interfaced with laboratory computers. One automated system is the Yellow IRIS Urinalysis Workstation,[¶] which includes a slideless sediment examination. Other systems include the Clinitek,* the Chemstrip Urine Analyzer,[†] and the Rapimat.[‡] These systems all utilize reflectance photometers for reading their respective reagent strips. Once the strip is placed in the analyzer, the microprocessor mechanically moves the strip into the reflectometer, turns on the light source needed, records the reflectance data, calculates the results, and removes the strip for disposal.

More recently available, the Clinitek Atlas is an automated urine chemistry analyzer that aspirates the specimen directly from the sample tube, which is then also centrifuged for the microscopic examination of the urine specimen. For chemical analyses, the specimen is aspirated from the sample tube and added to a strip containing nine reactive reagent pads (for chemical and physicochemical tests) and one nonreactive pad (for color) per specimen, supplied on a roll of plastic film to which are affixed 490 reagent strips. Use of this reflectance spectrophotometric instrument eliminates the need for "dipping" the reagent strip into the patient's urine specimen. It measures clarity, color, and specific gravity by refractive index. Samples are identified by bar code, and results may be interfaced to the laboratory computer for reporting.

REFERENCES

1. Department of Health and Human Services, Health Care Financing Administration: Clinical Laboratory Improvement Amendments of 1988. *Federal Register,* vol 60, no 78, April 24, 1995. Final rules with comment period.
2. Kaplan LA, Pesce AJ: *Clinical Chemistry: Theory, Analysis, and Correlation,* ed 3. St Louis, Mosby, 1996.
3. Skeggs LT Jr: An automated method for colorimetric analysis. *Am J Clin Pathol* 1957; 28:311.

---

*Coulter Electronics, Hialeah, Fla.
[†]Abbott Laboratories, Diagnostics Division, Irving, Tex.
[‡]Nova Biomedical, Waltham, Mass.
[§]Becton, Dickinson & Co, Franklin Lakes, NJ.
[¶]International Remote Imaging Systems, Inc., Chatsworth, Calif.

*Bayer Corp, Diagnostics Division, Tarrytown, NY.
[†]Boehringer Mannheim Diagnostics, Indianapolis, Ind.
[‡]Behring Diagnostics, Inc, Somerville, NJ.

BIBLIOGRAPHY

Bender GT: *Principles of Clinical Instrumentation.* Philadelphia, WB Saunders Co, 1987.

Burtis, CA, Ashwood, ER (eds): *Tietz Fundamentals of Clinical Chemistry*, ed. 4. Philadelphia, WB Saunders Co, 1996.

Physician's Office Laboratory Guidelines: Tentative Guidelines, ed 3. Villanova, Pa, National Committee for Clinical Laboratory Standards, 1995, POL ½-T3 and POL 3-R.

STUDY QUESTIONS

1. **Match each of the following terms (1 to 5) with its definition (A to E):**

   1. Discrete selective analyzer
   2. Continuous-flow analyzer
   3. Proportioning
   4. Dry-film technology
   5. Random access analyzer

   _____ A. Analyzer in which samples flow in sequence through a channel; each sample in the batch or run is subjected to the same analytic reaction.

   _____ B. A combining of predetermined amounts of reagent and sample.

   _____ C. Technology in which the reagents are already proportioned in the required amounts on slides and only the sample must be added.

   _____ D. Analyzer in which each sample undergoes analysis on a discretionary basis and only selected tests are run on each sample.

   _____ E. Analyzer that does all the selected determinations on a patient sample before it goes on to the next sample.

2. **List the sequence of the automation process for laboratory testing, beginning with test ordering by the physician.**

3. **What are the CLIA '88 regulations regarding use of control specimens in automated laboratory testing?**

CHAPTER 10

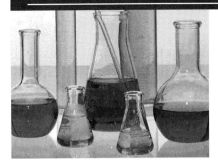

Introduction to Laboratory Computers

Learning Objectives

From study of this chapter, the reader will be able to:

➤ Be familiar with the terminology used to describe the components of a laboratory information system.

➤ Describe the parts of and uses for laboratory computers.

PURPOSE OF THE LABORATORY COMPUTER

Because the number of tests performed in the clinical laboratory has grown so dramatically over the years and because so much analytic information has been produced by these tests, the ability to process this information efficiently and accurately has become essential. This information is, of course, utilized for the benefit of the patient. We have seen that the quality assurance process requires the documentation of all work involved in patient care. The laboratory computer provides this service. It is a powerful tool for improvement of the quality of the work done as well as the productivity of the laboratorians employed to do the work. The advent of the microcomputer, under the control of microprocessors, has been responsible for the many changes in the design of laboratory analyzers and their interfaces with laboratory information systems (LIS).

The number of laboratory tests has increased in part as a result of the development of new diagnostic tests and also because of the increased use of automated analyzers. Many **laboratory information systems (LIS)** have been developed to assist in the delivery of the data. The laboratory computer system must be capable of delivering this information to the physician, the billing department, the patient record department, and other administrative support sites, and of ensuring that the data are communicated in a timely manner. In this way, the laboratory computer greatly influences the work done in the laboratory but also aids the users of the results outside the laboratory setting.

FUNCTIONS AND USES OF THE LABORATORY COMPUTER

An important function of the laboratory computer is to organize the various pieces of information and provide ready access to this information when it is needed. The information provided by each laboratory procedure should be maximized so that the patient receives the greatest benefit at the lowest cost. The functions

of laboratory computers include three categories: preanalytical, analytical, and postanalytical. Test ordering, printing specimen labels, and collecting the required specimens are included in the **preanalytical functions.** Generating work lists, doing the analyses, automatic entering of results via interfaces, quality control measures, and results verification are done as part of the **analytical functions** (process). **Postanalytical functions** include generating chart reports, printing result reports as needed, archiving patient results, workload recording, and billing.

Preanalytical Functions

Identifying and defining the patient in the computer system must take place before any testing is done. Most health care institutions assign a unique identification number to each patient and also enter other demographic information about the patient in the information database—information such as name, gender, age or birth date, and referring or attending physician. This is known as the **patient demographics.** This information is collected at the time of admission to the facility and entered into the hospital information system (HIS). The information is then transferred automatically and electronically from the HIS to the LIS.

Test ordering, or **order entry,** is an important first step in use of the laboratory information system. Specific data are needed during the order entry process: a patient number and a patient name, name of ordering physician or physicians, name of physician(s) to receive the report, test request time and date, time the specimen was or will be collected, name of person entering the request, tests to be performed, priority of the test request (such as stat or routine), and any other specimen comments pertaining to the request. Orders can be received most efficiently by the LIS through a computer-to-computer interface with the hospital information system, whereby physicians or nursing personnel directly order the test electronically. The laboratory can also receive a paper copy of the tests requested—the test request form or requisition, from which laboratory personnel enter the test request into the laboratory information system. The same data are needed on the paper form as are needed on the electronic order. The computer will generate collection lists, work lists, or logs with patient demographics and any necessary collection or analysis information. Work lists generated may include a loading list for a particular analyzer, for example. The LIS has numerous checks and balances built into it as a part of the order entry process.

Computerized order entry triggers the generation of specimen labels and prints those needed for the collection process. The patient demographic information will be printed on the labels (Fig. 10-1), along with special accession numbers in some institutions. These accession numbers will be represented in the bar-coding format for each of the patient's specimen labels. Bar coding greatly limits errors in specimen handling and improves productivity. For the greatest benefit, the specimen bar coding is also coordinated with the automated instruments used for testing, in which case the sampling is done directly from the primary collection tube (see Chapter 9).

After the specimen has been collected, it is sent to the laboratory for analysis.

Analytical Functions

The automated analyzers used must link each specimen to its specific test request; this is best done automatically through the use of bar codes on the specimen label but can be done manually by the laboratorian, who can link the sample at the instrument to the specimen number in the computer. Any results generated must be **verified** (approved or reviewed) by the laboratorian before the data are released to the patient report. Data useful to the laboratorian for this verification process include the display of "flags" signifying results that are outside the reference range values, the presence of **critical** or **panic values** (possible life-threatening values), values out of the technical range for the analyzer, or by failing other checks and balances built into the system. The use of automated analyzers is discussed in Chapter 9.

Quality assurance procedures, including the use of quality control solutions, are part of the analytical functions of the analyzer and its interfaced computer. CLIA '88 regulations require the documentation of all quality control data associated with any test results reported.

Postanalytical Functions

The end product of the work done by the clinical laboratory consists of the testing results produced by the particular methodology used, which are provided in the **laboratory report.** The data can be electronically transmitted to printers, computer terminals, or hand held pager terminals, giving rapid access to the test information for the user.

The Laboratory Report

An important use for the laboratory computer is to provide the physician with one comprehensive laboratory report that contains all the test information generated by the various laboratories that have performed analyses for a single patient. A paper report is still required by most accreditation agencies and by current medical practice. CLIA '88 regulations require that an LIS have the capacity to print or reprint reports easily when needed. The format of the report should be such that the test results are clear and unambiguous. Many questions need answering to establish or

```
         VALIDATION PATIENT
         9-999-999-3
PLC                02/28/94 11:05
DIGOXIN
 ‖‖‖‖‖‖‖‖‖‖‖‖‖       398291
                    AUPS
```

FIG 10-1. An example of a bar-coded specimen label. The six-digit specimen number (398291) is bar coded. The patient number, patient demographics, time/date, and test are written in human readable letters. (From Kaplan LA, Pesce AJ: Clinical Chemistry: Theory, Analysis, and Correlation, ed 3. St. Louis, Mosby, 1996, p 326.)

rule out a particular diagnosis, and the report should facilitate this process. The report should indicate any abnormality. It should answer these questions: What is the predictive value of the test for the disease in question? Is the result meaningful? What other factors could produce the result? What should be done next?

If the diagnosis has already been made, other uses can be made for the information on the report form, such as the management of the treatment plan for the patient. The physician must know the result of the most recent laboratory test, what clinically significant changes have occurred since the last test (through the retrieval of current and historical data), whether changes in therapy are indicated, and when the test should next be performed. This information constitutes what is known as an **interpretive report.**

An interpretive report form should give information about the range of reference values, flag any abnormal values, and provide these data in a readily accessible format.

Other Uses

The laboratory computer system also provides data for the hospital billing department, sends patient laboratory test data to the record room, and provides lists of available laboratory tests for the physician.

Special reports and lists can be generated by the computer. Lists of samples waiting to be tested, quality control data, lists of abnormal test results, and maintenance records all can be generated by the computer with considerable efficiency. The storage of preexisting data—all available tests, specimen requirements, quality control information (means, standard deviations, information included on report forms), instrument parameters—makes up the **database.**

Intralaboratory Communication

The computer stores information about laboratory policies, mission statements and specific objectives for the particular laboratory facility, and statements about laboratory medicine philosophy, in general. Procedure manuals with information about each test procedure, reference range statistics, the quality control systems used, test procedure reference materials, dates of adoption of new test methods, and evidence of other periodic review measures can be stored in the laboratory information system. The College of American Pathologists (CAP) accreditation standards, for example, require that laboratories establish methods for communication of needed information to ensure prompt, reliable reporting of results and that they have appropriate data storage and retrieval capacity.[1]

Extralaboratory Communication

Information regarding specimen requirements—procurement, transport, and processing—can be stored in an accessible form. Physicians ordering a test, nurses assisting in specimen collection, and others involved with the transport or handling of the specimen must have this information readily available.

Laboratory information systems often are interfaced with other information systems, most commonly the **hospital information system (HIS). Interfacing** is the use of a program allowing electronic communication between two computers. The HIS manages patient census information and demographics and systems for billing, and the more complex systems process and store patient medical information. The interfacing of the HIS and the laboratory computer facilitates the exchange of test request orders, information about the patient (patient census), the return of analytic results (the laboratory report), and the charges for the tests ordered and reported. When the data are verified, results can be retrieved by nurses or physicians in the patient care areas by use of terminals and printers. This linking of hospital and laboratory computer systems is not easy, and totally integrated systems require an institutional commitment to the process. A well-designed, easily accessible HIS-LIS database offers significant improvements in medical record keeping, patient care planning, budget planning, and general operations management tasks.

MAJOR COMPONENTS OF THE LABORATORY COMPUTER

Electronic computer systems are made up of **hardware,** the physical or "hard" parts of the computer, and **software,** the instructions that tell the computer what to do.

Hardware

Hardware for the computer consists of the physical components of the computer system. Central processing units, printers, and other terminals used for information input and output are examples of computer hardware.

Central Processing Unit

The **central processing unit (CPU)** is the central component of the computer. It functions as the brains of the system. The CPU is made up of a control unit, an **arithmetic logic unit (ALU),** and the **central memory.** The CPU carries out the instructions (program) given by the user.

Data Storage Devices

An important component is the data, or memory, storage section. This contains all the necessary instructions and data needed to operate the computer system. In addition, any short-term information, such as patient records and laboratory data, may also be stored temporarily in the memory. In addition to central memory, magnetic tapes and disks are used to store less frequently accessed data. These require more time for data retrieval but are considerably less expensive than central memory.

Central Memory, Random Access Memory. Central memory provides storage and rapid access. **Random access memory (RAM)** is a type of central memory and is commonly used to store data that are frequently altered, changed, or updated.

Magnetic Tapes. Magnetic tapes are the least expensive form of data storage. Access to information is generally slow. Data stored on tapes are sequential; all information, whether it is needed or not, must be serially passed over to find the needed information. Access time can be minutes, not seconds. The use of tapes is very common, however, for archival storage of data no longer needed on-line to the computer. Tapes are also used as a standard method for transporting information between computers.

Hard Disks. Hard disks, or a **hard drive,** are revolving disks, small record-like plates, with a magnetic surface that can be easily accessed. Data are stored in tracks, a series of concentric circles on the disk. Data are retrieved by positioning the reading head over the desired portion of the track, allowing a given piece of information to rotate under the head. Accessing information from disks takes milliseconds, not minutes. The transfer of information stored on a hard disk to another computer is usually not possible, and the cost of the disks and associated hardware is usually considerably higher than that of magnetic tape.

Floppy Disks. Floppy disks, also called **diskettes,** are used in many microcomputer-based instruments and word processors because of their low cost.

Input Devices

Input devices allow communication between the user and the CPU. There are several peripheral devices that allow this communication to take place. Some of these also function as output devices. The exchange of information between the computer and the user is called interfacing. Interfacing is accomplished through one of several kinds of devices. Most often the computer information is displayed on a video screen—the display screen.

Data input and output can be accomplished either by command line entry, also known as string entry, or by menu selection. Command line entry is the inputting of a series of individual commands or pieces of information in a single step to instruct the computer about the task to be done. Information about a patient identification number and a specific piece of information about a test result for that patient are examples of data that could be inputted by string entry. Instead of each piece of information being entered separately, the data are entered together ("strung" together). Individual command lines are separated from each other by commas. By entering a series of related commands, or inputs, as a single command, the user spends less time at the keyboard, the usual input device.

Menus are lists of programs or functions or other options offered by the system. A cursor is moved to the point on the list—for example, a list of tests—that is the option of choice and placed on the test desired. The use of a menu for data input is best when there are a limited number of choices to be made and also for persons who are new to the use of the computer.

Keyboard. Standardized codes called **ASCII (American Standard Code for Information Interchange)** allow the entire keyboard to be used to enter alphanumeric (letters and numerical symbols) as well as numerical data into the computer. More complex systems use function keys, which enter a series of commands, reducing the number of keystrokes required to carry out a function such as returning to a previous screen or terminating the data entry.

Cathode-Ray Tube. The **cathode-ray tube (CRT)** allows exchange of information between the user and the CPU on a specially designed television tube. The user can view on the display screen the commands given as well as the data exchanged.

Bar-Code Reader. **Bar-code readers** read a series of black lines (bars) on a label and convert these data to a sequence of numbers representing specific information (Fig. 10-1). This information can be patient identification, tests requested, or identification of a reagent for a test. Bar codes are being used on identification wristbands and hopefully will allow for better control of accuracy for patient identification purposes

and for labels for specimen containers and test requests.

Interfacing. Much laboratory time has been saved by the interfacing of the laboratory computer with the analytic testing instrument so that the test result can be entered directly into the computer information system. A port is used to permit the main computer to interface with the computer of the analytic instrument. The test result data are transferred directly over a single wire. The port is a memory location in the CPU that is connected to a series of wires. The wires are, in turn, connected to the instrument computer.

Other Input Devices. Additional input devices can enhance the exchange of information between user and computer. Touch screens allow interaction with the CPU through a menu. The position of touch on the screen determines the choice. A light pen (stylus) can be used to interact with a light-sensitive screen to indicate a menu choice. A mouse is a manual device that moves a cursor when the device is rolled along a flat surface. It also interacts with the computer through a menu.

Output Devices

Output is any information that the computer generates as a result of its calculations or processing. The CRT, printers, and instrument computers all can function as **output devices.** The computer directs the needed data from its central memory or from a storage device (magnetic tape or disk) to the specific output device. For the CRT, the output of the data generated is displayed on the screen. The printer is the usual output device of the computer system and produces a paper copy.

As laboratory results are entered and verified, a documented trail can be produced by the computer system. The organization of the data in the computer is called the database.

The computer has stored the data on when a test was ordered, when the specimen was collected, when the test was done in the laboratory, and when the test result was entered and verified. In addition, data are available about who ordered the test, who collected the specimen, and who ran the test in the laboratory. The names of the persons involved in the process are stored in the database of the computer. This documentation of data is an important part of the quality assurance program of the laboratory.

Printers. When the computer-generated data are printed on paper, they are called **hard copy.** The printed output data are placed on the patient's chart and added to the official (legal) medical record of the patient. The format or style of the printed report is determined by the kind of software program used. This allows for changes when needed.

One specific output function utilizing the printer is the generating of printed labels for specimen containers at the time of order entry for a test. Another use for printed output is the generation of a printed list of test requests along with their accession numbers. This list defines the workload for the laboratory for a given time period and thus is called a **work list.** This work list can be used in planning the day's work for specific areas within the laboratory. Computer-generated lists showing test results flagged for critical values or abnormal results can alert the laboratorian to transmit critical results to the physician or to ask to have a test repeated. Some computer systems will compare a patient result with a previous result for that patient. This is called a **difference check,** which serves to alert the laboratorian to an otherwise undetected error in analysis. This difference check can also signify a change in the condition of the patient and can alert the physician to this change.

Software

Instructions that direct the computer to perform its specific tasks are called the software or **program.** These instructions direct the various tasks to be done, using a predetermined order. Instructions that direct the collection of the data,

their assimilation, the various tasks that make use of the data, and the transfer of data are all included in the software program. The program also contains the information needed to communicate with the input and output devices being used.

Software programs are written in a specific language so that the computer can understand or accept it. Only by changing the program can any modification be made in the predetermined instructions for the operation of the laboratory information system.

FUTURE CONSIDERATIONS FOR LABORATORY COMPUTERS

New technologies for computers in the laboratory include the use of voice-recognition devices and portable electronic handwriting notebooks or tablets. Using voice recognition as input for the computer requires considerable computer power. These devices could be potentially easier to use than keyboards, but most are still in the developmental stage.

With the increased use of POCT, it has been difficult to interface results with the LIS; because many POCT devices are currently limited in their ability to interact with the LIS, results cannot be documented as regulations mandate. Often results are needed quickly, however, and the POCT results are utilized by clinicians without the proper documentation. When results are not in the LIS, they are not available for use by all clinical personnel. Interfacing POCT instrumentation with the LIS remains a problem.

Another challenge for computer technology is that of providing more information to the physician about the utilization of the various tests or interpretive data. Access to more clinical information and medical decision-making processes would also be beneficial to the physician.

Proposals have been made to utilize computerized medical charts as an effective cost-reduction scheme. By use of computerized medical charts, information pertaining to the patient could be transferred between users much more efficiently. This activity could be coupled with order entry and guidelines for medical practice. To date, the challenge of accomplishing this task is ongoing.

REFERENCES

1. Commission on Laboratory Accreditation: Laboratory Accreditation Manual, Inspection Checklist, Section 1, Laboratory general-computer services. Northfield, Ill,. College of American Pathologists, 1996.

BIBLIOGRAPHY

Aller RD, Elevitch FR (eds): *Clinics in Laboratory Medicine Symposium on Computers in the Clinical Laboratory*, vol 3. Philadelphia, WB Saunders Co, 1983.

Burtis CA, Ashwood ER (eds): *Tietz Textbook of Clinical Chemistry*, ed 4, Philadelphia, WB Saunders Co, 1996.

College of American Pathologists: Standards for laboratory accreditation. *Pathologist* 1982; 36:641.

Henry JB (ed): *Clinical Diagnosis and Management by Laboratory Methods*, ed 19. Philadelphia, WB Saunders Co, 1996.

Kaplan LA, Pesce AJ: *Clinical Chemistry: Theory, Analysis, and Correlation*, ed 3. St Louis, Mosby, 1996.

STUDY QUESTIONS

1. **Match the following terms (1 to 6) with their definitions (A to F):**

   1. Hardware
   2. Software
   3. Interface
   4. Database
   5. Program
   6. Difference check

   _____ A. Comparison of a patient result with a previous result for that same patient.

   _____ B. The physical or "hard" parts of the computer.

   _____ C. Instructions directing the computer hardware to do specific functions.

   _____ D. The instructions that tell the computer what to do.

   _____ E. Program allowing two computers to interchange data electronically.

   _____ F. Organization of the data in the computer.

2. **What are two common types of output devices?**

3. **What are four input devices?**

4. **Identify the following abbreviations:**
   A. CPU
   B. RAM
   C. LIS
   D. HIS

5. **What are three preanalytical functions of a laboratory computer?**

6. **What are three postanalytical functions of a laboratory computer?**

Prefixes, Suffixes, and Stem Words

Every specialty has a vocabulary of its own. The clinical laboratory is no different. Progress in learning the vocabulary of the laboratory and of medicine in general will come with experience, but some introductory information is important for anyone coming into the laboratory for the first time.

Most modern medical words are made up of parts derived from Greek or Latin, some with changes that have gradually been made over the years as the ancient words were adopted into English. All but the simplest medical terms are made up of two or three parts. For example, *pathology* is the study of disease. The root word is *pathos-*, from the Greek, meaning disease. The suffix *-logy* is from the Greek word *-logia,* from *logos,* meaning the study of. By examining the root or stem word along with the prefix or suffix, the meaning of most medical words can be understood.

Many of the common prefixes, suffixes, and stem words are listed below.

Prefix/Stem Word	Meaning
a-, an-	lack, not
ab-, a-	away from, outside of
ad-	to, toward
ambi-, ambo-	both
amyl-, amylo-	starch
angi-, angio-	vessel, vascular
ante-	before, preceding, in front of
arteri-, arterio-	artery, arterial
arthr-, arthro-	joint
aur-, auri-, auro-	ear

Prefix/Stem Word	Meaning
bi-	two, twice, double
bi-, bio-	life
brachi-, brachio-	arm, brachial
brady-	slow
bronch-, broncho-	bronchus, bronchial
cardi-, cardia-, cardio-	heart, cardiac
cephal-, cephalo-	head
cerebr-, cerebri, cerebro-	cerebrum, cerebral, brain
cervic-, cervico-	neck, cervix, cervical
chol-, chole-, cholo-	bile, gall
circum-	around, about
co-, com-, con-, cor-	with, together
col-, coli-, colo-	colon
contra-, counter-	against, opposite
crani-, cranio-	cranium, cranial
cyan-, cyano-	dark blue, presence of the cyanogen group
cyst-, cysti-, cysto-	gallbladder, urinary bladder, pouch, cyst
de-	undoing, reversal
dec-, deca-	ten, multiplied by ten
deci-	tenth, one tenth of
derm-, derma-, dermo-	dermis, dermal, skin
dextr-, dextro-	toward, of, or pertaining to the right
di-, dis-	two, twice, double
dipl-, diplo-	twofold, double, twin
dis-, di-	separation, reversal, apart from
dys-	abnormal, diseased, difficult, painful, unlike
en-, em-	in, inside, into
end-, endo-	within, inner, internal
enter-, entero-	intestine, intestinal
ep-, epi-	upon, beside, among, above
erythr-, erythro-	red
eu-	good, well, normal, true

Prefix/Stem Word	Meaning	Prefix/Stem Word	Meaning
ex-, e-, ef-	out, away, without	micr-, micro-	small, minute, one millionth
extra-	outside of, beyond the scope of	mon-, mono-	single, one, alone
ferri-	ferric, containing iron III	morph-, morpho-	form, structure
ferro-	ferrous, containing iron II	multi-	many, much, affecting many parts
fibr-, fibro-	fiber, fibrous		
gastr-, gastro-	stomach, gastric	my-, myo-	muscle
gluc-, gluco-	glucose	myel-, myelo-	marrow
glyc-, glyco-	sweet, sugar, glucose, glycine	nas-, naso-	nose, nasal
		ne-, neo-	new, recent
gyne-	female, woman	necr-, necro-	death
hem-, hema-, hemo-	blood	nephr-, nephro-	kidney
hemi-	half, partial	neur-, neuro-	neural, nervous, nerve
hepat-, hepato-	liver, hepatic	nitr-, nitro-	nitrogen
heter-, hetero-	other, another, different	non-	not, ninth, nine
hex-, hexa-	six	normo-	normal
hom-, homo-	common, like, same	nucle-, nucleo-	nucleus, nuclear
hydr-, hydro-	water, hydrogen	oo-	egg, ovum
hyp-, hypo-	deficiency, lack, below	orth-, ortho-	straight, direct, normal
hyper-	excessive, above normal	ost-, oste-, osteo-	bone
hyster-, hystero-	uterus, uterine, hysteria	ot-, oto-	ear
icter-, ictero-	icterus, jaundice	oxy-	oxygen
immuno-	immune, immunity	par-, para-	near, beside, adjacent to
in-, im-	not, in, into	path-, patho-	pathologic
inter-	between, among	peri-	about, beyond, around
intra-	within, inside	phag-, phago-	eating, feeding
is, iso-	equality, similarity, uniformity	pharyng-, pharyngo-	pharynx, pharyngeal
		phleb-, phlebo-	vein, venous
juxta-	near, next to	phon-, phono-	sound, speech, voice
kerat-, kerato-	horn, horny, cornea	phot-, photo-	light
ket-, keto-	presence of the ketone group	physi-, physio-	natural, physical, physiologic
kilo-	thousand	phyt-, phyto-	plant, vegetable
lact-, lacti-, lacto-	milk, lactic	plasm-, plasmo-	plasma, protoplasm, cytoplasm
lapar-, laparo-	flank, abdomen		
laryng-, laryngo-	larynx, laryngeal	pneum-, pneumo-	air, gas, lung, respiratory
latero-	lateral, to the side	poly-	multiple, compound, complex
leuk-, leuc-, leuko-, leuco-	white, colorless, leukocyte		
levo-	left, on the left	post-	after, behind
lith-, litho-	stone	pre-	before
lymph-, lympho-	lymph, lymphatic	pro-	front, forward, before
macr-, macro-	large, great, long	proct-, procto-	rectum, anus
mal-	wrong, abnormal, bad	prot-, proto-	first, primitive, early
mamm-, mammo-	breast	pseud-, pseudo-	false, deceptively resembling
medi-, medio-	middle, medial, median		
meg-, mega-, megal-	large, extended, enlarged, one million times as large as	psych-, psycho-	psyche, psychic, psychology
		pulmo-	lung, pulmonary
		py-, pyo-	pus

Prefix/Stem Word	Meaning
pyel-, pyelo-	renal, pelvic
pykn-, pykno-, pycn- pycno-	compact, dense
pyr-, pyro-	fire, heat
radio-	radiation, radioactivity
re-	again, back
ren-, reni-, reno-	kidney, renal
retro-	back, backward, behind
rhin-, rhino-	nose, nasal
rubr-, rubri-, rubro-	red
sarc-, sarco-	flesh, fleshlike, muscle
semi-	half
ser-, seri,- sero-	serum, serous
sub-	under, less than
super-	above, upon, extreme
supra-	upon, above, beyond, exceeding
syn-, sym-	together, with
tachy-	rapid, quick, accelerated
thorac-, thoraci-, thoracio-, thoraco-, thorax, thoracic	thorax, thoracic
thromb-, thrombo-	clotting, coagulation, blood platelets
thyr-, thyreo-, thyro-	thyroid
tox-, toxi-, toxo-	toxic, poisonous
trache-, tracheo-	trachea, tracheal
trans-	through, across
trich-, tricho-	hair, filament
un-	not, without
uni-	one
ur-, uro-	urine, urinary
uter-, utero-	uterus, uterine
vas-, vasi-, vaso-	vessel, vascular
ven-, vene-, veni-, veno-	vein, venous

Suffix/Stem Word	Meaning
-algia	a painful condition
-ase	enzyme
-ation	action, process
-blast	sprout, shoot, germ, formative cell
-cele	tumor, hernia, pathologic swelling
-cyte	cell
-desis	binding, fusing
-ectomy	surgical removal
-emia	blood
-ethesia	feeling, sensation
-gram	drawing, record
-graph	something written, recorded
-itis	inflammation
-logy	field of study
-lysis	dissolving, loosening, dissolution
-megaly	abnormal enlargement
-oma	tumor, neoplasm
-opia, -opy	defect of the eye
-osis	process, state, diseased condition
-pathy	disease, therapy
-penia	deficiency
-phil, -phile	having an affinity for
-plasty	plastic surgery
-rrhage, -rrhagia	abnormal or excessive discharge
-scope	viewing instrument
-scopy	inspection, examination
-stoma	mouth, opening
-stomy	operation establishing an opening into a part
-tomy	cutting, incision, section
-uria	of or in the urine

Abbreviations

ADH	antidiuretic hormone		**DAT**	direct antiglobulin test
AGN	acute glomerulonephritis		**DIC**	disseminated intravascular coagulation
AGT	antiglobulin test or reaction		**DNA**	deoxyribonucleic acid
AHG	antihuman globulin		**EA**	early antigen
AIDS	acquired immune deficiency syndrome		**EBV**	Epstein-Barr virus
AIN	acute interstitial nephritis		**EDTA**	ethylenediaminetetraacetic acid
ANA	antinuclear antibody		**EIA**	enzyme immunoassay
APTT	activated partial thromboplastin time		**ELISA**	enzyme-linked immunosorbent assay;
ASCLS	American Society for Clinical			enzyme-labeled immunosorbent
	Laboratory Science			assay
ASCP	American Society of Clinical		**EMB**	eosin methylene blue agar
	Pathologists		**ESR**	erythrocyte sedimentation rate
ASO	antistreptolysin O		**FIA**	fluorescence immunoassay
BAP	blood agar (plate)		**Hb**	hemoglobin
BT	bleeding time		**HBV**	hepatitis B virus
CAP	College of American Pathologists		**HCFA**	Health Care Financing Administration
CBC	complete blood count		**Hct (or Ht)**	hematocrit
CDC	Centers for Disease Control and		**HCV**	hepatitis C virus; formerly called non-
	Prevention			A, non-B hepatitis virus
CFU	colony-forming unit		**HDN**	hemolytic disease of newborn
CFU-C	colony-forming unit, culture		**Hgb**	hemoglobin
CFU-L	colony-forming unit, lymphoid		**HHS**	Department of Health and Human
CFU-S	colony-forming unit, spleen			Services
CLA	clinical laboratory assistant		**HIS**	hospital information system
CLIA '88	Clinical Laboratory Improvement		**HIV**	human immunodeficiency virus
	Amendments of 1988		**HLA**	human leukocyte antigen
CLT	clinical laboratory technician		**HMWK**	high-molecular-weight kininogen
COLA	Commission on Office Laboratory		**IAT**	indirect antiglobulin test
	Accreditation		**IDDM**	insulin-dependent (type 1) diabetes
CPD	citrate phosphate dextrose			mellitus
CPDA-1	citrate phosphate dextrose with		**IF**	intrinsic factor
	adenine		**Ig**	immunoglobulin
CPU	central processing unit		**IL**	interleukins
CQI	Continuous Quality Improvement		**IM**	infectious mononucleosis
CRT	cathode ray tube		**IU**	international unit
CSF	colony stimulating factor;		**IV**	intravenous
	cerebrospinal fluid		**JCAHO**	Joint Commission on Accreditation of
				Healthcare Organizations

L	liter		PCV	packed cell volume
LAP	leukocyte alkaline phosphatase		PEP	post-exposure prophylaxis
LIS	laboratory information system		PKK	plasma prekallikrein
LISS	low-ionic-strength saline solution		PMN	polymorphonuclear neutrophil
M	meter		PPM	provider-performed microscopies
Mac	MacConkey (agar)		PRP	platelet-rich plasma
MBC	minimal bactericidal concentration		PT	prothrombin time
MCH	mean cell hemoglobin		PTT	partial thromboplastin time
MCHC	mean cell hemoglobin concentration		PV	predictive value
MCV	mean cell volume		QA	quality assurance
MIC	minimal inhibitory concentration		QC	quality control
MKC	megakaryocyte		RAM	random access memory
MLA	medical laboratory assistant		RBC	red blood cell
MLT	medical laboratory technician		RCF	relative centrifugal force
mol	mole		RDW	red cell distribution width
MPV	mean platelet volume		RES	reticuloendothelial system
MSDS	material safety data sheets		RF	rheumatoid factor
MT	medical technologist		RhIG	Rh immune globulin
NA	numerical aperture		RIA	radioimmunoassay
NAD+	nicotinamide adenine dinucleotide, oxidized form		RTF	renal tubular fat
			SB	sheep blood (agar)
NADH	nicotinamide adenine dinucleotide, reduced form		SEM	scanning electron microscope
			SI	International System of Units (le Système International d'Unités)
NBS	National Bureau of Standards			
NCA	National Certification Agency for Medical Laboratory Personnel		SLE	systemic lupus erythematosus
			SPIA	solid-phase immunosorbent assay
NCCLS	National Committee for Clinical Laboratory Standards		TEM	transmission electron microscope
			TLC	thin-layer chromatography
NCEP	National Cholesterol Education Program		TQI	Total Quality Improvement
			TT	thrombin time
NIDDM	non-insulin-dependent (type 2) diabetes mellitus		VAD	vascular access device
			VDRL	Venereal Disease Research Laboratory (test for syphilis)
OFB	oval fat body			
OGTT	oral glucose tolerance test		vWD	von Willebrand's disease
OSHA	Occupational Safety and Health Administration		vWF	von Willebrand's factor
			WBC	white blood cell
PCT	postcoital test			

Reference Values

Selected reference values for common clinical laboratory tests follow. Values will differ slightly with individual laboratories and methodology. Reference values must be established for each laboratory.

▎HEMATOLOGY*

Values are for adults (unless indicated otherwise).

Hemoglobin	M	14.0-17.5 g/dL
	F	12.3-15.3 g/dL
Hematocrit†	M	40%-54%
	F	37%- 47%
RBC	M	4.5-5.9 × 10^{12}/L
	F	4.1-5.1 × 10^{12}/L
MCV	M/F	80-96.1 fL
MCH	M/F	27.5-33.2 pg
MCHC	M/F	33.4-35.5 g/dL (%)
RDW	M/F	11.5%-14.5%
WBC	M/F	4.4-11.3 × 10^9/L
		(over 21 years)
		6.0-17.5 × 10^9/L
		(12 months)

---

*Hematology reference values are taken from Beutler E et al: *Williams Hematology,* ed 5. New York, McGraw-Hill, Inc, 1995, unless indicated otherwise.

†Hematocrit values are from NCCLS: *Procedure for Determining Packed Cell Volume by the Microhematocrit Method: Approved Standard,* ed 2. Villanova, Pa, National Committee for Clinical Laboratory Standards, August, 1993, H7-A2.

Platelets	M/F	172-450 × 10^9/L
Reticulocyte count*		
Relative count	M	1.1%-2.1%
	F	0.9%-1.9%
Absolute count	M/F	50 × 10^9/L

Leukocyte differential cell count (M/F, age 21 and above)

	Mean % (relative count)	Mean absolute count × 10^9/L
Neutrophils	59	4.4
Band	3.0	0.22
Segmented	56	4.2
Lymphocytes	34	2.5
Monocytes	4.0	0.3
Eosinophils	2.7	0.20
Basophils	0.5	0.04

Erythrocyte sedimentation rate (ESR)†

	Less than 50 years	Over 50 years	Over 85 years
Male	0-15 mm/hr	0-20	0-30
Female	0-20 mm/hr	0-30	0-42

▎URINALYSIS‡

Specific gravity	
Random urine	1.001-1.035
Normal diet and fluid	1.016-1.022

---

*Reticulocyte count reference values are from Williams WJ et al: *Hematology,* ed 4. New York, McGraw-Hill Book Co, 1990.

†ESR reference values are from Henry JB (ed): *Clinical Diagnosis and Management by Laboratory Methods,* ed 19. Philadelphia, WB Saunders Co, 1996.

‡Urinalysis reference values are those established for the Fairview-University Medical Center, University Campus, Minneapolis, Minn.

Chemical screen

pH	5-7
Protein	Negative
Blood	Negative
Glucose	Negative
Ketones	Negative
Nitrite	Negative
Leukocyte esterase	Negative
Urobilinogens	To 1 EU/dL
Bilirubin (conjugated)	Negative

Sediment examination (12:1 concentration)

RBC	0-2/hpf
WBC	0-5/hpf (female > male)
Casts	0-2 hyaline/lpf
Squamous epithelial cells	Few/lpf
Transitional epithelial cells	Few/hpf
Renal tubular epithelial cells	Few/hpf
Bacteria	Negative
Yeast	Negative
Abnormal crystals	Negative

CHEMISTRIES, SERUM (ADULT)*

Alanine aminotransferase (ALT)	10-35 U/L
Alkaline phosphatase	
Male	30-90 U/L
Female	20-80 U/L
Aspartate aminotransferase (AST)	10-40 U/L
Bicarbonate	22-29 mmol/L
Bilirubin	
Total	0.3-1.2 mg/dL
Direct, conjugated	0.0-0.2 mg/dL
Calcium, total	8.5-10.2 mg/dL
Chloride	98-107 mmol/L

---

*Reference values are from Burtis CA, Ashwood ER (eds): *Tietz Fundamentals of Clinical Chemistry*, ed 4, Philadelphia, WB Saunders Co, 1996, pp 773-821.

Cholesterol	
Desirable	<200 mg/dL
Borderline/moderate risk	200-239 mg/dL
High risk	>240 mg/dL
Creatinine	
Male	0.7-1.3 mg/dL
Female	0.6-1.1 mg/dL
Creatinine clearance	
Male (under 40 yr)	90-139 mL/min/1.73 m^2
Female (under 40 yr)	80-125 mL/min/1.73 m^2
Creatine kinase (CK)	
Male	15-105 U/L
Female	10-80 U/L
Glucose (fasting)	70-105 mg/dL
Iron	
Male	65-170 μg/dL
Female	50-170 μg/dL
Total iron binding capacity (TIBC)	250-450 μg/dL
% saturation of iron	
Male	20%-55%
Female	15%-50%
pH (arterial blood)	7.35-7.45
Potassium	3.5-5.1 mmol/L
Protein, total	6.4-8.3 g/dL
Protein, albumin	3.9-5.1 g/dL
Sodium	136-145 mmol/L
Triglyceride (10-12 hr fast required)	
Male	40-160 mg/dL
Female	35-135 mg/dL
Urea	5-39 mg/dL
Urea nitrogen	7-18 mg/dL
Uric acid	
Male	4.4-7.6 mg/dL
Female	2.3-6.6 mg/dL

GLOSSARY

A

absolute cell count (absolute numbers) Concentration of a cell type expressed as a number per volume of whole blood, usually per liter; obtained by multiplying the relative percentage value by the total leukocyte count per liter.

absorbance Amount of light that is absorbed or retained and therefore not able to pass through or be transmitted through a solution.

absorbance spectrophotometry Methodology that utilizes Beer's law, whereby the amount of light absorbed by a solution is directly proportional to the concentration of the solution; this measurement can be made only by mathematical calculation from the transmission data obtained by use of a quantitative analytical method, such as spectrophotometry.

absorbance units Units of measure for light that is absorbed by a colored solution.

absorbed light Light that is not transmitted.

acceptable control range Statistically determined range of values within which a test result must fall to be considered acceptable; it is a means of quality control or assurance.

accuracy Correctness of a result, freedom from error, or how close the answer is to the "true" value.

accurate and precise technology (APT) "Easy" or automated quantitative tests or easy qualitative tests for which the manufacturer of the automated instrument has been granted special standing under CLIA '88 definitions of laboratory tests.

acholic stool Absence of bile; results in formation of colorless, chalky-appearing fecal specimens.

acid crystals Crystals seen in urine of an acidic pH, less than pH 7.0.

acid-base balance Maintenance of a constant balance between acids and bases; maintenance of constant pH.

acid-fast bacteria (AFB) Bacteria that retain staining dye and make the decolorization step difficult.

acid-fast stain Used to detect organisms that are difficult to decolorize, even with acid-alcohol solutions; typical organisms are those that cause tuberculosis or leprosy.

acidophilic Acid loving; on blood films, the cell components that stain with the acidic portion of Wright or Wright-Giemsa stain, such as hemoglobin and eosinophilic granules, which stain orange to pink.

acidosis Decrease in blood pH.

activated partial thromboplastin time (APTT) A test sensitive to heparin; useful in detecting deficiencies in intrinsic and common pathway factors.

active reabsorption A form of reabsorption that requires the expenditure of energy. This is usually against a concentration gradient, from a region of lower to one of higher concentration.

acute glomerulonephritis (AGN) Also postinfectious glomerulonephritis. A disease of the kidney glomerulus that is an immunologic sequela of a bacterial infection. Characteristics include, oliguria, edema, proteinuria, with red blood cell or granular casts, and hematuria.

acute interstitial nephritis (AIN)   An inflammation of the interstitial tissue of the kidney that is an immunologic, adverse reaction to certain drugs, such as sulfonamide or methicillin. The condition is characterized by fever, rash, proteinuria, and the presence of eosinophils in urine.

acute phase   Early in the course of a disease, when the disease is first suspected; blood is drawn (acute phase serum) when little or no antibody has had time to develop and is compared with antibody level in convalescent serum.

acute-phase reactants   Group of glycoproteins associated with nonspecific inflammatory conditions.

acute pyelonephritis   An infection of the pelvis and parenchyma of the kidney; usually the result of an ascending infection from the lower urinary tract.

additives, anticoagulants   Additives usually are anticoagulants that prevent coagulation of the blood specimen. Several different anticoagulants are available for different testing purposes. Some laboratory tests require the use of plasma or whole blood for the assay, and these must be anticoagulated during the collection process.

aerobes   Microbes that require oxygen for growth.

aerosols   Infectious particles that are airborne; fine mist in which particles are dispersed.

agar   A seaweed extract that is liquid when heated and solid when cooled; used as base medium for preparation of culture plates, slant tubes, and stab tubes.

agar disk diffusion tests   Tests that employ antibiotic-impregnated disks placed on an agar culture plate inoculated with the organism to be tested.

agar slant   Tubes of agar media that are solidified on a slant (the surface of the medium is on an incline); useful for particular cultures.

agglutination   Visible clumping or aggregation of red cells or any particles; used as an indication of a specific antigen-antibody reaction.

agglutinins   Antibodies that form visible clumps, or agglutinate, with their specific antigens.

agglutinogens   Antigens that form visible clumps, or agglutinate, with their specific antibodies.

aggregometer   Instrument that measures platelet aggregation in platelet dysfunction studies.

albuminemia   Decreased blood albumin.

albuminuria   Presence of albumin in urine.

aldosterone   Hormone that controls the sodium-potassium pump, the primary mechanism for sodium reabsorption in the kidney; regulator of blood sodium and potassium levels.

alignment   Microscope adjustment that ensures that the light path from the light source throughout the microscope and ocular is physically correct.

aliquot   One of a number of equal parts.

alkaline crystals   Crystals seen in urine of an alkaline pH; generally pH 7.0 and above.

alkalosis   Increase in blood pH.

alleles   Variants of a gene for a particular trait.

alloantibodies   Antibodies resulting from antigenic stimulation within the same species.

alpha hemolysis   Incomplete or partial hemolysis (appears green).

ambulatory patient   A patient not confined to bed; example, an outpatient or clinic patient.

American Standard Code for Information Interchange (ASCII)   Standardized codes allowing the keyboard of the computer to be used to enter alphanumeric as well as numerical data into the computer.

Americans with Disabilities Act (ADA)   Mandates that specific plans be developed for any person with a disability employed by a clinical laboratory, to ensure that the person is working in a safe atmosphere.

amorphous material   Crystalline material seen in the urine sediment as granules without shape or form.

anaerobes   Microbes that cannot grow in an atmosphere of oxygen; special steps must be taken to provide an oxygen-free atmosphere for incubation and growth of these organisms.

analog computation Measurement derived directly from an instrument signal.

analytical balance Instrument used to weigh substances to a high degree of accuracy (e.g., chemicals used in the preparation of standard solutions).

analytical functions Process whereby analytical analyses are carried out; includes generating work lists, doing the analyses, entering the results, quality control measures, and results verification.

analyzer In polarizing microscopy, a polarizing filter located above the specimen, between the objective and the eyepiece.

anemia A condition in which there is a decrease in hemoglobin in the blood and therefore in the amount of oxygen reaching the tissues and organs. May be the result of a decrease in the number of erythrocytes (decreased red cell mass), decreased hemoglobin concentration, or abnormal hemoglobin.

anion gap Concentration of unmeasured anions; calculated as the difference between measured cations and measured anions.

anisocytosis A general term indicating increased variation in the size of red cells in the blood film.

antibiotic resistance Exists if the growth of a microorganism is not inhibited by the presence of an antibiotic; the organism is resistant to the antibiotic.

antibiotic sensitivity or susceptibility Ability of the antibiotic to inhibit growth of a microorganism.

antibody Protein substance, found in the plasma or other body fluids, that is formed as the result of antigenic stimulation and is specific for the antigen against which it is formed. In blood banking, antibodies are present in commercially prepared serum, called antiserum.

antibody titer Amount of antibody present or required to produce a reaction with a particular amount of another substance; concentration of antibody.

anticoagulant Prevents coagulation of blood.

antidiuretic hormone (ADH) A hormone that regulates urine volume by increasing the amount of water reabsorbed by the kidney.

antigen Foreign (different from "self") substance that, when introduced into the body of a person lacking the antigen, results in an immune response and formation of a corresponding antibody. In blood banking, antigens are generally, but not always, found on the red cell membrane.

antigen-antibody ratio Number of antibody molecules in relation to the number of antigen sites per cell.

antihuman globulin (AHG) test (AGT) or reaction Method of detecting the presence of all human isoantibodies by using a specially prepared antiserum to human immunoglobulin and/or complement. May be a direct (DAT) or indirect (IAT) test. Also known as the Coombs' reaction or test.

antinuclear antibodies (ANA) Circulating immunoglobulins that react with the whole nucleus or nuclear components; frequently assayed by using indirect fluorescent antibody (IFA) techniques.

antiserum Serum containing antibodies. In blood banking, a special highly purified preparation of antibodies used as a reagent to show the presence of antigen on red blood cells.

anuria The complete absence of urine formation.

aperture iris diaphragm The part of the microscope located at the bottom of the Abbé condenser, under the lens but within the condenser body; controls the amount of light passing through the material under observation; can be opened or closed to adjust contrast by means of a lever.

aplastic Condition when the bone marrow is suppressed or unable to function normally in cell production.

Apt test Test for maternal hemoglobin ingestion in newborn infants.

arithmetic logic unit A component of the central processing unit (CPU) of a computer.

arthrocentesis Collection of synovial fluid from a joint by needle aspiration.

ASCII See American Standard Code for Information Exchange.

ascorbic acid (vitamin C) A strong reducing substance that may interfere with several of the reagent strip tests used in urinalysis, especially tests for blood and glucose.

atherosclerosis Condition of "hardening of the arteries," in which plaques of cholesterol, lipids, and cellular debris collect in the inner layers of the walls of large- and medium-sized arteries.

autoantibodies Antibodies directed against self-antigens.

autoclave Apparatus for effecting sterilization by using steam under pressure; when it is used with an automatic regulating pressure gauge, the degree of heat to which the contents are subjected is automatically regulated also.

automated cell counters Instruments designed to repeatedly and automatically count the numbers of formed cellular elements present in a blood specimen, usually the erythrocytes, leukocytes, and platelets.

automated differential counters Instruments designed to repeatedly and automatically determine the types and percentages of leukocytes present in a blood specimen.

automated hematocrit The hematocrit result obtained when a multiparameter instrument is used for hematology determinations. The result is computed from measured red cell volume.

automatic pipettes Devices used to repeatedly and accurately measure volumes of standard solutions, reagents, specimens, or other liquid substances.

automatic pipetting devices See automatic pipettes.

azotemia Significantly increased concentrations of urea and creatinine in the blood.

B

B lymphocyte Blood cell that matures in the bone marrow; undergoes transformation to plasma cell that produces antibodies or immunoglobulins.

bacilli Rod-shaped bacteria.

bacteremia Presence of bacteria in blood; bacteria can be cultured from the blood.

bacteriology The study of bacteria.

bacteriuria Presence of bacteria in the urine.

balance the centrifuge To make certain that weight is distributed evenly on opposite sides of the centrifuge to prevent breakage of contents being centrifuged.

bar-code readers Optical reading devices that convert a series of black lines into a sequence of numbers or letters for entry into a computer (e.g., names of patients, identification numbers, tests requested).

bar coding A sample recognition system whereby the bar codes—a series of black lines or bars on a label, for example—can be electronically read. Bar codes contain information such as name, hospital number, date, and other patient demographic data; see bar-code readers.

barrier precautions Personal protective devices (e.g., gloves, gowns) placed between blood or other body fluid specimen and the person handling it, to prevent transmission of infectious agents borne by specimens. See also personal protective equipment.

basic first aid Immediate care given after an injury, before treatment is started by trained medical personnel.

basophilia An increase in the number of basophils.

basophilic Base loving. The acidic cell components, such as nuclei and cytoplasmic RNA, that stain blue-violet by methylene azure in polychrome stains.

basophilic stippling The presence of dark blue granules evenly distributed throughout the red cell in Wright-stained blood films.

batch or run A collection of any number of specimens to be analyzed at any one time, plus control specimens, standard solutions, and so forth.

batch analyzers Analyzer that can test a batch of samples simultaneously for one particular analyte at a time; are designed to analyze a number of different analytes, but only one at a time.

bedside testing Capillary blood samples can be used to perform rapid testing procedures (many are utilizing commercial products) at the bedside; a common test is the glucose blood test, done for management of diabetes mellitus patients; see also point-of-care testing (POCT).

Beer's law, Beer-Lambert law In a solution, color intensity at a constant depth is directly proportional to concentration.

Benedict's qualitative test A copper reduction test for reducing sugars (substances) in urine; the basis of the Clinitest Tablet Test.

beta hemolysis   Clear or complete hemolysis.

bilirubin   Vivid yellow pigment; major byproduct of normal red blood cell destruction.

bilirubin glucuronide, direct bilirubin, conjugated bilirubin   Water-soluble form of bilirubin; formed by conjugation with glucuronic acid in the liver.

biochemical properties and reactions   Properties are characteristics (e.g., molecular weight, melting point) present in various types of chemicals; reactions involve the conversion of one chemical species, the reactant, to another chemical species, the product.

biohazard symbol   Symbol or term denoting any infectious material or agent that presents a possible health risk.

biohazard containers   All infectious materials are handled as potential biohazards. These special containers should be used for all blood, other body fluids, and tissues, and disposable materials contaminated with them; they should be tagged "Biohazard" or bear the standard biohazard symbol.

biohazard waste   See infectious waste.

biometrics   The science of statistics applied to biological observations.

biosafety cabinet   Protective workplace device used to control the presence of infectious agents in the air.

birefringence   Ability of an object or crystal to rotate or polarize light.

blank solution   Solution containing all the components, including solvents and solutes, except the compound to be measured.

bleeding time (BT)   The time required for cessation of bleeding after a standardized capillary puncture to a capillary bed; dependent on capillary integrity, numbers of platelets, and platelet function.

blood banking   The procedures involved in collecting, storing, processing, and distributing blood.

blood spot collection   Collection of capillary blood onto a filter paper; example, spot collections for neonatal screening programs.

blood transfusion   Technique of replacing whole blood and/or its components.

blood-borne pathogens   Infectious agents or pathogens carried by blood and blood products.

Board of Registry of the American Society of Clinical Pathologists (ASCP)   Offers an examination and certification for medical laboratory personnel.

body cavity fluids   Fluids normally found in small amounts in various cavities or body spaces (e.g., cerebrospinal, pleural, abdominal, pericardial, peritoneal, and synovial fluid). In certain conditions, such fluid is aspirated and assayed.

body tube   The part of the microscope through which the light passes to the ocular.

brightfield microscope   Illumination system used in the common clinical microscope.

broth media   Culture media that are in a broth or liquid form in a tube.

buffy coat   One of the three layers of normal anticoagulated blood. A thin grayish-white layer on top of the packed red blood cells, consisting of leukocytes and platelets, which normally makes up 1% of the total blood volume.

buret   Long cylindrical graduated tube with a stopcock delivery closing on one end, used to control the delivery of the flow of liquid from the device; used to deliver measured quantities of fluid or solutions.

C

calibrated cuvettes   Tubes or cuvettes that have been optically matched so that the same solution in each will give the same reading on the photometer.

calibration   Means by which glassware or other laboratory apparatus is checked to determine the exact units it will measure or deliver by relating them to a known concentration of an analyte.

calibration mark   Mark on volumetric glassware that indicates the point from which the volume is measured.

calculi   Kidney or renal stones.

CAP quality assurance program   Provided by CAP to assist a laboratory in organizing and managing its quality assurance program under CAP.

capillary blood (peripheral blood) collection Blood drawn from the capillary bed by means of puncturing the skin; example, a finger or heel puncture.

capillary pipette Small glass or plastic tube used to collect small amounts of capillary blood, usually directly from a capillary puncture.

capillary tube density gradient Method of cell enumeration whereby cells, upon centrifugation, settle in different layers because of their different densities; they are further expanded, stained, and magnified to derive the results of the counts.

carcinogens Substance that can cause the development of cancerous growths in living tissues.

casts Structures that result from solidification of Tamm-Horsfall mucoprotein in the lumen of the kidney tubules; they form a mold, or cast, of the tubule and trap other material that may be present when they are formed. Several types exist. They represent a biopsy of the kidney and are clinically significant.

catabolism The phase of metabolism in which fats are broken down for energy.

cathode ray tube (CRT), terminal, video display unit Television-like screen device used to monitor input, output, and general status of a computer system.

cell-mediated (cellular) response Involves actions of T lymphocytes and their subsets, together with plasma cells and macrophages.

Celsius scale Scale used to measure temperature in the metric system; outdated term for this scale is centigrade.

Centers for Disease Control and Prevention (CDC) Carries out mandated public health laws and reporting requirements.

central memory A component of the central processing unit (CPU) of a computer; provides storage and rapid access for information (data).

central processing unit (CPU) The part of the computer that controls and performs the execution of programs or instructions.

centralized laboratory A central location in a health care facility where all laboratory testing is done.

centrifugation Separation of a solid material from a liquid by application of increased gravitational force by rapid rotating or spinning.

cerebrospinal fluid (CSF) Extravascular fluid that surrounds the brain and spinal cord. Formed by the choroid plexus in the ventricles of the brain and found within the subarachnoid space, the central canal of the spinal cord, and the four ventricles of the brain.

cervical mucus test See Fern test.

chain of custody When results of laboratory testing are to be used in a court of law, a specific chain of documentation is required, whereby all steps of the testing are recorded, from specimen collection to the issuing of the results report.

chemical hygiene plan Outlines the specific work practices and procedures necessary to protect workers from any health hazards associated with use of hazardous chemicals.

chloride shift When carbon dioxide leaves the plasma and chloride diffuses or shifts out of the red cells to replace it; can take place when plasma and red cells are not separated in a timely manner.

chromasia Term used to describe the staining reaction of red cells in the Wright-stained blood film.

chromatography Method of analysis in which the solutes, dissolved in a common solvent, are separated from one another by differential distribution of the solutes between two phases (a mobile phase and a stationary phase).

chromosome Threadlike structure within the nucleus of each cell, made up of genes. Chromosomes exist in pairs in all cells except sex cells. Each species has a specific number of paired chromosomes.

chylomicrons Small droplets of lipoproteins that give blood specimens a characteristic milky appearance, when present.

CLIA '88 See Clinical Laboratory Improvement Amendments of 1988 (CLIA '88).

clinical immunology Study of antigen-antibody reactions in vitro.

clinical laboratory assistant (CLA) See clinical laboratory technician (CLT).

Clinical Laboratory Improvement Amendments of 1988 (CLIA '88) Standards set for all laboratories to ensure quality patient care; provisions include requirements for quality control and assurance, for the use of proficiency tests, and for certain levels of personnel to perform and supervise work done in the clinical laboratory.

clinical laboratory scientist (CLS) Formerly known as a medical technologist (MT); usually has earned a bachelor of science degree in medical technology or clinical laboratory science.

clinical laboratory technician (CLT) Category of laboratory personnel; this group usually has some formal laboratory training, as from a technical school or other vocational training program; CLTs usually have some limitations as to the complexity of laboratory testing they are trained to do.

clinical pathology Medical discipline by which clinical laboratory science and technology are applied to the care of patients.

clone Cell originating from a single ancestral parent cell.

clot Formation of a fibrin network; a thrombus.

clot retraction Clot becomes smaller.

clue cells Vaginal squamous epithelial cells that are covered or encrusted with *Gardnerella vaginalis*.

coagglutination To enhance visibility of agglutination, antibodies are bound to a particle.

coagulation Mechanism whereby after injury to a blood vessel, plasma coagulation factors, tissue factors, and calcium work together on the surface of platelets to form a fibrin clot.

coagulation cascade Process of coagulation, in which a series of biochemical reactions occur, converting inactive substances to active forms that in turn activate other substances; carefully controlled process responding to injury while maintaining normal blood circulation.

coagulation factors Proteins engaged in formation of a fibrin clot from fibrinogen.

coagulation system See coagulation cascade.

cocci Bacteria that are round.

coefficient of variation (CV) Used to compare the standard deviations of two samples; in percent, the CV is equal to the standard deviation divided by the mean.

cofactors Proteins that accelerate the reactions of the enzymes involved in the coagulation process.

College of American Pathologists (CAP) Professional organization of pathologists; one responsibility is to certify clinical laboratories.

colony forming unit, culture (CFU-C) Multipotential hematopoietic (myeloid) stem cell.

colony forming unit, lymphoid (CFU-L) Committed lymphoid stem cell.

colony forming unit, spleen (CFU-S) Uncommited pluripotential stem cell; also colony forming unit, lymphoid-myeloid (CFU-LM).

colony forming units (CFU) In microbiology, colony count; in hematology, a pluripotential, undifferentiated stem cell that is stimulated to proliferate and differentiate into colonies of a specific cell type.

colony stimulating factor (CSF) Factor required for hematopoietic stem cells to multiply and differentiate.

colorimetry Technique used to determine the concentration of a substance by the variation in intensity of its color.

commensal state Situation in which parasite and host exist together with no harm coming to the host.

Commission on Office Laboratory Accreditation (COLA) Provides accreditation for physician office laboratories; has been deemed HCFA-approved.

common pathway Final stages of the coagulation cascade, beginning with the convergence of the extrinsic and intrinsic pathways (factor X) and ending with formation of the fibrin clot.

community-acquired infection Infection from organisms residing or incubating in the patient before admission to a health care facility.

compatibility testing All of the tests performed before a transfusion to ensure that the transfused blood or component will benefit and not harm the recipient. These include tests on both recipient and donor blood, including a crossmatch between patient serum and donor red blood cells.

compensated polarized light Modification of the polarizing microscope in which a compensator (first-order red plate or filter) is inserted between the two crossed polarizing filters and positioned at 45 degrees to the crossed polarizer and analyzer to determine the type of birefringence. In the clinical laboratory, especially useful in examination of synovial fluid.

complement Group of serum proteins that can produce inflammatory effects and lysis of cells when activated.

complement fixation When complement is tied up or bound (fixed) to an antigen-antibody complex, it is no longer available to be activated.

complete blood count (CBC) Hematologic tests basic to the initial evaluation and follow-up of the patient. Generally includes measurement of hemoglobin, hematocrit, red blood cell count with morphology, white blood cell count with differential, and platelet estimate; specific tests vary with the facility.

components Portions of whole blood prepared for transfusion by physical means, especially centrifugation.

concentration of solution The amount of solute in a given volume of solution. May be expressed in different ways; example, moles of solute per volume of solution, with use of liter as the reference value.

condenser The part of the microscope that directs and focuses the beam of light from the light source onto the material under examination; positioned just under the stage, and can be raised or lowered by means of an adjustment knob.

confidence limits (confidence interval) A value used to express or estimate a statistical parameter; an example is when the reference range is set, using values 2 SD on either side of the mean, with 95% of the values falling above and below the mean; see also 95% confidence interval.

conjugated bilirubin, direct bilirubin, bilirubin glucuronide Bilirubin that has been conjugated with glucuronate in the liver; exists in plasma unbound to any protein, as contrasted to unconjugated bilirubin; is water soluble, and high blood levels are excreted in the urine.

Continuous Quality Improvement (CQI) See Total Quality Improvement (TQI).

continous-flow analyzer Instrument that constantly pumps reagent and sample through tubing and coil, forming a continuous stream.

control specimen Material or solution with a known concentration of the analytes being measured; used for quality control when the test result for the control specimen must be within certain limits in order for the unknown values run in the same "batch" to be considered reportable.

convalescent phase About 2 weeks after the acute phase of illness, convalescent serum is tested and the antibody titer compared with that of the acute phase serum; an important phase of serology testing is the manifestation of a rise in antibody titer during the course of a disease.

Coombs' test See antihuman globulin test.

cortex (kidney) Outer anatomical portion of the kidney; consists of the glomerular portions of the nephron and the proximal convoluted tubules.

coulometry Technique in which the charge required to completely electrolyze a sample is measured.

Coulter principle Means of counting particles and measuring their size or volume by impedance change caused by the particle in a current-conducting fluid (electrolyte); this principle is applied in many of the blood cell counters used in hematology laboratories (Coulter counter).

creatinine clearance Estimate of the function of the glomerular filtration rate; obtained by measuring the amount of creatinine in plasma and its rate of excretion in the urine.

crenated Appearance of red blood cells when present in a hypertonic solution (i.e., in urine of a high specific gravity). The cells appear shrunken, with little spicules or projections.

critical or panic values See panic or critical values.

crossmatch A procedure used to determine the compatibility of a donor's blood with that of a recipient after the specimens have been matched for major blood type. One part of compatibility testing.

crystalluria The presence of crystals in the urine sediment.

crystals, abnormal   Urinary crystals of metabolic or iatrogenic origin that are generally of pathologic significance and require chemical confirmation.

crystals, normal   Urinary crystals that may be found in normal urine specimens of an acid or alkaline pH; generally are not pathologic, and can be reported on the basis of morphologic appearance.

cyanide-nitroprusside reaction   Qualitative test used to confirm the presence of cystine crystals in urine.

cylindroids   A type of hyaline cast, with one end that tapers off to a tail or point.

cytocentrifugation   Special slow centrifugation method used to prepare permanent microscope slides of fluids (e.g., urine, other body fluids), resulting in better morphologic preservation than by other centrifugation or preparation methods.

cytocentrifuge   Uses a slow centrifuging speed, a low inertia, which rapidly spreads monolayers of cells across a special slide; used for critical morphologic studies.

culture   Growing of microorganisms or living tissue cells in special, artificial medium.

culture medium   Mixture of nutrients on which a microorganism is grown; see culture.

culture plate   Petri dish or plate in which the medium is placed; where a culture of an organism grows.

cuvette   Tube or receptacle used in a photometer for holding the sample to be measured.

cyanosis   Bluish discoloration of the skin and mucous membranes.

cysts   Inactive form of a microorganism, as a parasite cyst.

D

data   Information or results.

database   Systematic store of information (data) that can be accessed by the operator or user of a computer system.

decontamination   Process of eliminating something that has become contaminated or mixed with something that makes it impure; as cleaning a work surface after blood or other potentially infectious material has been spilled on it.

deionization   Process of removing ionized substances from water.

deionized water   See deionization.

density   Amount of matter per unit volume of a substance.

Department of Health and Human Services (HHS)   Department of the U.S. government under which the Health Care Financing Administration (HCFA) is managed. Responsible for implementation of laws and writing of regulations that provide details of how various laws are to be carried out; publishes details of proposed regulations in the *Federal Register,* an official government document.

derivatives   Blood products prepared from whole blood by more complex methods than components are. Also referred to as fractions.

dextrose   Glucose; a simple sugar.

diabetes mellitus   Chronic metabolic syndrome of impaired carbohydrate, fat, and protein metabolism that is secondary to insufficiency of insulin secretion or to the inhibition of the activity of insulin; characterized by increased concentration of glucose in the blood and urine.

diabetic coma   State of unconsciousness due to a high glucose concentration

diazo reaction   Coupling of a diazonium salt with another aromatic ring to give an azo dye.

difference check   Computer comparison of current patient result with a previous result for that same patient.

differential media   Media containing dyes, indicators, or other constituents that give colonies of particular organisms distinctive and easily recognizable characteristics.

differential stain   Stain used to differentiate specific cellular details in a microorganism; more than one stain is used to produce the end result. Gram stain is an example of a differential stain.

digital computation   Calculations that involve data available in the form of discrete units or numbers.

dilution factor Reciprocal of the dilution made; multiply the result by the reciprocal of the dilution to correct for the dilution used.

dilutions Weaker solutions made from a stronger solution. The term describes the relative concentrations of the components of a mixture; the preferred method is to refer to the number of parts of the material being diluted in the total number of parts of the final product.

diopter A metric unit of measure for the refractive power of a lens. The focus of a microscope is adjusted for the microscopist by means of the diopter adjustment in the ocular.

direct agglutination Showing visible agglutination when the constituent (antibody) being measured is present to react with the antigen, as with antigen-coated latex particles in latex agglutination assays.

discrete sample analyzer Instrument that compartmentalizes each sample reaction.

disinfectant Cleaning solution that removes pathogenic organisms but not necessarily bacterial or other spores; example, household bleach.

distilled water As water is boiled, the steam is cooled and condensed, and collected as distilled water; this process removes minerals of iron, magnesium, and calcium.

diuresis Any increase in urine volume, even if temporary.

documentation An important aspect of quality assurance; CLIA '88 regulations mandate that any problem or situation that might affect the outcome of a test result must be recorded and reported, with follow-up monitored.

dry film reagent technology Instruments or tests that use a dry film layered device that supplies the necessary reagents for the reaction to take place when the serum sample is added to it; the specimen (serum) provides the solvent (water) necessary to rehydrate the dry reagents on the film.

duplicate determinations Specimens are measured in duplicate to check technique used; a measure of precision or repeatability of the method.

dysmorphic Distorted or misshapen. Red cells in urine that are dysmorphic may indicate glomerular disease.

E

edema The abnormal accumulation of fluid in the interstitial spaces of tissues, resulting in generalized swelling.

effusion Abnormal accumulation of any of the extracellular fluids. Fluid escapes from the blood or lymphatic vessels into the tissues or body cavities (e.g., serous cavities: pericardium, peritoneum, or pleura) or the joints.

Ehrlich's aldehyde reaction Reaction of urobilinogen, porphobilinogen, and other Ehrlich-reactive compounds with *p*-dimethylaminobenzaldehyde in concentrated hydrochloric acid to form a colored aldehyde.

electrical resistance cell counter Cell counter that uses electrical resistance. Blood cells passing through an aperture through which an electrical current is being passed cause a change in the electrical resistance; this change is counted as voltage pulses.

electrolyte battery or profile Collection of tests for common electrolytes: chloride, bicarbonate, sodium, and potassium. These four electrolytes often are measured at the same time, because changes in the concentration of one almost always is accompanied by changes in one or more of the others.

electronic cell counting device Automatic instrument that counts cellular elements in the blood (usually erythrocytes, leukocytes, and platelets) repeatedly and accurately.

electrophoresis Movement of charged particles in an electrical field; technique used to separate mixtures of ionic solutes by the differences in their rates of migration in an electrical field.

employee "right to know" rule Designed to ensure that laboratory workers are fully aware of the hazardous chemicals being used in the workplace.

enrichment media Media that permit one organism to grow rapidly while inhibiting the growth of other organisms.

enumeration of formed elements Counting of cellular elements of the blood (usually erythrocytes, leukocytes, and platelets).

enzyme immunoassay (EIA)   Uses enzymes as immunochemical labels in detection of antigen-antibody reactions.

enzyme-linked (or labeled) immunosorbent assay (ELISA)   Immunoassay or test that uses an enzyme conjugated to antibodies or antigens to produce a visible end point; diagnostic test used to detect antigens or antibodies in a patient's specimen.

enzymology   The study of the various biological materials (proteins) that have catalytic activity; the study of enzymes present in the blood.

eosinopenia   A decrease in the absolute number of eosinophils below normal limits.

eosinophilia   An increase in the absolute number of eosinophils above normal limits.

epithelial cells   Cells that make up the covering of the various internal and external organs of the body, including the lining of the blood vessels.

equivalent (equiv) weight (or mass)   Mass in grams that will liberate, combine with, or replace 1 gram of hydrogen ion; generally is the molecular weight divided by the valence.

erythrocyte   Red blood cell, one of the formed elements of the peripheral blood; chief role is to transport oxygen to the tissues.

erythrocyte sedimentation rate (ESR)   Rate in millimeters at which the red blood cells fall, or sediment, in a given unit of time (usually 1 hour).

etiologic agent   Agent causing a disease.

eukaryote   Fungi, algae, protozoa; more complex than prokaryotes; contain membrane-enclosed organelles such as mitochondria, lysosomes, and a true membrane-enclosed nucleus.

exfoliated   Sloughed off tissue or cells.

exponents   Superscript numbers used to indicate how many times a number must be multiplied by itself.

exposures to hazardous chemicals   OSHA standards seek to minimize occupational exposures of this type.

extravascular component   Tissue surrounding the blood vessels.

extravascular fluid   Body cavity fluid other than blood or urine.

extrinsic system of coagulation   Coagulation pathway that is activated by tissue thromboplastin; necessary components are factor VII and calcium.

exudate   Effusion that results from inflammatory conditions, such as infections and malignancies, that directly affect the membranes lining a cavity.

eyepiece (ocular)   Microscope lens that magnifies the image formed by the objective.

F

facultative microorganism   Organism that can grow under either aerobic or anaerobic conditions.

facultative parasite   Parasite that can exist in a free-living state, as a commensal, or as a parasite; see commensal parasite.

false negatives   Those subjects who have a negative test yet do have the disease.

false positives   Those subjects who have a positive test but do not have the disease.

fastidious   Said of a microorganism that is sensitive to changes; usually requires protected culture conditions.

fasting blood glucose   Blood glucose test performed on a fasting specimen; see fasting state.

fasting state   Eight to twelve hours of refraining from consumption of food and liquids other than water. Example is when blood is collected after a 12-hour fast for some tests. Additional patient restrictions are sometimes also necessary, such as no smoking or administration of certain drugs during the fasting period.

federal regulations   Standards existing to meet objectives, such as safety regulations. For the clinical laboratory, see Clinical Laboratory Improvement Amendments of 1988 (CLIA '88).

Fern test (cervical mucus test)   Test used to determine ovulation in fertility studies and for contraception and rupture of membranes in pregnancy by observing the appearance of dried cervical mucus on a glass microscope slide.

fibrin   End product of coagulation. Forms a visible clot, a fibrin mesh, to entrap the blood cells. Is derived from fibrinogen, a plasma protein, by the action of thrombin.

fibrin clot   See fibrin.

fibrinogen, coagulation factor I   Plasma protein that is the substrate for thrombin action in the formation of fibrin. Manufactured by the liver; is not vitamin K-dependent; is the soluble precursor of the clot-forming protein, fibrin.

fibrinolysis   Destruction of the fibrin clot by plasmin activity to keep the vascular system free from clots; under normal conditions, coagulation and fibrinolysis are kept in balance.

fibrinolytic system   Functions to keep the vascular system free of fibrin clots or deposited fibrin; see fibrinolysis.

fibronectin   Assists in bonding platelets to substrate; is secreted by endothelial cells.

field diaphragm   The part of the microscope, located in the light port in the base of the microscope, through which light passes up to the condenser. It controls the area of the circle of light in the field of view when the specimen and condenser have been properly focused.

first morning urine specimen   First urine voided in the morning. It is generally the most concentrated specimen of the day, because less fluid or water is excreted during the night, yet the kidney has maintained excretion of a constant concentration of solid or dissolved substances.

fistula   An abnormal connection, such as between the colon and the urinary tract.

fixed angle-head centrifuge   A centrifuge in which the cups are held in a rigid position and at a fixed angle.

flame emission photometry   Atoms of certain elements, when sprayed into a hot flame, become excited and emit energy at wavelengths characteristic for those elements (commonly lithium, sodium, and potassium). Utilizes a device (flame photometer) to measure the intensity of the colored flame. Solution containing metal ions is sprayed into a flame, and the intensity and color of the flame are proportional to the amount of substance present in the solution.

flame photometer   Instrument used to measure the energy emitted by certain elements when they are sprayed into a flame in the photometer; see flame emission photometry.

flocculation   Clumping of fine particles to form visible masses.

floppy disks or diskettes   Diskettes that can store information not needed on a hard drive.

flow cytometers   Used to identify and enumerate the blood cells in a given patient sample; see flow cytometry.

flow cytometry   Enumeration and differentiation of blood cells by passing them through a focused beam of a laser.

fluorescent antibody (FA)   Assay that uses antibodies labeled with fluorescein compounds, which cause microscopic fluorescence as an indication of an antigen-antibody complex being formed.

fluorescent antinuclear antibody (FANA)   Screening assay for SLE; see fluorescent antibody.

focal length   Slightly less than the distance from an objective being examined microscopically to the center of the objective lens; practically, equal to the working distance.

Food and Drug Administration (FDA)   Issues certification and licensure requirements, which are an external control for clinical laboratory standards.

Forssman antibody   A heterophil antibody.

free bilirubin, unconjugated bilirubin, indirect bilirubin   Water-insoluble form of bilirubin that is carried through the blood bound to albumin.

fungemia   Presence of fungi in the blood.

G

galactosuria   The presence of galactose in urine.

galvanometer   Measures and records the amount of current (in the form of electrons) reaching it.

Gaussian curve or distribution   Particular symmetric statistical distribution, also known as a "normal" distribution; a statistical tool used to set reference ranges.

genitourinary tract specimens   Specimens collected from the genital or urinary tract (e.g., vaginal cervix and perineal area in women, anterior urethra in men).

genotype   Actual total genetic makeup. Often impossible to determine by laboratory testing, but requires additional family studies.

genus   Members of the same genus share common biological characteristics; the next larger classification after species.

germ tube   An appendage on yeast cells, the beginning of true hyphae.

gestational diabetes   Glucose intolerance that occurs during some pregnancies.

glitter cells   Large swollen neutrophilic leukocytes that appear in hypotonic urine with a specific gravity of about 1.010 or less. The cells show Brownian motion of granules in the cytoplasm, giving a glittering appearance.

glomerular filtrate   Ultrafiltrate of blood formed as blood is filtered through the glomerular capillaries of the glomerulus into Bowman's capsule. First step in urine formation; basically blood plasma without protein or fat.

glomerulus   Part of the nephron; made up of a tuft of blood vessels.

gluconeogenesis   Glucose from fat and protein that is provided to the blood.

glucose oxidase   Enzyme that allows for the oxidation of glucose to gluconic acid; the basis of the reagent strip tests for glucose in urine.

glucose tolerance test   Measures the response of the body to a challenge load of glucose; used to aid in the diagnosis of diabetes mellitus.

glucosuria, glycosuria   Abnormally high concentration of glucose in urine.

glycated hemoglobin   Hemoglobin derivative, also known as hemoglobin A_{1c}; formed when glucose and hemoglobin combine; tests used to monitor long-term blood glucose concentration in blood of diabetics measures diabetes control.

glycogenesis   Formation of glycogen from glucose.

glycolysis   Breakdown or oxidation of glucose.

glycosuria   Presence of glucose in the urine.

grades of chemicals   Varying qualities of production criteria that are placed on the manufacture of chemicals for laboratory use, depending on the use to which the chemical is put; the grade indicates the level of quality.

graduated pipette, measuring pipette   Cylindrical tube used to deliver a measured volume of liquid between two calibration (or graduation) marks on the tube; has several graduation or calibration marks on the tube, allowing a variety of measurements with the same device.

gram-molecular weight   One gram-molecular weight equals the sum of all atomic weights in a molecule of compound, expressed in grams.

gram negative   See Gram staining reaction.

gram positive   See Gram staining reaction.

Gram staining reaction (Gram stain)   With the Gram staining method, microorganisms retaining the violet (purple) color of the primary stain (crystal violet-iodine complex) are considered gram "positive"; microorganisms having the red-pink color of the counterstain (safranin) are considered gram "negative." Use of these properties serves to classify or differentiate organisms in microbiology; Gram stain is a differential stain.

gram-stained smear   Used routinely to determine Gram staining characteristics; see Gram staining reaction.

granulocyte   Leukocyte that contains prominent cytoplasmic granules; neutrophils, eosinophils, and basophils.

gravimetric analysis   Analysis by measurement of mass.

Griess test   A test for nitrite that involves a diazo reaction; basis of the reagent strip tests for nitrite in urine.

group A β-hemolytic streptococci   Microorganisms that account for most infectious "strep throat." Organisms are isolated from throat swabs by one of several methods (e.g., culture plates, rapid slide agglutination procedures).

gum guaiac   Phenolic compound that turns blue when oxidized. Commonly used as the chromogen in tests for the detection of occult blood in feces.

H

hand washing The most important means of interrupting the transmission of infectious pathogens.

Hansel's stain Stain containing eosin and methylene blue; used to stain for the presence of eosinophils.

hapten Nonantigenic, nonprotein substance that binds to protein, making a hapten-protein complex that is antigenic.

haptoglobin Protein-bound form of hemoglobin by which hemoglobin is carried through the bloodstream.

hard copy Computer-generated data printed on paper.

hard disks or hard drive Revolving disks in a computer with a magnetic surface that can be easily accessed; data are stored in tracks, a series of concentric circles on the disks.

hardware Physical elements of a computer system (e.g., central processing unit, printer, terminal).

hazard identification system Provides in words, symbols, and pictures information on presence of potential laboratory materials considered hazardous (e.g., flammable, health risk, chemical reactivity).

Health Care Financing Administration (HCFA) Agency of the U.S. Department of Health and Human Services; regulates and administers funding under the Health Insurance for the Aged Act of 1965 (Medicare); regulates reimbursement for Medicare-related activities. Medicare and Medicaid amendments to the Social Security Act authorize the regulation of specific laboratory services if the government is authorized to pay for these services to the aging and needy population of the United States. HCFA coordinates its regulatory functions with the Centers for Disease Control and Prevention (CDC).

hemagglutination (HA) Agglutination of red cells as indicator of antibody-antigen complex formation.

hematocrit Ratio of packed red blood cell volume to whole blood volume, expressed as a percent or ratio unit.

hematoma Collection of blood under the skin.

hematopoiesis Blood cell production.

hematuria Presence of red blood cells in urine.

heme An iron complex containing one iron atom. The iron-containing portion of the hemoglobin molecule.

hemocytometer Counting chamber used to perform manual cell counts.

hemoglobin Iron-containing protein portion of the red blood cells that carries oxygen to the tissues; four globin chains, each containing a hememoiety.

hemoglobin variants Different structural forms of hemoglobin, which vary in the content and sequence of amino acids in the globulin chains.

hemoglobinopathies Disorders in which the presence of structurally abnormal hemoglobins is considered to play an important role pathologically.

hemoglobinuria The presence of free hemoglobin in urine.

hemolysis Rupture of the red cell membrane and release of hemoglobin into the suspending medium or plasma; the plasma or serum appears reddish. In blood banking and other immunologic reactions, hemolysis is used as an indicator of an antigen-antibody reaction.

hemolysis, alpha In microbiology, partial destruction (lysis) of red blood cells in a blood agar plate; greenish color appears around the bacterial colony producing the alpha hemolysin.

hemolysis, beta In microbiology, complete destruction (lysis) of red blood cells around a colony on a blood agar plate; leads to a completely clear zone surrounding the colony producing the beta hemolysin.

hemolytic jaundice Type of jaundice that results from increased destruction of red cells.

hemolyzed serum Serum with lysed red blood cells in it; appears pink or red.

hemophilia Hereditary deficiency of plasma coagulation proteins; results in varying degrees of bleeding disorders, mild to severe, depending on the specific deficiency.

hemophilia A   Classic bleeder's disease; sex-linked deficiency of the coagulant component of factor VIII (antihemophilic factor); see Hemophilia.

hemophilia B   Christmas disease; sex-linked deficiency of factor IX; see Hemophilia.

hemosiderin   Iron-containing granules that may occur in urine after a hemolytic episode. Stain blue with Prussian blue stain for iron.

hemostasis/hemostatic mechanism   Cessation of blood flow from an injured blood vessel, with final intent to stop the bleeding. The state of equilibrium in which the supply is equal to the demand between all the fluid and cellular elements that make up the blood.

hemostatic plug   Result of activation of the hemostatic system; formation of platelet plug.

hepatic jaundice (hepatocellular jaundice)   Jaundice that results from conditions that involve the liver cells directly and prevent normal excretion of bilirubin, including failure in conjugation and failure in transport (regurgitation).

hepatitis B virus (HBV)   Virus that can be directly transmitted by the blood, causing hepatitis, an acute viral illness. Hepatitis is an inflammation of the liver that is endemic worldwide. Complete recovery is usual; some patients, however, remain carriers or can develop chronic hepatitis.

hepatitis C virus (HCV)   Previously known as non-A, non-B hepatitis virus. Can be transmitted directly by the blood, causing acute viral hepatitis. This infection does not show the serologic markers of hepatitis A or hepatitis B.

heteroantibodies   Antibodies resulting from exposure to antigenic material from another species.

heterophil antibodies   Antibodies stimulated by one antigen that react with entirely unrelated antigens on the red cells from different mammalian species; examples are Forssman, infectious mononucleosis and serum sickness antibodies.

heterozygous   Having different alleles for a given trait.

high-complexity tests   CLIA '88 regulations define a certain group of tests in this category; they require technical personnel of the highest degree of experience and training to be responsible for the testing.

high-power objective   Usually a 40× magnification objective, used for more detailed examination of wet preparations.

histiocyte   A cell of the reticuloendothelial system; called a macrophage when it has begun to phagocytose.

Hoesch test   Inverse aldehyde reaction, used for the detection of porphobilinogen in urine.

homozygous   Having identical alleles for a given trait.

horizontal-head centrifuge   A centrifuge in which cups holding tubes of material to be centrifuged occupy a vertical position when the centrifuge is at rest, but assume a horizontal position when the centrifuge revolves.

hospital information system (HIS)   Main hospital database; contains the base of information about the patient, established when the patient was first admitted or registered by the hospital or clinic. This database can be accessed by the laboratory information system (LIS) as necessary.

household bleach   See disinfectant.

human chorionic gonadotropin (hCG)   Hormone produced by the placenta during pregnancy; constituent measured in most rapid pregnancy tests.

human immunodeficiency virus (HIV)   Virus that can be transmitted by the blood and some body fluids; can cause HIV infection or acquired immunodeficiency syndrome (AIDS).

humoral response   Involves antibodies produced by the B lymphocytes along with complement.

hyaluronate (hyaluronic acid)   High-molecular-weight mucopolysaccharide found in synovial fluid, responsible for its normal viscosity. Secreted by the synovial fluid cells that line the joint cavity.

hyperglycemia   Increase in concentration of blood glucose.

hyperkalemia   High concentration of potassium in the serum or blood.

hypernatremia   High concentration of sodium in the serum or blood.

hypertonic   Solution or diluent that is more concentrated than that inside of the red cell.

hyphae Tube-like projections, a part of the basic structure of molds; also called mycelium.

hypochromic Said of red cells with decreased hemoglobin content, which appear very pale and show an increased area of central pallor on the peripheral blood film.

hypoglycemia Low concentration of glucose in blood.

hypokalemia Low concentration of potassium in the serum or blood.

hyponatremia Low concentration of sodium in the serum or blood.

hypotonic Solution or diluent that is less concentrated than that inside of the red cell.

hypoxia Lack of oxygen.

I

iatrogenic The result of medication or treatment; inadvertently caused by the physician.

icterus See jaundice.

immune antibodies Result from stimulation by a specific foreign antigen.

immune response Any reaction demonstrating specific antibody response to antigenic stimulus.

immunoassays Assays utilizing antigen-antibody reactions to detect the presence of a specific constituent.

immunofluorescence Technique used for rapid identification of an antigen by treating it with a known antibody tagged with a fluorescent dye and by observing the resulting characteristic antigen-antibody reaction; will appear luminous in ultraviolet light projected, using a fluorescent microscope.

immunoglobulins (Ig) Antibodies; proteins of the gamma globulin type; produced by B lymphocytes (plasma cells).

Immunohematology The study of antigen-antibody reactions and their effects on blood. Includes blood transfusion medicine and blood banking.

immunoprophylaxis Recommended after exposure to blood that is known to contain or might contain hepatitis B antigen; immune globulin is given in a single dose as soon as possible after the exposure, within 24 hours if practical.

impaired glucose tolerance When there is an abnormal glucose tolerance test but no measured hyperglycemia; a midway position between normal and a state of diagnosed diabetes mellitus.

input devices Allow communication between the user and the CPU.

in situ monitoring Monitoring in place or on site.

in vitro antigen-antibody reactions Reactions between antigens and antibodies in a test tube or on a slide (outside the living body; *in vitro* is a Latin term meaning "in glass").

incidence The number of subjects found to have a disease within a defined period of time, such as within a particular year.

indirect agglutination Assays that show agglutination when no positive constituent is present.

indwelling lines Devices used to administer therapeutic products (e.g., fluids, medications, blood products) to patients over long periods. With careful training, it is also possible to collect blood samples from these lines. Also called vascular access devices (VAD).

infection control Set policy or program within a health care institution to prevent exposure to biological hazards.

infection control program Program whereby laboratory sets up specific steps to prevent contamination from biohazardous specimens in the collection steps, transportation to the laboratory, and processing and testing steps.

infectious waste Waste that contains biohazardous specimens, such as blood and blood products, contaminated materials, or other potentially infectious products.

informed consent Legal consent granted by the patient whereby he or she is made aware of, understands, and agrees to the nature of the testing or services to be done.

infusion set Allows collection of blood from patients with small, fragile, or rolling veins.

inoculate To place the specimen on the medium in the plate or tube.

inoculating loop or needle   Metal loop or needle attached to a long handle, used to inoculate culture media with specimens or to transfer colonies for subculture. Metal loops must be flamed between uses. Disposable varieties of these loops are available.

inoculum   What is being inoculated onto the medium—plate or tube; usually the specimen is the inoculum; in antimicrobial susceptibility tests, the isolated organism to be tested is prepared in a specific way, depending on the methodology being used.

input device   Any device allowing data or instructions to be placed into a computer system.

insulin shock   State of unconsciousness due to a low blood glucose concentration.

interfacing data   Communications link that allows the transfer of data between the user and the computer system or between another processor and the computer system.

interleukins (IL)   Hematopoietic growth factors that contribute to the control of hematopoiesis.

internal standard   Chemical compound of known amount added to a specimen and carried through all steps of an analytical procedure to provide a basis for accurate quantitation, despite variations in the procedural steps; is similar chemically and structurally to the substance being assayed; frequently used in gas chromatography and high-pressure liquid chromatography assays.

International Bureau of Weights and Measures   Responsible for maintaining the standards on which the SI system of measurement is based; see also International System of Units.

International Committee on Nomenclature of Blood Clotting Factors   Establishes and maintains standardized terminology for the various coagulation factors.

international normalized ratio (INR)   The PT ratio that would have been obtained if the WHO international reference standard preparation was used as the source of thromboplastin in the PT assay; compares the patient's PT to a mean, normal PT; ensures that results for PT tests done in any laboratory can be compared.

international sensitivity index (ISI)   Mathematical indicator of the responsivenes of the PT testing systems to deficiencies of vitamin K coagulation factors; WHO reference standard is assigned an ISI of 1.0.

International System of Units   (SI units, from Système International d'Unités); standard international language of measurement.

interpretive report   Reporting of laboratory results in a usable format, including information about reference ranges or flagging of abnormal values, so that the physician can find the results for the requested analyses in an efficient, concise manner.

interpupillary distance   The distance between the two oculars of a binocular microscope; must be adjusted for the microscopist.

intravascular component   Platelets and coagulation proteins that circulate in the blood vessels.

intravascular devices   Devices used to obtain specimens of blood from blood vessels.

intravascular hemolysis   Hemolysis or abnormal destruction of red blood cells in the bloodstream.

intrinsic system of coagulation   Utilization of plasma contact factors to initiate coagulation, beginning with the activation of factor XII; all necessary factors required are contained in the circulating blood.

ionic concentration   In urinalysis, a measure that is related to specific gravity. The principle of the reagent strip test for specific gravity; substances must ionize in order to be measurable with this method.

ionized calcium   Calcium that participates in the coagulation process; necessary to activate thromboplastin and to convert prothrombin to thrombin.

ion-selective electrodes   Indicator electrodes used in potentiometry devices to respond to specific ions in the solution.

iris diaphragm   The part of the microscope located at the bottom of the Abbé ondenser, under the lens but within the condenser body; controls the amount of light passing through the material under observation; can be opened or closed to adjust contrast by means of a lever.

isoantibodies Antibodies resulting from antigenic stimulation within the same species.

isolated colonies When streak plates are properly made, isolated, or individual, colonies may be seen in specific sections of the plate; enables pure cultures to be made.

iso-osmolar Two solutions having the same solute concentratiom, such as the glomerular filtrate and plasma, are normally iso-osmolar with each other.

isotonic Situation when the concentration of fluid or diluent outside the red cell is the same as it is inside the red cell.

J

jaundice Accumulation of bilirubin pigment in the tissues and blood; skin and sclera of eyes become jaundiced, or yellow.

jaundiced serum Increased concentration of bilirubin in the blood (serum) and accumulation of bilirubin pigment in the tissues; serum appears brownish yellow.

Joint Commission on Accreditation of Healthcare Organizations (JCAHO) Voluntary organization, not governmental, made up of representatives from various health care associations (e.g., hospital, physician, dentist). Mission of JCAHO is to enhance the quality of health care provided to the public, and the organization is dedicated to improving the process to carry out this mission. One important function of JCAHO is accreditation of U.S. hospitals. Standards and guidelines are set for hospitals, and accreditation is carried out and monitored through a continual process of site visits, surveys, and reports. The organization also monitors other health care facilities (e.g., mental health facilities, nursing homes, home health agencies, hospices, managed care and ambulatory care organizations).

K

kernicterus Results when unconjugated bilirubin passes into the brain and nerve cells and is deposited in the nuclei of these cells; can result in cell damage and death.

ketoacidosis Acidosis resulting from the presence of increased ketone bodies.

ketogenic diet A diet containing more than 1.5 g of fat per 1.0 g of carbohydrate; this will result in ketone accumulation with ketosis and ketonuria.

ketonemia Increased concentration of ketones in the blood.

ketonuria Increased concentration of ketones in the urine.

ketosis Increased concentration of ketones in blood and urine.

kilogram (kg) Standard unit for measurement of mass (and weight).

L

labile factor Factor V; essential for prompt conversion of prothrombin to thrombin in clotting mechanism; is involved in common pathway of both intrinsic and extrinsic clotting pathways.

laboratory information system (LIS) Computer system designed for use by the clinical laboratory; includes collection of patient information, generation of test results, assembly of data output, production of ancillary reports, and storage of data.

laboratory medicine Medical discipline by which clinical laboratory science and technology are applied to the care of patients.

laboratory procedure manual Collection of information about the specific procedures for all analytical assays performed by the laboratory; includes information about specimen requirements and special collection or processing details, test request information, procedural information (how to perform the test, reagents used for the assay, control specimens used), calibration of instruments, quality control data, details about reference values and reporting of results, and any information about bibliographical resources.

laboratory report Information about results of various assays performed by the laboratory; should be presented in a usable format; see interpretive report.

Landsteiner's rule In the ABO blood group system, if the A or B antigen is lacking on the red cell, the corresponding antibody will be found in the serum.

larvae Immature form, as in parasite larvae.

latex agglutination Particles of latex are used to visualize an antigen-antibody agglutination reaction; test latex particles are coated with a specific antibody and clump together (agglutinate) when the specific antigen is present in the specimen being assayed.

latex-microparticle enzyme immunoassay (MEIA) An immunoassay technology.

lattice formation In process of agglutination, results in the visible aggregation or clumping reaction.

LE (lupus erythematosus) factor Present in blood of persons with SLE; has ability to depolymerize the nuclear chromatin of PMNs, making them capable of being ingested by an intact PMN (thus creating the LE cell).

leukemia Progressive malignant disease of the blood-forming organs, characterized by abnormal proliferation of leukocytes and their precursors in body tissues. Peripheral blood cells and bone marrow cells are changed quantitatively and qualitatively.

leukoblastic reaction The presence of white blood cell forms more immature than bands in the peripheral blood.

leukocyte White blood cell; one of formed elements found in peripheral blood.

leukocyte differential Classification and recorded percentages of various types of leukocytes as seen on a stained blood film or as obtained from an electronic counting device.

leukocyte esterase Enzyme present in the azurophilic or primary granules of the granulocytic leukocytes; presence of this enzyme in urine indicates urinary tract infection.

leukocytosis An increase in the white cell count above the normal upper limit.

leukoerythroblastotic reaction The presence of younger forms of leukocytes and red cells than are normally found in peripheral blood.

leukopenia A decrease in the white cell count below the normal lower limit.

Levey-Jennings control chart See quality control chart.

light absorbed Light that is absorbed by a colored solution; measured as absorbance units or optical density (OD).

light transmitted Light that passes through a colored solution; measured as percent transmittance units (%T).

light-emitting diode (LED) Readout device found in digital computerized equipment; a semiconductor device visualized as a glowing readout.

linear graph paper Graph paper with a linear scale on both axes.

linkage (linked genes) Genes for different traits located on the same chromosome, positioned so closely that they are inherited as a unit.

lipemic serum Serum with presence of fats or lipids; appears white or milky.

liter (L) Standard unit of volume.

lithiasis Kidney stone formation.

low-power objective Usually a 10× magnification objective; used for the initial scanning and observation in most routine microscopic work.

lymphocytosis An increase in the absolute number of lymphocytes above normal limits.

lysin Antibody that causes lysis.

lysis Hemolysis of the red cells, rupture of the red cell membrane, and release of hemoglobin; an indicator of an antigen-antibody reaction.

M

macrophage Any phagocytic cell of the reticuloendothelial system. Thought to be derived from both monocytes and histiocytic cells.

malabsorption Inadequate, incomplete, or impaired absorption from the gastrointestinal tract; may be associated with presence of increased fat in the feces.

mass per unit mass See weight per unit weight.

material safety data sheets (MSDS) Information about the hazards of each chemical are provided by the supplier or manufacturer of the chemical; any hazardous chemicals used in a laboratory should be accompanied by this information.

mean (X-bar) Statistically calculated mathematical average value for a valid series of numbers, as for a series of test results, for example; the series of values is totaled and divided by the number in the series; also called the X-bar.

measurement of mass or weight Gravimetric analysis; commonly, measurement of weight by using various types of balances for preparation of laboratory reagents and standard solutions.

meconium Viscid, elastic, greenish black material composed of amniotic fluid, biliary and intestinal secretions, and epithelial cells; passed from the intestine by newborn infants within the first 24 hours after delivery.

median The middle value of a body of data; the point that falls halfway between the highest and lowest in position.

median cubital vein Vein in the antecubital area, most commonly used as site for venipuncture collection of venous blood.

medical laboratory assistant (MLA) See clinical laboratory technician (CLT).

medical laboratory technician (MLT) See clinical laboratory technician (CLT).

medical technologist (MT) See clinical laboratory scientist (CLS).

medulla (kidney) Central anatomical portion of the kidney; consists of the loop of Henle, the distal convoluted tubules, and the collecting tubules.

melena Black or tarry fecal specimens; dark color is due to the presence of blood, which is changed to a black substance as it passes through the gastrointestinal tract.

meniscus Curvature in the top surface of a liquid.

menu Programs or functions (options) offered by a system.

meter (m) Standard unit for measurement of length or distance.

metric system System of weights and measures based on a decimal system, or divisions and multiples of tens; based on a standard unit of length, the meter.

microalbuminuria The presence of very small amounts of albumin in the urine.

microorganisms Microscopic organisms; organisms seen only with the use of a microscope (e.g., bacteria, viruses, fungi, protozoa).

micropipette, micropipettor Device used to measure very precise, very small volumes; micropipettes are usually calibrated to contain a specific volume, and the entire contents is part of the measurement.

microsampling Obtaining very small amounts of blood or other body specimens (e.g., capillary blood, cerebrospinal fluid); usually requires micromethods for assay.

milliequivalent Relates to the equivalent; see milliequivalent weight.

milliequivalent weight The equivalent weight in milligrams equals one milliequivalent (mEq).

milligram-molecular weight Molecular weight expressed in milligrams.

millimole (mmole) One milligram-molecular weight is equal to a millimole (mmole).

minimum bactericidal concentration (MBC) Minimum concentration of antimicrobial agent needed to kill an organism.

minimum inhibitory concentration (MIC) Minimum concentration of antimicrobial agent needed to prevent visually discernible growth of a bacterial or fungal suspension.

mode The value that occurs most commonly in a mass of data.

moderate-complexity tests CLIA '88 regulations place most laboratory tests in this category. Complexity is based on the analyte tested and the method or instrumentation used to perform the test.

molarity Gram-molecular mass or weight of a compound per liter of solution.

molecular diagnostics The use of principles of basic molecular biology in the practice of laboratory medicine.

monoclonal antibody Highly specified antibody derived entirely from a single ancestral antibody-forming parent cell. Produced by hybridization; used in diagnostic testing.

multiple-reagent strips Plastic strips that contain one or more chemically impregnated test sites on an absorbant pad. When a chemical reaction occurs, it is indicated by a color change. The basis for chemical screening in urinalysis, for example. Also referred to as dipsticks.

myeloid Of or pertaining to the bone marrow. The granulocytic leukocytes come from the myeloid series of development and include neutrophils, eosinophils, basophils, and monocytes.

mycelium See hyphae.

mycology The study or science of fungi.

myoglobinuria The presence of myoglobin in the urine.

N

National Bureau of Standards (NBS) Agency of the U.S. government. Maintains and supplies standard reference materials needed for the preparation of primary standard solutions; develops reference methods and reference materials.

National Certification Agency for Medical Laboratory Personnel (NCA) Offers an examination and certification for medical laboratory personnel.

National Cholesterol Education Program (NCEP) Program established to set standards for the detection and classification of individuals at high risk for coronary heart disease (CHD).

National Committee for Clinical Laboratory Standards (NCCLS) Nonprofit educational organization that sets voluntary consensus standards for all areas of clinical laboratories.

natural antibodies Exist without antigenic stimulus; examples are anti-A and anti-B in ABO groups.

negative birefringence Pattern of birefringence seen when a crystal appears yellow when the long axis of the crystal is parallel to the slow wave of vibration of a full-wave compensator and blue when the long axis is perpendicular to the slow wave.

negative exponent Indicates the number of times the reciprocal of the base is to be multiplied by itself; indicates a fraction.

negative predictive value (PV) Indicates the number of patients with a normal test result who do not have a disease compared with all patients with a normal (negative) result.

neonatal physiologic jaundice Type of jaundice that results from an enzyme deficiency in the immature liver of the newborn.

neonatal screening programs Approved testing laboratories test for specific diseases or pathologies in newborns; capillary blood is usually collected onto filter paper and sent to the reference laboratory for testing; see also blood spot collections.

nephelometry Measurement of light that has been scattered when it strikes a particle in a liquid; the nephelometer measures the amount of light scattered.

nephron Working unit of the kidney, where urine is formed; includes glomerulus, Bowman's capsule, proximal and distal convoluted tubules, and loop of Henle.

nephrotic syndrome An abnormal kidney condition characterized by heavy or massive proteinuria (albuminuria), decreased blood albumin (hypoalbuminemia), and edema.

neutropenia A reduction of the absolute neutrophil count below normal limits.

neutrophilia An increase in the absolute number of neutrophils present in blood above normal limits.

95% confidence interval Numerical limits within which a sample must fall to be part of the normal distribution of values; determined statistically, and is the basis for quality control "rules" for the acceptance or rejection of certain results; based on a gaussian curve, whereby 95% of the population have observations within ± 2 standard deviations.

nocturia The excretion of over 400 mL of urine at night.

nomenclature of blood clotting factors International Committee on Nomenclature of Blood Clotting Factors ascertains consistency in terminology used; standardizes the complex nomenclature for the various clotting factors.

nonglucose reducing substances (NGRS) Substances other than glucose (including several sugars) that may be present in the urine and that have the ability to reduce heavy metal from a higher to a lower oxidation state. NGRS are not detected by the reagent strip tests specific for glucose.

normal flora Organisms that inhabit the human body normally and do not cause disease.

"normal" range or value See reference range or value.

normality Number of equivalent weights per liter of solution.

normochromic Said of red cells with normal hemoglobin content.

nosepiece The part of the microscope on which the objectives are mounted. Usually on a pivot to allow for a quick change of objectives.

nosocomial infection Infection acquired in a hospital or health care facility.

numerical aperture (NA) Index or measurement of the resolving power of a microscope. Also an index of the light-gathering power of a lens that describes the amount of light entering the objective. As the numerical aperture increases, resolution decreases.

O

objective The major part of the magnification system of the microscope. Most commonly used microscopes have three objectives: low power, high power, and oil immersion. Usually mounted in a rotating nosepiece that enables a quick change of objectives.

obligate parasite A parasite that cannot survive without its designated host.

obstructive jaundice, posthepatic jaundice, regurgitative jaundice Type of jaundice that results from obstruction of the common bile duct by stones, tumors, spasms, or stricture.

occult blood Blood not observable by the naked eye; requires use of a chemical test to be detected.

Occupational Health and Safety Act of 1970 Created the Occupational Health and Safety Administration within the U.S. Department of Labor to set levels of safety and health for all workers in the United States. A federal agency.

Occupational Health and Safety Administration (OSHA) See Occupational Health and Safety Act of 1970.

ocular (eyepiece) The part of the microscope that magnifies the image formed by the objective.

oil-immersion objective Generally a 100× magnification lens with a relatively short working distance of 1.8 mm. Requires the addition of a special immersion oil placed between the objective and the slide or coverglass. Cannot be used with wet preparations.

oliguria Abnormally small excretion of urine; less than 500 mL/24 hours.

opportunistic pathogen Organism that does not usually cause disease in persons with an intact immune system but does cause disease in immunocompromised persons.

optical density (OD) Term used to express the amount of light being absorbed when being passed through a solution; see absorbed light.

optical methods, cell counters Automated cell counters with focused laser beams whereby cells cause a change in the deflection of a beam of light, which is converted to measurable pulses by a photomultiplier tube.

oral glucose tolerance test (OGTT) Oral glucose is consumed and blood tested for glucose concentration; test measures the ability of a person to respond appropriately to a heavy load of glucose.

order entry The first step in the laboratory information system is the test ordering or order entry.

organized sediment The biological part of the urine sediment; includes cells, fat of biological origin, casts, organisms, and microorganisms.

OSHA standards See Occupational Health and Safety Act of 1970.

orthostatic proteinuria Proteinuria that is present when persons are engaged in normal activity but disappears when they lie down or recline.

osmolarity Number of osmoles of solute per liter of solution.

osmosis The passage of a solvent through a membrane from a dilute solution into a more concentrated one.

osmotic fragility   Test to determine the ability of the red blood cells to withstand hypotonic or hypoosmotic solutions. Measure of the resistance of the red cell membrane to rupture; cells with membrane defects (hereditary spherocytosis) have increased fragility.

output/output device   Any device that allows information generated by a computer system to be used (e.g., results of calculations for a laboratory assay). Information output can be printed, displayed, or transferred to another processor.

ova   Eggs, as in parasite eggs.

oval fat body (OFB), renal tubular fat (RTF) body   Renal epithelial cell (and possibly macrophage) filled with fat droplets.

P

packed cell volume (PCV)   The hematocrit. A macroscopic measurement of the percentage volume of packed red cells.

panic or critical values   Possibly life-threatening laboratory values that must be noted and communicated to the physician as quickly as possible; automated instruments flag or highlight these results for the laboratory personnel.

parasitism   Result of parasite injuring its host by its actions.

parasitology   The study or science of parasites.

pathogens   Microorganisms that cause disease.

pathologist   A licensed physician with special training in clinical and/or anatomical pathology.

patient demographics   Information about the patient, such as name, gender, age or birth date, referring or attending physician.

Patient's Bill of Rights   Document drawn up by a health care institution that declares certain rights for all patients being cared for in that facility. Being considerate of these rights constitutes good patient care. In the laboratory context, the Patient's Bill of Rights must be considered in collecting the various patient specimens needed for testing.

percent   Parts per hundred parts.

percent solution   Somewhat outdated expression of concentration based on parts per hundred parts (e.g., 10% sodium chloride, which is 10 g NaCl diluted to 100 mL with deionized water; currently expressed as 10 g/dL).

percent transmittance   Amount of light that passes through a colored solution compared with the amount of light that passes through a blank solution.

percent transmittance units   Units used to measure the amount of light transmitted through a solution.

pericardial fluid   Extravascular fluid that surrounds the heart.

peripheral blood film   Blood smear prepared on a glass microscope slide using circulating peripheral blood. Blood is usually obtained by venipuncture or finger puncture.

peritoneal fluid   Extravascular fluid that surrounds the abdominal and pelvic cavities.

peroxidase   Enzyme that catalyzes release of free oxygen from hydrogen peroxide. Peroxidase activity of the heme portion of the hemoglobin molecule is the basis of the reagent strip tests for blood.

personal protective equipment   OSHA requires facilities to provide their personnel with protective equipment, such as protective clothing, gloves, eyewear, protective shields and barriers, and respiratory devices, for their safety in the workplace.

Petri dish or plate   Shallow, flat glass or plastic plate with a loose-fitting deep cover, used to hold culture media.

pH   Unit that describes the acidity or alkalinity of a solution.

phagocytosis   A process in which a cell engulfs, and disposes of, foreign material.

phase contrast   Microscope illumination system that uses a special condenser with an annular diaphragm with a matched absorption ring in the corresponding objective. Used to give additional contrast in wet preparations; especially useful for counting platelets and observing urinary sediment.

phenotype   Observable genetic makeup that can be determined by direct testing (i.e., blood type).

phlebotomist Person trained in drawing blood. Primarily trained to draw blood by venipuncture but also trained to perform capillary collections and to do skin punctures of various types. Drawing blood specimens from indwelling lines is an additional technique performed by a trained phlebotomist.

photoelectric cell, photodetector Electronic device that measures the intensity of light being transmitted by a solution; produces electrons in proportion to the amount of light reaching it.

photometry Technique used to determine the quantitative concentration of a substance by measuring the variation in its color intensity by use of a photometer.

physical properties In urinalysis, color, transparency, odor, foam, and specific gravity of a urine specimen.

physician office laboratory (POL) A laboratory in a physician's office or clinic where tests are done only on the patients coming to the practice or group.

physiologic jaundice Can result from a deficiency of an enzyme that transfers glucuronate groups onto bilirubin or from liver immaturity; can result in jaundice that occurs in some infants during the first few days of life; also called neonatal jaundice; see jaundice.

plan for evacuation Routes for exiting the laboratory site in an emergency must be readily available to all persons working in the laboratory area.

plasma Liquid portion of blood after it has been anticoagulated and centrifuged or otherwise allowed to settle.

plasma cell, plasmacyte Derivative of the B lymphocyte. Large, with a round or oval eccentric nucleus. Specialized for production of antibodies; rarely is seen in the peripheral blood.

plasmin Proteolytic enzyme that breaks down fibrin; is generated by the activation of a plasma precursor, plasminogen.

platelet adhesion, platelet adherence Test that measures the ability of platelets to adhere to glass surfaces; essential requirement for primary hemostasis.

platelet aggregation Massing or clumping of platelets with one another; test for platelet function.

platelet plug Formation of an aggregate or mass of platelets that physically plug or slow down the flow of blood at the site of an injury to a blood vessel; result of activation of the hemostatic system.

pleural fluid Extravascular fluid that surrounds the lungs.

pluripotential stem cell (PSC) Stem cell that is uncommitted to any specific cell line; stimulation results in differentiation and maturation.

point-of-care testing (POCT) Tests performed at the bedside of the patient or near the site where the patient is; a decentralized form of laboratory testing—the laboratory testing comes to the patient.

polarize To bend or rotate light.

polarized light Light that is propagated so that radiation waves occur in only one direction rather than at random.

polarizer A filter that allows the passage of light waves in only one orientation.

polarizing microscope Microscope illumination system that employs two crossed polarizing lenses, extinguishing the passage of light through the microscope. Used to detect objects or crystals that bend or polarize light, making them visible when viewed with crossed polarizing filters.

polychromasia Many colors. A property of red cells that show a faint blue or blue-orange color when stained with Wright stain, because of the presence of both blue RNA and red hemoglobin in young red cells.

polyclonal antibodies Antibodies derived from multiple ancestral clones of antibody-producing cells; characteristically produced in infectious diseases.

polydipsia Excessive thirst.

polyphagia Excessive, constant hunger.

polyuria Excessive urination.

porphobilinogen An unstable intermediary product in the synthesis of heme; a significant increase in the urine can be seen in acute intermittent hepatic porphyria.

porphyrias A group of inherited disorders that are characterized by an increased production of porphyrins; some forms result in the presence of porphobilinogen in urine.

positive birefringence Pattern of birefringence seen when a crystal appears blue when the long axis of the crystal is parallel to the slow wave of vibration of a full-wave compensator and yellow when the long axis is perpendicular to the slow wave.

positive exponent Indicates the number of times the base is to be multiplied by itself.

positive predictive value (PV) Indicates the number of patients with an abnormal test result who have a disease compared with all patients with an abnormal result.

postanalytical function Includes functions that occur after the analysis itself, such as generating chart reports, printing result reports as needed, archiving results, and billing.

postcoital test (PCT) Test that evaluates cervical mucus; scored on a scale of 1 to 15 by assessment of spinnbarkeit, ferning, consistency, and pH.

posthepatic jaundice See obstructive jaundice.

postprandial Directly after a meal; a postprandial blood specimen is one collected directly after a meal.

postprandial specimen, 2-hour Blood that is drawn 2 hours after a meal.

postrenal azotemia Azotemia resulting from obstruction whereby urea is reabsorbed into the circulation; see azotemia.

post-exposure prophylaxis (PEP) For HIV exposure, the degree of risk for infection must be assessed and the worker followed by the health care facility's infection control department and offered post-exposure prophylaxis immediately.

potentiometry Technique in which the potential difference between two electrodes is measured under equilibrium.

pour plates A specimen is inoculated in a liquid medium, which is then mixed and poured into a culture plate, where it solidifies.

preanalytical functions Functions in testing protocol that occur before the actual analyses—test ordering, specimen collection, and so forth.

precipitation (precipitate) Visible result of an antigen-antibody reaction between a soluble antigen and its specific antibody.

precipitin An anitbody that reacts with a soluble antigen to form a precipitate.

precision, reproducibility Measure of the closeness of the results obtained when analysis on the same sample is repeated; agreement between replicate measurements.

predictive value (PV) Means or ability to predict the results of an analysis of the same data by using another test instrument or measurement; contributes to the validity of a test.

prerenal azotemia Azotemia resulting from poor perfusion of the kidneys; see azotemia.

prevalence The proportion of a population that has a disease.

primary culture The initial or first culture done with a specimen.

primary hemostasis Involves platelets and the vascular response.

primary response First antibody response to foreign antigen.

proenzymes Enzyme precursors or zymogens.

proficiency testing (PT) or survey Program under which samples are sent to a group of laboratories for analysis; results are compared with those of other laboratories participating in the program. Included as a component of quality assurance programs.

proficiency testing programs See proficiency testing (PT) or survey.

program Set of commands or steps that instruct the computer to perform a certain task.

program for infection control See infection control.

prokaryote Small bacterium containing DNA in a single, circular chromosome.

proportioning A combination of predetermined amounts of reagent and sample in an automated laboratory instrument.

proportion   Two or more ratios having the same relative meaning but with different numbers.

protective immunity   Provided by antibodies that after formation will protect from subsequent exposure to the antigen.

protective isolation   Measures used to protect a patient from infectious agents.

protein error of pH indicators   Color change of a pH indicator due to the presence of protein rather than hydrogen ion concentration.

protein-free filtrate   After preparation of a specimen to remove the protein, the filtrate, free from protein, remains.

proteinuria   Presence of protein, usually albumin, in urine.

prothrombin, coagulation factor II, prethrombin   Produced by the liver; is vitamin K-dependent.

prothrombin time (PT)   Time it takes for the plasma to clot after an excess of thromboplastin and an optimal concentration of calcium have been added; measures functional activity of the extrinsic and common pathways of coagulation.

protoplasts   Unusually long rod-shaped forms of bacteria with central swelling; the result of damage to the cell wall by antibiotics.

provider-performed microscopies (PPM)   Specific microscopies (mostly wet mounts) usually performed by the physician or provider for his or her own patients; these tests are a special subcategory of the moderately complex CLIA '88 tests.

prozone phenomenon   An excess of antibody; can result in a false-negative reaction.

pseudocasts   False casts. Structures in the urine sediment that appear like, and might be mistaken for, casts.

pseudohyphae   False hyphae. Elongated yeast cells that may be branched and have terminal buds and resemble the mycelia of true fungi.

Public Health Service Act   Act under which Medicare and Medicaid are licensed.

puncture-resistant sharps containers   Used for disposal of sharps such as needles, lancets, and broken glass.

pure culture   Culture in which each colony is from a single isolated originating bacterial cell.

pyuria   Presence of pus (leukocytes) in the urine; indicates a possible urinary tract infection.

Q

quality assurance (QA)   Comprehensive set of policies, procedures, and practices necessary to make sure that a laboratory's results are reliable. QA includes record keeping, calibration and maintenance of equipment, quality control, proficiency testing, and training.

quality assurance indicators   Indicators that monitor the performance of a laboratory and are evaluated as part of CQI; see continuous quality improvement.

quality assurance program   Plan to carry out policies and practices necessary to comply with quality assurance standards set by accreditation agencies to make certain that a laboratory's results are reliable and that these results are used in the best interest of the patient. See also total quality improvement (TQI).

quality control (QC)   Set of laboratory procedures designed to ensure that a test method is working properly and that the results meet the diagnostic needs of the physician. QC includes testing control samples, charting the results, and analyzing them statistically.

quality control chart   Visual documentation of information derived from using control specimens; values for control specimen assays used for a particular substance are plotted on the chart on a regular basis and are statistically analyzed for trends of change.

quality control program   Plan to carry out procedures established to make certain that laboratory assay methods are working properly and that assay results meet the diagnostic needs of the physician; makes use of control specimens and standard solutions.

quality control specimen   See control specimen.

quantitative analysis   A very precise means of measurement of the quantity of a substance.

quantitative transfer Process of transferring the entire amount of a weighed or measured substance from one vessel to another; usually used in the process of reagent preparation, in which the weighed substance (chemical) must be transferred in its entirety to a volumetric flask for dilution with deionized water.

quantitative urine culture methods Traditional method of detecting urinary tract infection, in which urine is cultured on an appropriate medium and identified.

R

random access analyzer Instrument that does all the selected determinations on one sample before going on to the next sample.

random access memory (RAM) Central memory in the central processing unit (CPU) of a computer; commonly used as a means of storage of information that is frequently altered, changed, or updated.

rapid streptococcal antigen detection Basis for rapid tests for detection of "strep throat," caused by group A β-hemolytic streptococci.

ratio Amount of something in proportion to an amount of something else; always describes a relative amount.

reactive lymphocytes Altered lymphoctes associated with viral infections, especially infectious mononucleosis; also referred to as atypical or variant lymphocytes.

reagent Any substance employed to produce a chemical reaction.

reagin antibodies Antibody-like proteins that react in some serologic tests for syphilis.

recovery solution A measured amount of a substance being quantitated is added to a specimen; theoretically, the amount of substance added should be recovered at the end of the determination if the method is an accurate one.

red blood cell indices In hematology, the calculated values for red cell measurements, such as mean cell volume (MCV), mean cell hemoglobin (MCH), and mean cell hemoglobin concentration (MCHC).

reducing sugars Sugars (including glucose) that have the ability to reduce copper ions from Cu^{++} to Cu^+ in the presence of alkali and heat.

reference laboratory Laboratory setting where specimens are sent that require more complex testing methodologies and for tests that are infrequently ordered.

reference range, normal range, normal values, reference values Range of values that includes 95% of the test results for a healthy reference population; see Gaussian curve.

reflectance photometry or spectrophotometry Photometric technique whereby light reflected from the surface of a colorimetric reaction is used to measure the amount of unknown colored product generated in the reaction; a beam of light is directed at a flat surface, and the amount of light reflected is measured.

refractive index A measure of solute concentration. The ratio of the velocity of light in air to the velocity of light in solution.

refractometer Temperature-compensated instrument used to measure refractive index.

relative centrifugal force (RCF) Expression of the number of revolutions per minute and the centrifugal force generated; method of comparing the forces generated by various centrifuges, taking into account the speed of rotation and the radius from the center of rotation.

relative numbers (cell count) The concentration of a cell type expressed as a percentage.

reliability Ability of a laboratory assay to produce consistent results when testing is repeated successively.

renal azotemia Azotemia resulting primarily from diminished glomerular filtration; see azotemia.

renal threshold Level above which a substance cannot be reabsorbed by the renal tubules and is thus excreted into the urine.

renal tubular fat (RTF) See oval fat bodies

reproducibility See precision, reproducibility.

resolution Limit of usable magnification; tells how small and how close individual objects can be and still be recognized.

reticulocyte   Young red blood cell that has just extruded its nucleus. Characterized by the presence of RNA; becomes a normal, mature red cell when all the RNA is lost; stains with a supravital stain.

reticuloendothelial system (RES)   A functional system of the body involved primarily in defense against infection and in disposal of the products of the breakdown of cells by phagocytosis.

Rh immune globulin (RhIG)   Concentrated and purified form of anti-D antibody, used to immunosuppress Rh-negative women who deliver Rh-positive babies, to prevent sensitization of the mother by her child's red blood cells.

Rh negative   Red blood cells lacking the D antigen (d/d).

Rh positive   Red blood cells containing the D antigen (D/D or D/d).

rhabdomyolysis   Acute destruction of muscle fibers.

rheostat   Control used to adjust the amount of light entering a microscope.

rheumatoid factor (RF)   Autoantibodies present in the serum of patients with clinical features of rheumatoid arthritis; circulating complexes of immunoglobulins, known collectively as rheumatoid factor.

rhinitis   Inflammation of the mucous membranes of the nose, usually accompanied by swelling of the mucosa and nasal discharge.

rickettsiology   The study or observation of rickettsia.

rounding off a number   To bring a digit (number) to the chosen number of significant figures.

Rous test   A wet Prussian blue stain for iron; used to confirm the presence of hemosiderin in the urine sediment.

S

safety manual   Current compilation of all safety practices and procedures, kept in a readily available format for use by all persons in a specific laboratory setting; anything that could pose a potential safety hazard for persons in the laboratory must be described in this manual.

safety program   Required by OSHA for every clinical laboratory.

sampling procedure   Only a very small amount of sample is usually used in laboratory measurements; sampling difficulties can lead to fluctuations and variations in results reporting; affects reliability of the procedure.

scanning electron microscope (SEM)   A type of electron microscope that looks at the surface of a specimen and produces a three-dimensional image by striking the sample with a focused beam of electrons.

secondary hemostasis   Response by coagulation proteins.

secondary response   Response to second exposure to the same antigen; rapid amounts of detectable antibody in the serum or plasma.

sediment   Solid material that has settled out of suspension (e.g., urinary sediment).

selective media   Substances present in these media selectively inhibit growth of certain microorganisms and permit growth of others.

semilogarithmic graph paper   Graph paper with a logarithmic scale on one axis and a linear scale on the other; allows the plotting of a straight line when percent transmittance readings are plotted against concentration.

sensitivity   The proportion of cases having a specific disease or condition that give a positive test result.

sensitivity to antimicrobial agents   The situation thats exists when an organism's growth is inhibited in the presence of certain antibiotics (antimicrobial agents).

sensitization   Process in which an individual is made sensitive to a foreign antigen through exposure. Once sensitization has occurred, the individual responds to a repeated exposure with an accentuated immune response.

septicemia, sepsis   Bacteria in the blood or toxin produced by the bacteria is causing harm to the patient.

serial dilutions   Progressive dilutions of a substance in a series of tubes in predetermined ratios to give concentrations of a specific amount.

serologic pipette   Much like a graduated pipette, but is graduated to the end of the delivery tip; allows for a faster delivery and is less precise for this reason.

serologic reaction   The observed reaction when an antigen-antibody reaction has taken place.

serology   The division of immunology specializing in detection and measurement of specific antibodies that develop in blood (serum) during a response to exposure to a disease-producing antigen.

serotonin   Vasoconstricting substance.

serous fluids   The fluid within the closed cavities of the body (e.g., pleural, pericardial, peritoneal).

serum   The fluid portion of blood that remains after coagulation. Preferable to plasma when typing or otherwise testing blood for compatibility.

serum separator collection tubes   See serum separator gel.

serum separator gel   Additive used to assist in obtaining serum after centrifuging a whole blood specimen. A special silicon gel layer is added to the collection tubes that moves to form a barrier between the cells and serum during centrifugation; the gel hardens to form an inert barrier, allowing easy serum separation or removal after the centrifugation process.

sharps containers   Used disposable needles and other sharp objects must be safely discarded in these containers, which are made of rigid plastic, metal, or stiff paperboard. The containers must be conveniently located, easily recognizable, and marked as a biohazard. All skin lancets, needles, scalpel blades, and bleeding time devices must be discarded properly in a sharps container, with extreme caution.

shift cells   Nucleated red cells or polychromatic macrocytes (reticulocytes) in the peripheral blood.

shift to the left   The release into the peripheral blood of immature cell forms that are normally present only in the bone marrow.

significant figures   Digits of whole numbers or in decimal form, beginning with the leftmost nonzero digit and extending to the right; numbers should contain only digits necessary for the precision of the determination or measurement; the digits of a number that are known to be reliable.

simple stain   One stain that colors everything in the cell the same color.

single dilution   When one unit of original specimen is diluted to a final volume of 2, 5, or 10, etc.; when a concentrated specimen or solution needs a single dilution, usually expressed as a ratio; examples are 1:2, 1:5, and 1:10.

skin puncture   Capillary puncture for blood microsampling, such as finger puncture or heel puncture.

slide agglutination   Used in assay to determine antigen-antibody reaction; usually employs latex agglutination.

slant culture, tube   The surface of the medium is inclined at an angle.

software   Series of instructions or commands that direct the operation of a computer system.

solute   Substance dissolved in a solution; usually the substances being measured in clinical laboratory analyses are the solutes, these being dissolved in blood.

solvent   Substance in which a solute is dissolved; usually deionized water in laboratory reagents.

species   Basic unit of the biological world; used in nomenclature.

specific gravity   Ratio of the density of a solution to the density of an equal volume of water at a constant temperature; depends on the weight and number of particles in a solution.

specificity   The proportion of cases with absence of a specific disease or condition that gives a negative test result.

spectrophotometer   Device that quantitatively provides the relationship between the intensity of the color of an unknown solution and that of a standard solution; see photometry.

spectrophotometry   Quantitative measuring technique in which the color of a solution of an unknown concentration is compared with the color of a similar solution of known concentration.

spermatozoa   Mature male germ cells.

spores   An inert stage of a microorganism that the organism can revert to in a hostile environment.

spring-activated skin puncturing device   Device used to collect capillary blood that makes a clean, rapid incision of a consistent depth.

spun microhematocrit method Hematocrit measurement method that utilizes a high-speed centrifuge in a relatively short centrifugation time.

stab tube A tube of medium that is inoculated by stabbing or passing through the medium with an inoculating needle, leaving the specimen behind in the medium.

stable factor Factor VII; presence monitored by thrombin time.

standard calibration curve Plotting of percent transmission or absorbance readings on graph paper for several known standard solutions of varying concentrations will enable construction of a "standard curve" for a particular assay.

standard deviation (SD) Statistical measurement of the degree of variation from the mean of a series of measurements; measure of precision or reproducibility.

standard precautions Recommended safety policies used for handling all biologic (patient) specimens. Potential infectivity of any patient's blood or body fluids is unknown; therefore all blood and body substances (fluids) are considered equally infectious; also called universal precautions.

standard solution Reference material of the substance being assayed that is of fixed and known chemical composition and can be prepared in a pure form for use in the laboratory; certified reference material that is generally accepted or officially recognized as the unique standard for the assay, regardless of the purity of the analyte content.

steatorrhea Presence or increased quantities of fat in the feces.

stem cell The common progenitor or uncommitted pluripotential stem cell from which all types of blood cells are derived.

stercobilin Pigment derived from bilirubin; responsible for normal color of the feces.

stercobilinogen Colorless degradation product of urobilinogen; is formed in the intestine and oxidized to the colored pigment stercobilin.

Sternheimer-Malbin Stain A crystal violet and safranin stain commonly used in the microscopic analysis of the urine sediment.

sterile Free from living microorganisms.

sterilization Killing or destroying all microorganisms.

streak plate Culture plate prepared by inoculating so as to spread out colonies as much as possible, so that single, isolated colonies may be observed after incubation.

subculture A colony from the primary culture plate that is picked up with an inoculating loop or needle and transferred to a second medium for further culturing.

supportive media Media that contain nutrients that allow most nonfastidious organisms to grow at their normal rates.

synovial fluid Extravascular fluid that surrounds the joints of the body.

syringe and needle collection system Separate syringes and needles of appropriate size and gauge are used to collect some blood specimens. Blood in the syringe is carefully added to the appropriate collection tube containing the necessary additive.

T

T lymphocyte Blood cell that is derived from the thymus; functions in cell-mediated responses; makes up the majority of the lymphocytes in the peripheral blood.

Tamm-Horsfall protein Mucoprotein secreted by the renal tubular cells and not derived from the blood plasma. This protein forms the matrix of urinary casts.

taxonomy Biological classification system of microorganisms on the basis of their natural relationships and, from this, giving them suitable names.

telescoped sediment Urine sediment that contains all, or most, types of casts (hyaline, cellular, granular, and waxy) in one sediment.

test tube culture Culture medium dispersed in test tubes, such as slants or liquid broth.

therapeutic drug monitoring Testing of blood level of a drug to monitor or keep track of its medical effectiveness in treatment of a disease.

thin-layer chromatography Method of chromatography often used to do therapeutic drug monitoring tests; the stationary phase is a thin layer of an adsorbent coated on a glass plate or sheet of plastic; the mobile phase is a solvent or a solvent mixture.

throat swab Sterile fibrous material (commonly dacron or rayon) fixed to a stick; used to collect material from the back of the throat for culture or rapid detection tests for diagnosis of "strep throat."

thrombin Activated form of factor II that acts as a serine proteolytic enzyme to cleave fibrinogen and form fibrin; is a reagent to test platelet aggregation.

thrombin time (TT) Measurement of the time required for change of fibrinogen to fibrin.

thrombocyte, platelet One of the formed elements in the peripheral blood; chief function is its role in coagulation of blood.

thromboplastin Substance with ability to convert prothrombin to thrombin.

thrombosis Formation of a thrombus or fibrin clot.

thrombus Result of activation of the hemostatic system; formation of platelet plug.

timed urine collection Urine collected over time (e.g., 2, 12, or 24 hours). Collection commonly is preserved by refrigeration between voidings, and is used when a quantitative assay is needed. It is important to adhere to specific time requirements and be certain that the collection time is noted on the container. Entire timed collection must be sent to the laboratory in the container.

titration Quantitative volumetric technique of measuring the concentration of an unknown solution by comparing it with a measured volume of a solution of known concentration.

to-contain pipettes Pipettes calibrated to contain a specific amount of liquid; to ensure that all the liquid is emptied from the pipette, it must be rinsed well with a diluting solution.

to-deliver pipettes Pipettes calibrated to deliver a specified volume when filled properly and the liquid is allowed to drain completely into a receiving vessel.

tolerance Form of resistance to an antimicrobial agent. In volumetric glassware, the degree of acceptable variability of volume delivery from that stated on the glassware; the tolerance increases with the capacity of the pipette.

torsion balance Laboratory balance commonly used to weigh chemicals; is assembled as a single flexible structure by means of highly tensed torsion bands of watch-spring alloy; has no knife edges to dull, or other loose parts.

Total Quality Improvement (TQI) Internal monitoring programs to improve the quality of services performed by the clinical laboratory.

Total Quality Management (TQM) See total quality improvement (TQI).

tourniquet Elastic strip or cuff that can be tightened when applied around the arm, usually just above the elbow; allows the vein to become more prominent so that venipuncture can be more easily done.

toxicology Study of the origin, nature, and effects of poison. Toxicologic analyses are used to detect the amounts of substances that could be poisonous or toxic at certain concentrations.

transfer needle See inoculating loop or needle.

transfusion reaction Any adverse effect of transfusion; generally characterized as hemolytic, febrile, allergic, or circulatory overload.

transmission-based precautions Precautions coming from the CDC that apply to patients (1) with known specific infection or suspected to be infected with specific microorganisms spread by airborne, droplet, or contact routes or (2) during the incubation period of certain easily transmitted diseases.

transmission electron microscope (TEM) A type of microscope that illuminates the specimen with a beam of electrons produced by an electron gun; the electrons are accelerated by a high voltage potential and passed through a condenser lens system (usually two magnetic lenses). The electron microscope allows for significantly greater magnification (up to 50,000 times magnification) than the brightfield microscope.

transmitted light Light that is not absorbed.

transudate   An effusion formed as the result of filtration through a membrane.

traumatic tap   The presence of blood in a body fluid specimen, such as cerebrospinal fluid, as a result of bleeding at the site of entry as the fluid is collected. First tube appears bloody while subsequent tubes show lesser concentrations of blood.

triple-beam balance, "trip" balance   Three-beamed balance. Each beam provides a different weighing scale; scales are provided with movable weights. Used commonly in preparation of laboratory reagents.

trophozoite   Motile form of a parasite.

true negatives   Those subjects who have a negative test and who do not have the disease.

true positives   Those subjects who have a positive test and who have the disease.

tuberculosis control   OSHA requires use of special masks and/or respirators for persons who are exposed to patients with known or suspected pulmonary tuberculosis.

turbidimetry   Measurement of the loss in light intensity transmitted through a solution because of the light being scattered as a result of the turbidity of the solution.

type 1, or insulin-dependent, diabetes mellitus (IDDM)   Insulin injection is required because insufficient amounts of insulin are secreted by the pancreas.

type 2, or non-insulin-dependent, diabetes mellitus (NIDDM)   The activity of the insulin present is not sufficient; patients are usually not dependent on insulin injections.

typing   Testing of suspensions of red cells with known antibody solutions (antisera) to determine the identity of antigens, known as the blood type.

U

ultracentrifuge   High-speed centrifuge; generally used for research.

ultrafiltrate of plasma   Filtrate of plasma over a membrane, whereby extremely small particles such as proteins are restricted, or not filtered.

unconjugated bilirubin, indirect bilirubin, free bilirubin   Water-insoluble form of bilirubin that is formed as a breakdown product from heme by the reticuloendothelial system and carried in the bloodstream bound to albumin. Because of its insolubility, this form cannot be excreted by the kidney or found in the urine.

unexpected antibody   Antibody that results from specific antigenic stimulus. In blood banking, the result of stimulation from pregnancy, transfusion, or injection of red cells. Also referred to as an immune antibody.

universal precautions   See standard precautions.

Universal Blood and Body Substance Technique (UBBST)   See standard precautions.

Unopette system   Commercially available disposable self-filling pipette and diluent-reservoir system used to measure and dilute blood for testing purposes.

unorganized sediment   The chemical part of the urine sediment, includes crystals of chemicals and amorphous material.

urea nitrogen/creatinine ratio   Useful relationship in diagnosis of renal function disorders. Normal ratio for a person on a normal diet is between 12 and 20.

uremia   Abnormally high concentration of urea nitrogen in the blood.

urinalysis   The physical, chemical, and microscopic analysis of urine.

urinary system   Consists of two kidneys and two ureters plus the bladder and the urethra.

urine   Fluid composed of the waste materials of blood; formed in the kidney and excreted from the body by way of the urinary system.

urobilin   An orange-yellow pigment found in normal urine Urobilin in an oxidation product of the colorless urobilinogen.

urobilinogen   Group of colorless chromogens that are formed in the intestine from the reduction of bilirubin by the action of bacteria present in the normal bacterial flora; normal product of bilirubin metabolism.

urochrome A yellow pigment, found in normal urine.

uroerythrin A red pigment found in normal urine.

V

vacuum tube and needle collection system Blood collection system consisting of evacuated collection tubes with appropriate additives, double-ended needles, and needle holders; allows blood collection directly from the vein into the tube.

valence Expression of the total combining power of an element whereby it can combine chemically with atoms of hydrogen or their equivalent.

variance (or error) Fluctuation in the measurement of a substance; factors causing variance can be limitations of the procedure itself or can be related to the sampling mechanism.

vascular access device (VAD) Device or indwelling line used to administer therapeutic products over a long period; see indwelling line.

vascular component Activity of the blood vessels themselves.

vasoconstriction Constriction of blood vessels; most immediate response of the body to bleeding.

venipuncture Process of collecting blood from a vein.

venous blood Blood collected from a vein by venipuncture.

verified Results must be verified, or approved or reviewed, before the data are released to the patient report.

virology The study or science of viruses.

visible spectrum The range of light that is visible to the human eye, generally from wavelengths of 380 to 750 nm.

visual colorimetry Determination or comparison of color intensity of a solution by use of the human eye; has all but been replaced by photoelectric colorimetry and spectrophotometry instrumentation.

voided midstream urine specimen Noncatheterized urine specimen collected after the first few milliliters have been deposited in the urinal or toilet; the urine is free flowing, and the midportion of the collection is saved in a specimen container.

volume per unit volume Measured volume of a liquid added to a specific volume of another liquid (v/v); usually expressed as milliliters per milliliter (mL/mL) or milliliters per liter (mL/L).

volumetric glassware Glassware that has been manufactured of good-quality glass and calibrated under strict conditions to hold, contain, or deliver a specific volume of liquid (e.g., volumetric pipette, flask, buret).

volumetric (or transfer) pipette Extremely accurate, single-line pipette used to measure specimens, controls, and standard solutions, or anything requiring precise measurement.

von Willebrand's disease (vWD) Deficiency of vWF; prolonged bleeding time results; see vWF.

von Willebrand's factor (vWF) Subendothelial factor (factor VIII:vWF); acts as the glue necessary for optimal platelet-collagen binding to occur; factor is required for normal platelet adhesion to endothelium.

W

waived laboratory tests CLIA regulations specify that the FDA has cleared these tests; that is, the tests are so simple that the likelihood of erroneous results is negligible, or no risk is posed to the patient if the tests are performed incorrectly.

waste disposal program OSHA standards mandate implementation of a specific plan for disposal of medical wastes to prevent transmission of infectious agents and accidental exposure to possibly hazardous material.

Watson-Schwartz test Test for urobilinogen and porphobilinogen, based on the Ehrlich aldehyde reaction; basis of the Multistix reagent strip test for Ehrlich reacting substances.

wavelength of light Linear distance traveled by one complete wave cycle of a particular beam of radiant energy.

weight (mass) per unit volume (w/v) Measured weight of a substance added to a specific volume of a diluent, usually deionized or distilled water. The usual way is as grams per liter (g/L) or milligrams per milliliter (mg/mL).

weight per unit weight (w/w)   Mass per unit mass; used when the desired chemical to be weighed is a solid and is mixed with or diluted with another solid.

Western blot technology   Antigenic proteins or nucleic acids are separated by gel electrophoresis and transferred or blotted onto membrane filter paper antiserum from the patient is allowed to react with the filter paper, and by use of labeled anti-antibody detectors, the specific antibody bound to its homologous antigen is detected.

wet reagent chemistry   Assay utilizing wet reagents. Traditional manual chemistry assays use wet reagent chemistry. Compare with dry reagent technology.

white blood cell differential   Determination of the percentage of each white blood cell type present in a peripheral blood film.

Wintrobe hematocrit method   A macromethod for hematocrit determination, which has been generally replaced by the microhematocrit or calculated hematocrit.

work list   Defines the workload for a laboratory for a defined time period—for the day, for example.

working distance   In microscopy, the distance from the bottom of the objective to the material being studied.

Wright stain   A mixture of eosin and methylene blue used to observe cellular morphology of blood cells in examination of blood films; a polychromatic Romanovsky-type stain.

Wright-Giemsa stain   Variation of Wright stain. See Wright stain.

X

xanthochromia   Yellowish discoloration; used to describe the supernatant spinal or other serous fluid, indicating the presence of previous hemorrhage. Strictly speaking, xanthochromia represents a yellow color; however, the term is applied to pale pink to orange or yellow in describing fluids.

xenoantibodies   Antibodies resulting from exposure to antigenic material from another species.

Z

Zymogens   Enzyme precursors or proenzymes.

ANSWERS TO STUDY QUESTIONS

CHAPTER I

1. C
2. A. 4
   B. 1
   C. 2 or 3
   D. 5
   E. 2
3. (1) waived, (2) moderately complex, (3) highly complex, (4) provider-performed microscopies
4. B, C
5. A. 2
   B. 3
   C. 1
   D. 4

CHAPTER 2

1. B
2. To ensure that all laboratory workers are fully aware of possible hazardous situations present in their workplace that might be detrimental to their safety and well-being.
3. A, B, C, and D
4. To avoid direct contact with patient specimens in general; precautions used should recognize the infectious potential of any patient specimen.
5. Hepatitis B vaccine and the vaccination series of injections.
6. Hand washing
7. The material safety data sheet (MSDS) for the particular chemical must be consulted. This information includes specific details about the chemical—hazardous ingredients, physical data, fire and explosion data, and health hazard and protection information. An MSDS is provided by all chemical manufacturers and suppliers for each chemical that they sell or manufacture and must be available in the laboratory where the chemicals are in use, in the event that this information is needed.
8. To confine or isolate any possible hazardous waste from all workers—laboratory personnel, custodial personnel, and housekeeping personnel.

CHAPTER 3

1. D
2. B
3. B
4. D
5. A
6. A. 2
   B. 1
   C. 3
7. Refrigeration at 4° C.
8. First-morning, well-mixed, uncentrifuged specimen tested at room temperature.
9. At starting time (8 AM, for example), note time, empty bladder, and discard this urine. Collect all subsequent voidings into a container, up to and including collection at 8:00 the following morning. Store collection in refrigerator between collections.
10. The tubes are numbered sequentially as collected from the hub of the collection needle. If there has been a traumatic tap, the first tube collected will be pink-red, with subsequent clearing in later tubes as the fluid is collected.

CHAPTER 4

1. A. 2 (meter = m)
   B. 3 (gram = g)
   C. 1 (liter = L)
2. A. 0.1 m
   B. 200 mm
   C. 50 cm
   D. 20 cm
   E. 0.010 m
3. A. 0.025 g
   B. 0.5 g
   C. 0.1 kg
   D. 2000 g
   E. 10,000 mg
4. A. 0.2 L
   B. 200 mL
   C. 0.5 mL
   D. 0.6 L
   E. 5000 μL

5. 77° F

6. 4° C

7. 99.05 to 100.05 mL

8. A. 3

   B. 1

   C. 2

9. The MSDS, material safety data sheet, contains information about possible hazards in the use of the chemical and about safe handling, storage, and disposal of the chemical.

10. To ensure that the entire amount of weighed or measured substance is used in the preparation of the solution or reagent.

11. A. 3

   B. 1

   C. 2

12. $N_{acid} \times V_{acid} = N_{base} \times V_{base}$

$$N_{base} = \frac{0.1000N \times 1.0\ mL}{0.5\ mL} = 0.20N$$

CHAPTER 5

1. a

2. 400×

3. At the bottom of the condenser, under the lenses but within the condenser body. It is used to control the amount of light presented to the objectives; this adjusts the numerical aperture of the condenser so that it more nearly matches the NA of the objective.

4. Over the light port, in the base of the microscope. It controls the area of the circle of light in the field of view when the condenser has been properly focused, and is used in the alignment of the microscope.

5. A. 2

   B. 1

   C. 3

6. A. 3

   B. 2

   C. 1

   D. 2

   E. 1

   F. 3

CHAPTER 6

1. A. Concentration

   B. Beer's law

2. 380 to 750 nm

3. The substance must be colored in itself or be capable of being colored.

4. The wavelength of light.

5. The green wavelength is being transmitted; all other wavelengths are being absorbed by particles in the solution.

6. A. 2

   B. 3

   C. 1

7. A. 2

   B. 1

8. Used for analyses in POCT, for home testing for blood glucose in diabetics, and for analyzers using dry-film technology (chemistry and urinalysis) used in many physicians' offices and clinics.

CHAPTER 7

1. A. 2

   B. 5

   C. 4

   D. 1

   E. 3

2. A. 63.2

   B. 15.57

   C. 10.02

   D. 26

   E. 24

3. $V_1 \times C_1 = V_2 \times C_2$

   x mL × 5 = 1000 × 2

       5x = 2000

        x = 400 mL

4. A. 1024

   B. 1/27 or 0.037

   C. 1000

5. Measure 1 mL serum and dilute with 9 mL saline; this gives a total volume of 10 mL. The serum to total volume ratio is designated as 1:10.

6. Weigh 5 g NaCl and dilute to 100 mL with deionized water, using a 100-mL volumetric flask.

7. Molecular weight of NaCl = 58.5.

$$Molarity = \frac{g/L}{mol.\ wt.} = \frac{20}{58.5} = 0.34M$$

8. Molecular weight of NaCl = 58.5

   Molecular weight × molarity = g/L = 58.5 × 0.5

                = 29.3 g NaCl diluted to 1000 mL (1 L)

9. Use the formula: $V_1 \times C_1 = V_2 \times C_2$

       x mL × 2M = 50 mL × 5M

          2x = 250

           x = 125 mL

10. Molecular weight of $CaCl_2$ is 111.

$$\text{Equivalent weight} = \frac{\text{Gram molecular weight}}{\text{Valence}} = $$

$$\frac{111}{2} = 55.5 \text{ g}$$

1 L of a 1N solution would contain 55.5 g/L. A 0.5N solution would contain only half as much chemical per liter of solution, or 27.8 g. A proportion could be set up to solve this:

$$\frac{55.5 \text{ g/L}}{1N \text{ solution}} = \frac{x \text{ g/L}}{0.5N \text{ solution}} = 27.8 \text{ g/L}$$

However, only 500 mL of this solution is needed. Therefore another proportion could be set up:

$$\frac{27.8 \text{ g}}{1,000 \text{ mL}} = \frac{x \text{ g}}{500 \text{ mL}} = 13.9 \text{ g/500 mL}$$

CHAPTER 8

1. Quality assurance is an overall and continuing process by which a hospital or health care facility monitors all areas that contribute to providing the highest quality and most appropriate care for the patient.
2. CLIA '88
3. Quality assurance programs monitor test requesting procedures; patient identification, specimen procurement, and labeling; specimen transportation and processing procedures; laboratory personnel performance; laboratory instrumentation, reagents, and analytic test procedures; turnaround times; and, ultimately, the accuracy of the final result.
4. A. 2
   B. 6
   C. 3
   D. 1
   E. 5
   F. 4
5. A. Sensitivity

   Test A = 77% $\dfrac{10}{10 + 3} \times 100 = 76.9$ or 77%

   Test B = 91% $\dfrac{10}{10 + 1} \times 100 = 90.9$ or 91%

   B. Specificity

   Test A = 91% $\dfrac{10}{10 + 1} \times 100 = 90.0$ or 91%

   Test B = 77% $\dfrac{10}{10 + 3} \times 100 = 76.9$ or 77%

6. A. 15.2 (or 15 rounded off)
   B. 15
   C. 18

7. 95%
8. A standard solution is one that contains a known, exact amount of the substance being measured in the sample.
9. A. 3
   B. 1
   C. 2
10. Allows observation of trends leading toward trouble with a procedure—reagents, standards, and so on—by visually displaying what the same control solution is reading on a regular basis; any values falling "out of control" can be easily identified.

CHAPTER 9

1. A. 2
   B. 3
   C. 1, 4
   D. 5
   E. 5
2. The process includes test ordering, sample collection and transport to the laboratory, sample processing and analysis by the laboratory, quantitating the result, and test reporting (see Fig. 9-1).
3. For laboratories doing moderately complex or highly complex testing, a minimum of two control specimens (negative or normal and positive or increased) must be run in every 24-hour period when patient specimens are being run.

CHAPTER 10

1. A. 6
   B. 1
   C. 2
   D. 5
   E. 3
   F. 4
2. Printer and display on screen via a cathode ray tube (CRT)
3. Keyboard, interface with another computer, light pen or stylus, mouse
4. A. Central processing unit
   B. Random accesss memory
   C. Laboratory information system
   D. Hospital information system
5. Test ordering, printing specimen labels, and specimen collection
6. Generating chart reports, printing result reports, archiving patient results, workload recording, and billing

INDEX